THE LIFE AND TEACHING OF NĀROPA

Translated from the original Tibetan with a Philosophical Commentary based on the Oral Transmission

BY

HERBERT V. GUENTHER

OXFORD UNIVERSITY PRESS

LONDON OXFORD NEW YORK

OXFORD UNIVERSITY PRESS

London Oxford New York
Glasgow Toronto Melbourne Wellington
Cape Town Ibadan Nairobi Dar es Salaam Lusaka Addis Ababa
Delhi Bombay Calcutta Madras Karachi Lahore Dacca
Kuala Lumpur Singapore Hong Kong Tokyo

UNESCO COLLECTION OF
REPRESENTATIVE WORKS
TIBETAN SERIES

The translation in this volume has been accepted in the Tibetan Translations Series of the United Nations Educational, Scientific and Cultural Organization (UNESCO)

FIRST PUBLISHED BY THE CLARENDON PRESS, OXFORD, 1963
FIRST ISSUED AS AN OXFORD UNIVERSITY PRESS PAPERBACK, 1971
PRINTED IN THE UNITED STATES OF AMERICA

This reprint, 1974

CONTENTS

INTRODUCTION

In the history of Tibetan Buddhism the Indian Nāropa (A.D. 1016–1100) occupies a unique position. To the present day his life is held up as an example to anyone who aspires after spiritual values, which are never realized the easy way but only after years of endless toil and perseverance. It took Nāropa twelve years of ardent devotion and indefatigable service to his Guru Tilopa (A.D. 988–1069) to attain his goal: the overwhelming experience of the Real in direct knowledge. Apart from this, Nāropa also marks the beginning of a new and rich era of Buddhist thought in Tibet, while at the same time he is the culmination of a long tradition. None of his contemporaries or successors in India can compare with him in depth of experience.

Nāropa's biography, which has been translated here from hitherto unknown sources, contains a number of strictly historical data, but it is pre-eminently an account of the inner development of this scholar-saint. This makes it of particular interest.

Nāropa (Nāḍapāda, Nāroṭapa) was born in the Fire-Male-Dragon year (A.D. 1016) in Bengal. He is said to have been of royal parentage, his father being the 'king' Ži-ba go-cha (Śānti-varman) and his mother the 'queen' dPal-gyi blo-gros (Śrīmatī). Since in ancient-Indian usage the term 'king' is merely an administrative title and does not denote the rank of a European monarch, and since the genealogical tree of his royal ancestry occurs in other combinations in other texts, this designation is merely a long-winded way of pointing out that he belonged to the gentry.

When he had reached the age of eleven (A.D. 1026) he went for study to Kashmir, at that time the main seat of Buddhist learning. He stayed there for three years and having acquired a solid knowledge of the essential branches of learning he returned home in A.D. 1029. A large number of scholars went with him and for a further three years he continued his studies in their company. But then in A.D. 1032 he was forced to marry. His wife came from a cultured Brahmin family. The marriage lasted for eight years, then it was dissolved by mutual consent. His wife seems to have gone by her caste name Ni-gu-ma, and according to the widely practised habit of calling a female with whom one has had any relation 'sister' she became known as 'the sister of Nāropa'.[1] She engaged in literary activities and her works, which show a marked affinity to those of Nāropa, are preserved in the Tibetan bsTan-'gyur under her name Ni-gu-ma. Nāropa went to Kashmir in the same year that the marriage was dissolved (A.D. 1040). He stayed there for three years and then proceeded to Pullahari/Puṣpahari where he stayed another six years. This place became famous in the history of Tibetan Buddhism because it was there that Mar-pa later received the last instruction from Nāropa. In A.D. 1049 Nāropa went to Nalanda where he took part in a religious-philosophical debate. He was successful in this and was elected abbot, a post he held for eight years. The year A.D. 1057 was decisive for his spiritual development. He resigned from his post and set out in search of Tilopa who had been revealed as his Guru in a vision. After an ardent search which almost ended in suicide he met Tilopa and served him for twelve years until the latter's death in A.D. 1069. Nāropa himself died in the Iron-Male-Dragon year (A.D. 1100).[2] His mortal remains were preserved in the Kaṇika (Kaṇiṣka) monastery at Zangskar.[3]

The vision which induced Nāropa to resign from his post and to abandon worldly honours, was that of an old and ugly woman who mercilessly revealed to him his psychological state. Throughout the years he had been engaged in intellectual activities which were essentially analytic and thereby had become oblivious of the fact that the human organ of knowledge is bi-focal. 'Objective' knowledge may be entirely accurate without, however, being entirely important, and only too often it misses the heart of the matter. All that he had neglected and failed to develop was symbolically revealed to him as the vision of an old and ugly woman. She is old because

[1] George Roerich, *The Blue Annals*, ii. 730. In Thkv ii. 1, part iv, fol. 3*a*, Ni-gu-ma is stated to have been the wife of Nāropa.

[2] In Alfonsa Ferrari, *mK'yen brtse's Guide to the Holy Places of Central Tibet*, p. 169, Nāropa's death year is given as A.D. 1040. This is physically impossible because by that time Mar-pa could never have told him that he had a disciple of extraordinary gifts, Mi-la-ras-pa, who was born in A.D. 1040.

[3] Oral communication by Mr. H. Lee Shuttleworth, I.C.S. (retd.).

all that the female symbol stands for, the emotionally and passionately moving, is older than the cold rationality of the intellect which itself could not be if it were not supported by feelings and moods which it usually misconceives and misjudges. And she is ugly, because that which she stands for has not been allowed to become alive or only in an undeveloped and distorted manner. Lastly she is a deity because all that is not incorporated in the conscious mental make-up of the individual and appears other-than and more-than himself is, traditionally, spoken of as the divine. Thus he himself is the old, ugly, and divine woman, who in the religious symbolism of the Tantras is the deity rDo-rje phag-mo (Vajravārāhī) and who in a psychological setting acts as 'messenger' (*pho-ña*).[1]

It is characteristic of Nāropa's unemotional and intellectualist attitude that he makes each sign of ugliness a topic of analysis. But the vision has effected a subtle change in him. He becomes aware of the futility and fleeting character of what we are wont to call the world, from within, and in this awareness dimly realizes that every object that emerges into the focus of attention has meaning beyond the set of 'facts' in which it figures. He is all of a sudden confronted with his own possibilities.

This vision which is both a summons and an anticipation of what is to be won, is soon followed by eleven others. Each of them shows him in symbolic form what he has to do in order to establish the integrity of his being. Above all he has to get rid of his ordinary pre-occupations which are the product of his being divided against himself. But it is precisely this dividedness which prevents him from understanding the meaning of the symbols and as a consequence each succeeding vision is more terrible than the preceding one. The gradual process of undermining his one-sided attitude culminates in his complete break-down, and in utter despondency he is about to commit suicide. Exactly at this stage he meets Tilopa who assures him that after this process of dismantling and destruction a constructive phase can be entered upon.

[1] This aspect has a great similarity to what the Swiss psychologist C. G. Jung calls the 'anima'. The subject-matter is discussed in detail in Dnz 49*a* sq.

This means that after the breaking of every mental habit, one's prejudices, antipathies, and petrifications, a sense of wholeness is being recovered. The world of 'blunt facts' has lost its hold over man, but he has not become blind to them, rather does he illumine it from and transfigures it into a world of infinite value and meaning. What formerly was a source of conflict and bondage now becomes one of contentment and genuine freedom. This constructive phase is initiated by the intuitive understanding of certain symbolic acts or by an explanation of the 'maturing confirmations' (*dbaṅ*, *abhiṣeka*) which are an inner experience. Having thus become mature and fit to be entrusted with the teaching which will enable him to live by the perception of worth as a constant factor in ordinary consciousness, altering judgement and conduct, during the course of twelve years of toil Nāropa received twelve instructions which form the essence of the 'Oral Transmission' (*sñan-rgyud*, *karṇatantra*) and the core of Tantric philosophy as a guide to conduct.

Although the historicity of Tilopa cannot be doubted—he was born in the Earth-Male-Mouse year (A.D. 988) and died in the Earth-Female-Hen year (A.D. 1069)—he is more than the individual who happened to become Nāropa's Guru. In a certain sense Tilopa is Nāropa's total-self which summons him to find himself. The way in which Tilopa and Nāropa met at a critical stage of the latter's life—'ever since you met me in the form of the leper woman we have never been apart, but were like a body and its shadow. The various visions you had were the defilements of your evil deeds and so you did not recognize me'—points to this interpretation. Moreover, it is a maxim of the Guru-disciple relation that the Guru must never be conceived of in mere human form.[1] To do this would inevitably reinforce the ordinary attitude of the disciple which both the Guru and he himself, though not clearly understanding, are at pains to overcome. Therefore not any odd person is qualified to act as a Guru, nor is any odd person accepted as a disciple. On the part of the disciple there must be the need for instruction, deeply felt, and the Guru must have experienced within himself what he is going to teach. Only if these conditions

[1] sGam-po-pa, viii. 19*a*.

are fulfilled, can a profitable relationship exist out of which that which is to be of the highest value for the individual's further life will be born.[1]

This first English translation of the life and teachings of Nāropa is based on an old Tibetan edition, which I was able to study during my repeated stays at bKra-śis śugs-gliṅ dgon-pa in Lahoul. An identical copy, at places more legible than the one preserved in the lamasery, is with my Guru Lama Dam-chos rin-chen. The text is printed in the 'old' orthography. The style is rather concise, sometimes even cryptic. The blocks seem to have been prepared in a hurry, judging from minor omissions and repetitions.

The author mentions his name at the end of his work, also the place where he wrote it. He is lHa'i btsun-pa Rin-chen rnam-rgyal of Brag-dkar. He was a contemporary of the famous saint gTsaṅ-pa sMyon-pa'i He-ru-ka who according to tradition was one of the disciples of dPal Phag-mo gru-pa (A.D. 1110–70), who in turn was a disciple of sGam-po-pa (A.D. 1079–1153). The work thus belongs to the late twelfth century. It is likely that this text is the first authoritative Tibetan account of Nāropa's life that has been written. The author states that he has faithfully recorded the transmission by the 'siddha king' (siddha being the name for a person who has attained the highest realization) who is dPal Phag-mo gru-pa.

Nāropa's life seems to have been a favourite theme for composition. There exists another version which leaves out the 'Oral Transmission' teachings, the topics of Nāropa's studies and the meeting between him and Mar-pa. Instead it elaborates his earthly career and the occasions of his visions in a highly ornate style, without, however, adding anything that might be of interest for, or further an understanding of, Nāropa's significance. This text was edited together with a German translation by Albert Grünwedel.[2] The text itself is insignificant, because it contains nothing of philosophical interest. The translation is a faithful picture of the

[1] A long discussion occurs in sGam-po-pa, v. 2*a* sq.; 24*a* sqq.; x. 40*b*; xix. 2*a* sq. The problem is treated of in all works dealing with the Guru-disciple relation such as Tsoṅ-kha-pa, xiii. 20*a* sqq.; Zl 8*b* sq., and many others.

[2] *Die Legenden des Nā-ro-pa*. The title of the original, of which a handwritten copy was reproduced by A. Grünwedel with considerable distortions, is *mKhas*

translator's tragic illness. Part of it is what a psychiatrist calls 'word-salad' and unintelligible even to a German speaking person; the remainder is intelligible nonsense. For example: 'recognize your very nature as a mother knows her child' is in Grünwedel's translation 'the interest was added to the capital of the knowledge of the essential which had been won by former habit' (p. 143). Or, 'thinking that his training would be incomplete without this ordination' is rendered by Grünwedel as 'therefore he thought: "I have not become perfected on the funeral pyre"' (p. 55).

A new translation was, therefore, necessary, and lHa'i btsun-pa Rin-chen rnam-rgyal's text is of the utmost philosophical importance. He outlines the whole of Tantric thought and training, which are in fact inseparable.

It would not have been possible for me to give a translation of a Tibetan text which would convey its real meaning if I had not had the constant advice of learned Lamas. First of all I have to thank Lama Dam-chos rin-chen who lent me this text and explained its significance as well as the practices involved. I am equally indebted to Guru brTul-žugs gliṅ-pa who enabled me to support the oral instructions with quotations from the rare bKa'-brgyud-pa works, some of them, as for instance the 'Oral Transmission Texts' of gTsaṅ-pa He-ru-ka, existing only in manuscripts. Above all I have to thank my teachers and friends, the Incarnate Lamas Kathog dbOn sprul-sku and gNas-naṅ dPa'-bo rin-po-che, and dge-bśes Ṅag-dbaṅ ñi-ma of sGo-maṅ grva-tshaṅ (Drespung monastery, Tibet).

I also wish to express my gratitude to Mangalchand Thakur, Esq., and to Captain Pratapchand Thakur, whose unbounded hospitality made it possible for me to pursue my studies in the solitudes of Lahoul; to the Readers and Publishers of the Clarendon Press for their patience and coöperation; and, last, but not least, to my wife, Dr. Ilse Guenther, who prepared the manuscript and the index.

grub mñam-med dpal-ldan Nā-ro-pa'i rnam-par thar-pa dri-med legs-bśad bde-chen 'brug-sgra 'The well-narrated immaculate life-story of the incomparable sage Nāropa or the voice of the thunder of Great Bliss'. The author, who acknowledges his indebtedness to the bKa'-brgyud-pa Gurus, is Śākya'i btsun-pa dBaṅ-phyug rgyal-mtshan, who seems to belong to the fifteenth century. Grünwedel's statements concerning this book and its author are pure fancies.

PART I

THE BIOGRAPHY

THE WONDROUS LIFE OF THE GREAT SCHOLAR NĀROPA CROWN-JEWEL OF ALL PHILOSOPHER-SAINTS

PRAISE to the Guru, the Deva, and the Ḍākinīs!
In the vast expanse of space,[1] the boundless path divine,
The Dharmakāya embodied as the lordly ruler rDo-rje-'chaṅ (Vajradhara)[2]
Appears as (the sun, that) bright jewel in the sky, which represents
The five Sambhogakāyas, each an integral unity of the noetic and communicative,
Whose myriad rays, the Nirmāṇakāyas of Śes-rab bzaṅ-po (Prajñābhadra)[3],
Have opened the lotus of Nāropa's mind to these Kāyas Three.
Praise then to him who throughout the world has spread
The honeyed spirituality transmitted by word of mouth,
The Essence of all Sūtras and all Tantras.

Praise to Nāropa on his seat of lotus, sun, and moon,
On the lion throne of fearlessness, the embodiment of Buddhahood,
Who interprets the fundamental doctrine, the flawless gem Nam-mkha'i sñiṅ-po (Gaganagarbha),
Who has realized the transcending awareness of those who are exalted in renown supreme (the Buddhas),
Who is Kun-tu bzaṅ-po (Samantabhadra), Chos-kyi rgyal-mtshan (Dharmadhvaja), and bsTan-pa 'dzin-pa (Śāsanadhara).[4]

[1] This is a rather free translation of the original term *kloṅ-yaṅs*. *kloṅ* corresponds to Sanskrit *ūrmi* and signifies undulating movement. It is used exclusively with reference to Reality which is not a frozen absolute, but vibrating in all our experiences of it.

[2] rDo-rje-'chaṅ (Vajradhara) is for the bKa'-brgyud-pa and dGe-lugs-pa followers the symbol representation of the Dharmakāya which is pure noeticness (*ye-śes chos-sku, jñānadharmakāya*).

[3] This opening verse reveals the whole metaphysical background of Mantrayāna. See Note A, p. 265.

[4] These are names which Nāropa had at different stages of his spiritual development.

Devoutly worshipped by (the sun,) the friend of lotus flowers,
brilliant in his ornaments of rays and lord over the three worlds,
By Asuras, Gandharvas, Nāgas,
By Śiva, Īśvara, Viṣṇu, by men and those that are not men;
Obedient to his Guru's word; refuge sublime for all that lives, the Lord himself,
Belonging to the family of the Awakened[1]
May he shine as the gods' crown-jewel.

Devout and reverent, with body, speech, and thought, from deep within my heart
I salute those who from Nāropa stem, his spiritual fold and lineage;
I offer up my body with its endowments mystic, secret, and expressed;
I confess the evil I have done from time without beginning and shall do;
I rejoice at the good deeds of saints and common people;
I pray that the Doctrine be proclaimed 'til the world is void of beings; and
That renouncing Nirvāṇa, (Buddhas and Bodhisattvas) may stay 'til then;
And all the good, done by myself and others, however great or small,
Into enlightenment may turn.

With pure intent that others may benefit thereby
I beg the Guru, the protecting deity and all Ḍākinīs
To let me relate, though it be small as a drop of water,
The miracles and wondrous life of 'Jigs-med grags-pa (Abhayakīrti).[2]

May future generations who loathe all worldly things and strive
For the ultimate with all their might, lend me their ears.

[1] 'The family of the Awakened' is the lineage of the Buddhas. See my *Jewel Ornament of Liberation*, p. 6.

[2] This was the name which Nāropa had when he renounced his post of abbot at Nalanda and set out in search of his Guru.

Many prophecies have come down to us about this great scholar Nāropa, the sublime and noble spiritual son of the exalted incarnate being Tilopa. rGyal-ba rDo-rje-'chaṅ (Jina Vajradhara) sang:

Great bliss is he and the supreme origin thereof,
The teacher of the path that leads to enlightenment.
The supreme protector of all beings,[1] endowed
With the eye of spirit, triumphant over foes;
Explaining the fundamental Doctrine, he relapses
Into worldliness no more.

rDo-rje rnal-'byor-ma (Vajrayoginī=Vajravārāhī) said:

He is the son of bDe-mchog 'khor-lo[2] who is the father
Of all Buddhas in the present, the future and the past;
And of their mother rDo-rje Phag-mo.
He is their son, the glorious Nāropa.

'Khor-lo sdom-pa (Cakrasaṃvara):

Ineffable is Nāro, the undispersed spirituality of Buddha,[3]
Nāropa is perfect incarnate Buddhahood.

The venerable Tilopa:

I am 'Khor-lo sdom-pa (Cakrasaṃvara),
My pupil is Buddhahood in human form,
That man sublime, Nāropa the great scholar.

[1] Lit.: 'six kinds of beings'. They are: men, animals, spirits, denizens of hell, gods, and demons.

[2] bDe-mchog 'khor-lo is a contraction of bDe-mchog and 'Khor-lo sdom-pa, two different names for the same deity. bDe-mchog is the translation of Sanskrit *saṃvara* analysed as *saṃ* and *vara* 'bliss supreme', and 'Khor-lo sdom-pa that of Cakrasaṃvara 'Integration of Cakras', the *cakras* being focal points of experience. See also below, p. 164. rDo-rje Phag-mo (Vajravārāhī) is the consort of Cakrasaṃvara. She is also known as rDo-rje rnal-'byor-ma (Vajrayoginī). A special form of her, visualized by Nāropa, is known as Nā-ro mkha'-spyod-ma (*khecarī*). For a pictorial representation see Raghu Vira and Lokesh Chandra, *A New Tibeto-Mongol Pantheon*, i, pl. 26.

[3] *spros-bral, niṣprapañca* is a difficult term. It denotes a state which is beyond imaginative activity and hence cannot be formulated in words. The absence of imaginative activity does not mean, however, that this state is a blank tablet; it is rather the sum total of all possible contents which in imagination become separate and conflicting. In a certain sense *niṣprapañca* is synonymous with *vipaśyana*, a cognitive experience which develops out of a state of pure sensation. sGam-po-pa, vii. 13*b* uses this term as meaning 'when there is no longer any external reference'. Similarly x. 16*b* and elsewhere. See also Phntm 4*b*.

And also:

Nāropa who remembered all he heard
Was with me for twelve years. To him I gave
My intuitive understanding of the ultimate.
All future generations must rely on him
If they would realize the ultimate.

The great scholar Nāropa himself said:

My mind is the perfect Buddha
And my word the perfect doctrine,
My body is the holy congregation.
Nāropa in whom the three jewels are perfected,
Should not be sought elsewhere, Here am I.

And in a Vajragīti is stated:

He who is known as rDo-rje sems-dpa' (Vajrasattva)[1]
Should teach and live in humble form
For the benefit of living beings.

When a Guru, who fulfils the prophecies like the great scholar Nāropa, has appeared as a spiritual teacher endowed with the marks of Buddhas and Bodhisattvas of the tenth spiritual level, and has come into this world for the sake of sentient beings, the most important task is to worship him.

It is indeed hard to relate the life and describe the immense treasure-house of virtues of the glorious great scholar Nāropa who is the noble and venerable lord-protector of all sentient beings and the Guru of the three worlds, the Buddha of the three divisions of time.

[1] In this context the term means something like 'incarnate spirituality'. In Sphyd 21*a*, Padma dkar-po explains this term to the effect that *rdo-rje* (Vajra) or the bliss of the indivisibility of the relational and functional structures that make up man (*sku, gsuṅ, thugs*), is noetic capacity (*śes-pa*), while *sems-dpa'* (Sattva) or the three worlds together, is the object (*śes-bya*). Their unity is invariable. Padma dkar-po here anticipates that which has been cogently pointed out by modern existentialist philosophy, that all human experience is intentional in structure. John Wild, *The Challenge of Existentialism*, p. 189, points out: 'Every phase of these relational structures, the objective as well as the subjective, is given with the same evidence. There is no more reason for denying the one than the other. Hence idealism, which attempts to reduce the object to a state of the subject, and pan-objectivism, which attempts to reduce the subject to an object, must be rejected. Both are always found together in an intentional structure of some type.'

There are three parts in this biography which tells how Nāropa developed the Doctrine outwardly by hearing and pondering over the texts; how inwardly he sought and found the Guru by unflagging perseverance and by undergoing hardships for the sake of entering the path of the secret Mantra[1] and of comprehending the ultimate; and how he attained the highest realization. These three parts are:

I. His miraculous and significant birth;
II. His becoming disgusted with the world and embracing a religious life;
III. His performing great acts of self-denial, in particular, after having set out on the Mantra path.

[1] Tsoṅ-kha-pa, iii. 12*a* and mKhas-grub, iii. 1, 5*b* say that 'it is secret because it is not divulged to anyone who is not a suitable person'. This has nothing to do with that sort of secretiveness with which Mantrayāna is often charged, rather it is the expression of a wise deliberation: the scalpel in the hand of a skilled surgeon is a helpful instrument, in the hand of an ordinary man a murderous weapon.

I

NĀROPA'S BIRTH

This part has four chapters:

(i) The place;
(ii) The noble line into which he was born;
(iii) The special characteristics of his royal parents;
(iv) The miraculous details of his birth.

(i) Our universe which is called sToṅ-gsum mi-mjed (Trisāhasrasahalokadhātu), has twenty-five levels,[1] one above the other, and lies in the hands of the primordial Buddha Gaṅs-can mtsho. On its thirteenth level there are four continents of which the best is our human world. Here in the midst of some hundred thousand towns, in the city 'Dzam-bu in Śrīnagara, a district of Bengal in the East of India, there stood the palace of a king who possessed the means of exquisite enjoyments on earth. Here Nāropa was born.

(ii) In this country there were many classes: royalty, nobility, Brahmins, citizens, common people and so on. Among them the most excellent man, Nāropa, the central pillar of a renowned family—like a tree firmly rooted in the soil—was born in the royal line of the Śākya clan. Long ago, though still in this aeon, the clan was led by Maṅ-pos bkur-ba (Mahāsammata). His successors in the direct line were the kings 'Od-mdzes (Roca), dGe-ba (Kalyāṇa), dGe-mchog (Varakalyāṇa), bSo-sbyoṅ-'phags (Upoṣadha), sPyi-bo skyes (Mūrdhaja), mDzes-pa-can (Cāru), Ñe-mdzes-'od (Upacāru), mDzes-ldan-dpal (Cārumant), Legs-skyes (Sujāta), Goutama, Bu-ram-śiṅ (Īkṣvāku), bSod-nams skyes (Puṇyajāta), dBaṅ-phyug grags-pa (Īśvarakīrti), bSod-nams rtse-mo (Puṇyaśikhara), Ye-śes rgyal-mtshan (Jñānadhvaja), bSod-nams grub

[1] Ordinarily twenty-four levels are counted, as may be gleaned from *Abhidharmakośa*, iii. 2 (Louis de la Vallée Poussin's translation). The number twenty-five seems to be due to a peculiar mode of counting, adding the total as a separate item to the available number.

(Puṇyasiddha), bSod-nams bkra-śis (Puṇyamaṅga),blaSod-nams grags-pa (Puṇyakīrti) and Ži-ba go-cha (Śāntivarman).

(iii) Nāropa's father was the great king Ži-ba go-cha (Śāntivarman). He was born with all the major and minor lucky marks, of excellent character, and with great discriminating awareness light shone from his body at times. He married dPal-gyi blo-gros (Śrīmatī), daughter of the great king sKal-ldan grags-pa (Śrīmatkīrti), whose virtues had been earned in former lives. Together they exhorted their subjects to live worthily.

The royal couple, who fasted and made acts of atonement on all suitable occasions, always worshipped the Most Sublime. They had renounced evil and devoted themselves exclusively to good deeds. They had only one daughter, the princess dPal-gyi Ye-śes (Śrījñānā). When in spite of all their attempts no son was born, they invited from his solitude the spiritual advisor Grags-pa'i blo-gros (Yaśomati) and asked him to ascertain by his supernatural insight the cause of their failure. He declared: 'You should take refuge in the Triple Gem, and because of the infallibility of the Most Sublime you should develop an enlightened attitude,[1] say your prayers and make lavish offerings to the Guru who is the Most Sublime, to the tutelary deity, the Ḍākas[2] and the protectors of the doctrine. By doing this with genuine devotion and reverence you will achieve what you desire.' He then went back to his solitude.

The royal couple therefore ordered many exquisite places of worship to be built, and when they worshipped lavishly and prayed with devotion and reverence, the glorious Nāropa, remembering that he needed a special body to realize enlightenment in a single lifetime, entered the womb of his royal mother Śrīmatī.

That night she experienced in a dream the radiant vision of the indivisibility of nothingness and bliss,[3] by which the whole country was revealed in a brilliant light. The next morning, when she told

[1] See in particular my *Jewel Ornament of Liberation*, pp. 112 sqq.

[2] According to the *Śrī-Ḍākārṇavamahāyoginītantrarāja*, *ḍāka* is synonymous with *jñāna*, the mystic's illumination and transcending awareness. The anthropomorphism is symbolic, rather than factual. Dkt 58*b* explains this term as 'an understanding awareness travelling over the spaciousness of Reality'.

[3] For an explanation of my choice of the term 'nothingness' instead of 'emptiness', and of 'void' as a translation of *stoṅ-ñid*, *śūnyatā*, see Note B, p. 265.

her husband of the dream, the king was delighted and said: 'A sentient being has taken temporary residence in your womb. It will through the mercy of the Most Sublime become a superior being'. And so the royal couple continued to make the choicest offerings to the Most Sublime, until the child was born.

(iv) In the early morning of the tenth day of the first half of the ninth month, which happened to be the fourth month of the Fire-Male-Dragon year (A.D. 1016), under the lunar mansion of *sa-ga* (Viśākhā, Alpha Librae), the voice of the thunder resounded in the sky, the earth trembled and a miraculous omen of rays of light was seen.

When a boy, who had all the major and minor lucky marks on his body, had been born, the royal couple in their deep devotion sent for the Brahmin gSaṅ-ba'i blo-gros (Guhyamati) who, after having examined the newly born prince, declared:

A great miracle indeed! This boy sublime
Is like the son of Śuddhodana.
If he embraces not religious life, he will be lord of all the earth;
He will be like Prince Siddhārtha.

Thus he prophesied and spoke many blessings, naming the boy Kun-tu bzaṅ-po (Samantabhadra).

From earliest childhood the prince had a keen mind and great wisdom. He was not afflicted with the shortcomings of ordinary children, and put his trust in the Most Sublime. As he had supernatural insight, he sometimes spontaneously related incidents of his former lives and also declared that in the future he would have such and such qualities in this world and would perform such and such deeds. He had come, indeed, as the sublime being that had been spoken of in the prophecies.

Although his parents greatly favoured the sublime doctrine, they feared that with only one son their line might die out. The king therefore did his best to prevent the young prince from learning to read and write. Nevertheless the boy did so in secret and had no difficulty in becoming a scholar. Since he led a life which was illumined solely by the light of the Dharma, he became famous in all the regions of the world.

II

NĀROPA BECOMES DISGUSTED WITH THE WORLD AND EMBRACES THE RELIGIOUS LIFE

THIS part has four chapters:

(i) Receiving ordination as a lay disciple and mastering the five branches of learning;[1]

(ii) Marrying Dri-med-ma (Vimalā) in order to please his parents;

(iii) Renouncing the world again and by having become fully ordained making the doctrine of the Victorious One shine like the sun; and

(iv) Spreading the Buddhist religion from the Vajra-seat and defeating heretics.

(i)

Since Nāropa belonged to the Awakened Family[2] there did not appear to him anything that might not have been the Dharma. At the age of eight he spontaneously felt disgusted with the world and realized that it is transitory.[3] Constantly concerned with the noble doctrine, he was often moved to tears; wherever he saw an attendant he taught him that everything must die and will not last for ever. He showed great respect to those whom he thus urged to follow the Dharma. He always rewarded those whom he saw doing good, but when he witnessed a man doing evil his heart shrank with sadness. Since his mind was set solely on the Dharma, he told his parents: 'For the sake of the Dharma I must go to Kashmir and study there'. And he sang:

Salutation to the Three Gems Divine!
Inspired by them, I beg you my father to listen to my words.

[1] They are: arts, medicine, grammar, epistemology, and rhetoric.

[2] See above note one, p. 3.

[3] Usually it is a spiritual friend who opens our eyes to the transitory character of all that we wish to believe to be permanent. It is the first step in transcending the world. See my *Jewel Ornament of Liberation*, pp. 41 sqq.

Every act is of misery the root
If it accord not with the Dharma.

'So I shall not stay here but will go to Kashmir for the sake of the Dharma.'

When his mother clasped him to her bosom and refused to let him go, he sang:

Salutation to the Three Gems Divine!
Mother, hold not back your son, give him to the Dharma.
Mother, though parents are great benefactors, when their work
Agrees not with the Dharma the world continues ever.
Hard indeed is it to gain a human body
Hence not to follow Dharma causes me distress.
If you really love your son, do your best
For him in accordance with the Dharma.

Then his mother began to weep, but out of love she said: 'My dear son, so that you may be happy I shall for a while give you to the Dharma, but return to us quickly so that we, your parents, may also be happy'. Thus she gave him permission to go and when he was eleven he arrived in Kashmir.

There he was ordained as a lay disciple with the abbot Nam-mkha'i grags-pa (Gaganakīrti) and his name became Nam-mkha'i sñiṅ-po (Gaganagarbha).

This is how he studied arts, medicine, grammar, epistemology, and rhetoric:

He studied and mastered art in the Dus-'khor (Kālacakratantra), the sDom-'byuṅ (Samvarodayatantra) and the Śa-ri-bus žus-pa'i mdo; and medicine in the 'Bum and its commentaries, the Tshaṅs-pa-la gsuṅs-pa, the lHa'i dbaṅ-po-la gsuṅs-pa, and the Phyi-naṅ-gi draṅ-sroṅ-la gsuṅs-pa. In grammar he studied the Kun-tu bzaṅ-po, the Kalāpa, the Candrapa, and the four basic languages.[1] Then he mastered the Tshad-ma kun-las btus-pa (Pramāṇasaṅgraha) and the seven auxiliary texts of which three

[1] They are: Prākrit, Apabhraṃśa, Paiśācī, and Sanskrit. See for instance Tsoṅ-kha-pa, iv. 1*a*.

explain the body of the text and four its limbs; the Tshad-ma snaṅ-ba by kLu-sgrub (Nāgārjuna), the mṄon-sum rjes-dpag by 'Phags-pa lha (Āryadeva), and many other works. He studied and mastered the sÑan-ṅag don-rgyan so-gñis-kyi mdo, the Mu-tig 'phreṅ-ba by kLu-sgrub (Nāgārjuna) father and son, the sÑan-ṅag me-loṅ (Kāvyādarśa) composed by the jewel among poets, the teacher dPa'-bo (Vīrya = Aśvaghoṣa),[1] and many other works.

He stayed in Kashmir for three years and became an outstanding scholar in the five branches of learning. He then returned home with thirteen scholars: Ye-śes sñiṅ-po (Jñānagarbha), Śākya bśes-gñen (Śākyamitra), Legs-ldan 'byed (Bhavya), Zla-ba grags-pa (Candrakīrti), Śes-rab 'byuṅ-gnas, Nag-po-pa (Kṛṣṇācārya), Kun-dga' sñiṅ-po (Ānandagarbha), Ratnākaraśānti, Yan-lag med-pa'i rdo-rje (Anaṅgavajra), Ye-śes zabs (Jñānapāda), Candrahari, sPrin-gyi śugs-can (Meghavegin) and mṄon-śes-can (Abhijña).[2]

For three years Sūtras and Mantras were studied and explained in the lecture halls. In the Sūtras he followed the order of The Deeper Understanding of the Hidden Meaning, and mastered the mṄon-par rtogs-pa'i rgyan (Abhisamayālaṅkāra), the rGyud bla-ma (Uttaratantra), the mDo-sde rgyan (Mahāyāna-sūtrālaṅkāra), the dbU-mtha' rnam-'byed (Madhyāntavibhaṅga), and the Chos-ñid rnam-'byed (Dharma-dharmatā-vibhaṅga). As to the order of The Doctrine of Nothingness, which is the substance of the Buddhist teaching, he mastered the rTsa-śe (Prajñāmūla= Mūlamadhyamakakārikā), the sToṅ-ñid bdun-cu (Śūnyatāsaptatikārikā), the Rigs-pa drug-cu (Yuktiṣaṣṭikā), the Žib-mo rnam-dag (Vaidalyasūtra), the rTsod zlog (Vigrahavyāvartanī), and the Rin-chen 'phreṅ-ba (Ratnāvalī), that is the six works of the Mādhyamikas.

In Mantra literature he studied and mastered from the Kriyā-

[1] The *Kāvyādarśa* is written by Daṇḍin. Our author confuses various important authors.

[2] The scholars mentioned here are important in the history of Buddhist thought. For the time being, however, it must be left undecided whether they were contemporaries of Nāropa. As is so often the case, persons of various periods are lumped together because there exists a spiritual affinity between them.

tantra the bSam-gtan phyi-ma (Dhyānottara-paṭalakrama), from the Caryātantra the rNam-snaṅ mṅon-byaṅ (Vairocanābhisambodhitantra), from the Yogatantra the sByoṅ-skyil bcu-gñis (Sarvadurgatipariśodhanatejorājasya Tathāgatasya Arhato Samyaksambuddhasya kalpaikadeśa), and other texts. From the Anuttarayoga Mother Tantras he mastered the dGyes-pa rdo-rje (Hevajratantrarāja) of the complete Kye-rdo-rje (Hevajra) in 500,000 verses and the condensed Tantra of the brTag-gñis (Hevajratantra); and from the bŚad-rgyud (explanatory works on Tantras) the Gur (Vajrapañjara) and the Sampuṭikā. He also studied and mastered the basic work in fifty chapters of the bDe-mchog (Abhidhāna-uttaratantra), the sDom-pa 'byuṅ-ba (Samvara-udbhava); the bŚad-rgyud: Heruka sṅon-'byuṅ (Heruka-abhyudaya), the Phag-mo sṅon-'byuṅ (Ḍākinī-sarvacittādvayācintya-jñānavajravārāhyabhibhavatantrarāja), the Kun-spyod bla-ma, the mṄon-spyod bla-ma, the mKha'-'gro-ma dra-ba'i rgyud, the mKha'-'gro rgya-mtsho (Śrī-Ḍākārṇavamahāyoginītantrarāja), and other texts.

Thereafter teachers and disciples set the Dharmacakra in motion in order to bring those who are to be educated, to spiritual maturity. That is, according to the mental capacity and spiritual interest of the three classes of sentient beings they taught the Śrāvakayāna, the Bodhisattvayāna, and the Mantra-Vajrayāna. The message of these three Yānas was continuously heard. Moreover, since for full three years the Dharma comprising grammar, epistemology, and other branches of learning was taught, the whole country was filled by the Dharma.

One day, thinking that there had been enough study, Nāropa's father said:

> What noble doctrine violates a parent's word?
> So settle down to living in a house.

When the king, displeased with his son, thus began to upbraid him, all the scholars whom the excellent Gaganagarbha had invited were dismissed with many exquisite presents. Yet feeling kindly towards his parents the scholar-prince said with a smile.

Salutation to the Three Gems Divine!
Inspired by them I beg you
My parents, to listen to me.
What is the use of great faith
If it be not in the noble doctrine?
Why fondle a son if he is not pleased?
How shall I practise Dharma if unmindful
Of transitoriness and death?
Father and mother, if with me you are displeased
Let me return with the scholars to Kashmir.

His parents replied: 'Listen, you are a worthy and holy man; teach us the Dharma, but let the other scholars go'. To this he agreed. But after the scholars had left, when he was pondering over the Dharma, his parents said: 'Dear son, you have preached and practised the Dharma enough. If our noble line is not to come to an end, it is time you found a wife'.

'Oh my father and mother, listen', said the prince, 'what will happen to the Dharma if I marry? How shall I become enlightened when I add to the world? Long ago, Śākyamuni renounced married life, became a seeker after truth and thereby repaid all that had been done for him by his mother and father. I will do the same. Please give me permission'.

'If you do so, you are likely to deprive us, your parents, of the very life we breathe', they answered and angrily showed their determination not to give in. Then the sublime Gaganagarbha thought: 'If I do not marry, my parents' life will be endangered. But if I do I shall plunge into something horrible and no longer be able to follow the path of the Dharma. If I go against the Dharma, though I am a scholar in the five branches of learning, I must be a man of little sense'. Aloud he said: 'I shall live a married life in such a way that it does not go against the Dharma'. His parents were delighted, took him by his hands and said:

Well done, indeed, most noble son.
You have pleased your parents.
We are overjoyed.

And they bowed many times to him.

(ii)

The prince declared: 'If I am to live a married life which is not against the Dharma, any girl will not suit me; therefore, if I have to marry she must be as follows', and he sang:

Salutation to the Three Gems Divine.
Inspired by them I sing:
No one recognizes that all things
Are his parents, none the less
Seek a girl unprejudiced, clean, by birth
Hindu, by name Dri-med-ma (Vimalā)
And spiritually of the Mahāyāna family.
Let me know when you have found her.

And he added that he would not dare to disobey his parents if they should find such a girl for him. Then he noted down the qualities he wanted in his wife, and gave the list to his father, who said to himself: 'Really, this is only a device to avoid marriage; where shall I ever find such a girl?' and he went for the night into his chamber of mourning.

The next day the chief minister Ye-śes spyan-ldan (Jñānacakṣumant) said to the king: 'Your Majesty, have I done anything wrong?'

'No, but I have only one son, and when I asked him to get married because I was afraid that our line might die out, he answered that he did not want to marry, and that if he were forced to do so he would have a girl from a Hindu family, who was unprejudiced and clean, had an enlightened mind, practised love and compassion, was sixteen years old and named Dri-med-ma (Vimalā). Where shall I find such a girl? That is why I am plunged in despair.'

'Your Majesty, do not worry. Your son is an excellent being who has accumulated merit (and for this reason everything will turn out properly). Do not torment yourself by thinking whether you will find such a girl or not.'

'I am sure she cannot be found. Anyhow, do your best.'

The chief minister then chose another as his companion, to whom he confided his conversation with the king.

After a year's search they came one evening to 'Dam-bu-ka, a village of Hindus, in Bengal in the East of India. Tired from walking they sat down at a well. A Brahmin girl approached, wearing the sacred cord and with her hair tied in a knot, and looked around with wide-open eyes. As there was no one to draw the water, she did so herself without hesitation. Then the chief minister said: 'We are thirsty, give us some water.' When he saw that she gladly offered them the water, which could only mean that she belonged to the Mahāyāna family of compassion, and that she thoroughly rinsed the drinking bowl, so revealing her sense of cleanliness, he asked her: 'Who are your father and mother? What is your name, how old are you, and to which caste do you belong?'

The girl looked at the minister for a long time. Seeing that he was tired and worried, hoarse, pale, and worn, she was filled with compassion and with tears in her eyes replied: 'My father is the Brahmin sKar-rgyal (Tiṣya), my mother the Brahmini Ni-gu and my brother the Brahmin Na-gu. I myself am called Dri-med sgron-ma (Vimaladīpī). I am sixteen years old, by caste a Brahmini and by religion Hindu.' And she looked apprehensive. The minister thought that her name, caste, and behaviour corresponded in every particular to the qualities the king had detailed, and in order to find out whether she would be willing or not to marry the prince he asked her: 'Have you ever heard about Samantabhadra, the great scholar and son of king Śāntivarman?'

'I have heard about him.'

'Would you like to become his wife?'

'Go and ask my father. I will go if he is willing. I will ask him as well. But if he does not give his permission I cannot gainsay his word.'

When the minister asked about her father she said: 'Tomorrow before sunrise my father will come out to make a secret Brahmin offering. He will be followed by another Brahmin who limps, carries a stick, and wears his hair in a knot. Ask my father without this man hearing anything.'

With these words the girl went home.

The next morning everything happened as related, and the two ministers approached the Brahmin Tiṣya saying: 'You must give your daughter Vimaladīpī as wife to prince Samantabhadra, son of our king Śāntivarman.' Tiṣya retorted: 'Your king belongs no doubt to an excellent family, but we are high caste Brahmins and not Buddhists. Since you are Buddhists I cannot give my daughter'. And he went back into the house.

The two ministers shouted: 'If you do not give us your daughter we will commit suicide in front of your house', and lying down on the steps they stayed there many days. Then the people began to inquire: 'Why are you doing this?'

'We want Vimalā to marry our prince Samantabhadra. This Brahmin Tiṣya, however, won't hear about giving his daughter in marriage and does not care if we lose our lives.'

The people pitied them, reviled the Brahmin Tiṣya and demanded: 'Allow Vimalā to marry.' When the Brahmin was thus forced to agree, the two ministers joyfully returned to their country. When they told king Śāntivarman about their mission, he was delighted and sent expensive presents to the Brahmin Tiṣya. He sent the ministers back with a large retinue to invite the Brahmin. When they reached Tiṣya's house he gladly entrusted his daughter to them, and his son rejoiced. The girl was moved to deep faith, respect, and devotion for her betrothed prince Samantabhadra. The ministers returned with the noble princess Vimaladīpī, and the prince married her when he was seventeen.

But Nāropa thought: 'I asked for a girl with certain qualities, thinking she could never be found. One should remember that in this world nothing is impossible'. And to his parents he showed a smiling face.

Then the excellent Gaganagarbha instructed his wife in the doctrine of the Mahāyāna. Vimalā listened with fervent conviction, never forgetting (the message of this doctrine). Having become his disciple she served him in everything.

(iii)

Feeling disgusted with his home life which was nothing else but Saṁsāra, the excellent Gaganagarbha yearned to renounce the world. So he said to Vimalā: 'We have lived together for eight years, but I loathe such a life. Even as a child I always wanted to leave home, but there were always difficulties. It would have meant disobeying my parents. Now, however, I am going to leave home. You may either follow the Dharma or marry anyone you like.'

'You cannot just discard me by reproaching me with not being a Buddhist', his wife said. 'Considering that it is uncertain when death will come, there is no safety anywhere. I shall not hinder you practising the Dharma but will do whatever possible to help. So renounce the world saying that I have faults.'

The excellent Gaganagarbha then informed his parents: 'Women are full of guile, and Vimalā, of course, has countless faults. I cannot live with her any longer.' King Śāntivarman invited the Brahmin Tiṣya to talk the matter over. Then they both asked Gaganagarbha to continue living with Vimalā. He replied:

> Countless are woman's defects.
> My elephantine mind has fallen
> Into the poisonous swamp of guile.
> So I must renounce the world.

Both parents then asked Vimalā what she had to say. She declared: 'It is true, I have countless faults:

> Having not a single virtue
> I merely beguile him.

We should therefore be separated.'

After due deliberation both parents decided on a divorce. Princess Vimalā became a companion in the Dharma, and the excellent Gaganagarbha went to the hermitage dGa'-ba'i tshal (Ānandārama). He was then twenty-five.

The abbot Saṅs-rgyas skyabs (Buddhaśaraṇa) and the teacher Ye-śes 'od (Jñānaprabha) ordained him a Śramaṇera (novice) and renamed him Saṅs-rgyas ye-śes (Buddhajñāna). He stayed with them for three years. He studied and mastered the 'Dul-ba luṅ-gži (Vinayavastu), the rGya-che rol-pa (Lalitavistara), the Las brgya-pa (Karmaśataka), the Dran-pa ñer-bžag (Smṛtyupasthāna), the sKye-rabs (Jātakamālā), and the mDo-rtsa (Vinayasūtra). He also visited many learned men such as the former scholars he had invited, and under them he studied and mastered the basic Tantra in 25,000 verses and the condensed Tantra in eighteen chapters with 1,800 verses of the gSaṅ-ba 'dus-pa (Guhyasamājatantra), belonging to the Father Tantra group, and also the bSad-rgyud: the lHa-mo bži žus (Caturdevīparipṛcchā), the dGoṅs-pa luṅ-bstan (Sandhivyākaraṇatantra), the rDo-rje 'phreṅ-ba (Vajrāvalīnāmamaṇḍalasādhana), the Ye-śes rdo-rje kun-las btus-pa (Śrī-jñānavajrasamuccaya) and the lHa'i dbaṅ-pos žus-pa'i rgyud. He also studied the dMar-nag-'jigs gsum-gyi rgyud, and in particular the third and seventh sections.

Although a novice he was not yet a Bhikṣu (monk). Thinking that his training would be incomplete without this ordination he went to Puna in Kashmir, like a man who is thirsty and determined to get water. He was then twenty-eight. Surrounded by many Bhikṣus, headed by the abbot Chos-kyi bla-ma (Dharmaguru), the teacher Chos-kyi ye-śes (Dharmajñāna), and the instructor in the secret doctrine Chos-kyi byaṅ-chub (Dharmabodhi) he was ordained as a Bhikṣu. His name became Chos-kyi rgyal-mtshan (Dharmadhvaja). He remained three years in Kashmir.

Under the guidance of the abbot and his other teachers he studied the commentary on the Dus-'khor (Kālacakratantra), the Dri-med 'od-gsal (Vimalaprabhā), and also the Mahāmaya and the gDan-bži (Śrī-catuḥpīṭhamahāyoginītantraraja).

Then he went to Pullahari. By his explanations and realizations he spread the Buddhist doctrine far and wide. Round him gathered innumerable Bhikṣus who all developed various qualities. Some had deeply moving experiences and an intuitive understanding of reality; others developed supersensible cognitions and acquired miraculous powers, while still others became most erudite in the five branches of learning. Thus his fame and glory spread everywhere. People started saying that here is a man who thoroughly understands the doctrine of the Buddha, and he was most famous under his name the Elder bsTan-pa 'dzin-pa (Śāsanadhara). He spent six years at Pullahari and wrote several works about the gSaṅ-ba 'dus-pa (Guhyasamājatantra), he composed the rGyud phyi-ma'i 'grel-pa, the gSaṅ-ba'i sgron-ma, and the Rim-lṅa bsdus-pa gsal-ba. He wrote the Mu-tig-'phreṅ-ba, a commentary on the bDe-mchog rtsa-rgyud (Abhidhāna-uttaratantra) and the sDom-'byuṅ (Samvara-udbhava). He also composed the brGyan-gyi 'phreṅ-ba, a commentary on the Kye-rdo-rje (Hevajratantra), and many works on the Sūtras and Mantras.[1]

He then joined the university of Nalanda where scholars spread the message of the Buddha. They knew the Sūtras, the Vinaya, the Abhidharma, and the mystic diagrams in equal perfection. There were at Nalanda 500 scholars of whom eighty-four were most famous, and among these four stood out in particular. At the eastern gate Śes-rab 'byuṅ-gnas was foremost in immediate and intuitive understanding of the profound and radiant nature of reality; at the southern gate Nag-po-pa (Kṛṣṇācārya) in discipline; at the western gate Ratnākaraśānti in his knowledge of grammar, epistemology, spiritual precepts, and logic; and at the northern gate Dzetari (Jetari) in his realization that rejection and attainment are the same when all obstacles have been overcome.

When this latter head of the department died and no other scholar could be found to fill his post, the 500 pandits resolved: 'There is none more worthy than the Elder bStan-pa 'dzin-pa.' Unanimously they requested him to accept the post. At first he declined. But then they said: 'Our Elder who presided over the department at the northern gate has gone to another realm. In the whole world we shall not find a substitute for him, only you have such wide knowledge, so kindly accept the post.' And when all the Bhikṣus with folded hands begged him for nine days to accept, he graciously consented; and so they installed him at the northern gate.

According to the Indian custom when a new scholar was installed, it was the rule to hold a debate between the Buddhist scholars and those of other philosophical systems. An announcement was made that a debate would be held in a fortnight, and all the scholars assembled in order to tear any professed doctrine to pieces. In the middle court of the university of Nalanda a throne was erected for the king, presiding over the conference. To his

[1] With the exception of the Pañcakramasangrahaprakāśa none of the works mentioned here seem to have come down to us. See Note C, p. 266.

right and left the scholars, Buddhist and Hindu, were seated. First the Elder bsTan-pa 'dzin-pa debated with the Buddhists for half a month, but nobody could defeat him. Then the Hindus held forth for another fortnight, discussing grammar, epistemology, spiritual precepts, and logic. Contending with all sorts of spiritual powers and miraculous faculties, the Elder won a complete victory over his opponents. The king Phyogs-kyi go-cha (Digvarman) then addressed the assembly: 'I am the impartial patron of both parties. But in this contest to vindicate the truth nobody could defeat the Elder bsTan-pa 'dzin-pa and an unusual faith in the liberating power of the Victorious One (the Buddha) has been created everywhere'.

(iv)

At that time the staff of Nalanda requested the Elder bsTan-pa 'dzin-pa to become their abbot and they conferred upon him the name 'Jigs-med grags-pa (Abhayakīrti).

The venerable Abhayakīrti defeated all the non-Buddhist scholars and he composed the following verses:

> With the iron hook of grammar, the lore of knowledge, logic
> And spiritual precepts,
> I, the Elder Abhayakīrti
> Have scattered the opponents as a flock of sparrows.[1]
> With the axe of grammar, the lore of knowledge, logic
> And spiritual precepts
> I have felled the opponents' tree.
> With the lamp of certainty in logic and precepts
> I have burnt the darkness of my foes' ignorance.
> With the sacred jewels of the three disciplines[2]
> Have I removed the dirt of impurity.
> With instruction's battering ram
> Have I conquered the vicious city of bewilderment.
> At Nalanda in the presence of the king

[1] Lit.: thrown as food to the birds.

[2] i.e. the three types of ethics and manners (*śīla*) among the beings of this world (Kāmadhātu), the behaviour resulting from meditation (Rūpadhātu), and from following the Path. See *Abhidharmakośa*, iv. 13*cd*.

Have I felled the ever trembling tree of the heretics.
With the razor of the Buddha's doctrine
I have shaved the hair of my opponent heretics,
And have raised the banner of the Buddha's doctrine.

At that time 100 learned Hindu teachers shaved their heads, were converted to Buddhism, and were followed three days later by another 600. The inmates of Nalanda university hoisted the great banner, beat the big drum, blew the conch of the Dharma and were full of joy and happiness. The great king Digvarman showed his faith in and respect for the venerable Abhayakīrti, bowed many times to him, and touched the latter's feet with his head saying, 'I am happy to be your patron'.

After the defeat of the heretical doctrines this great scholar spread the Buddha's message for eight years.

III

HOW NĀROPA PERFORMED GREAT ACTS OF SELF-DENIAL

THIS part has six chapters:

(i) Purifying the Wish-Fulfilling Gem, Being-in-itself as being-oneself,[1] from positive and negative attributes;

(ii) Uncovering the Wish-Fulfilling Gem as the path to maturity through the understanding of symbols;

(iii) Walking the path of freedom by suffering the torment of the acts of self-denial;

(iv) Setting those who may be taught on the paths of maturity and freedom by virtue of the realization of ten signs and eight qualities;[2]

(v) Attaining a spiritualized ('rainbow') existence or Vajrakāya during his lifetime and realizing the transcending awareness revealing Reality as it is;

(vi) Handing over to the venerable Mar-pa the Oral Transmission together with its explanation and spreading the Buddhist Doctrine in Tibet through him.

(i)

This chapter has three sections:

(*a*) Having twelve minor visionary experiences whilst seeking the Guru with ardent faith and unflagging zeal;

(*b*) The attempt at suicide and the resolution to meet the Guru in a subsequent life;

(*c*) Being accepted as a disciple after meeting Tilopa.

[1] *rgyud, tantra/santāna*. This term is a comprehensive one inasmuch as it refers to Being-in-itself or the transcendent totality of truth and to being-oneself, the self-conscious existence of the individual who is aware of the transcendent and can reach it only through this awareness of his own existence.

[2] Usually one speaks of 'five signs and eight qualities', which refer to meditative experiences. The peculiar way of counting 'ten' signs and their significance is explained below in their proper context. See pp. 60 sqq.

(*a*)

The twelve minor visionary experiences begin with the exhortation by rDo-rje rnal-'byor-ma (Vajrayoginī) to go to Tilopa in order to attain the highest realization and to spread the intrinsic message of the Doctrine.

Once when 'Jigs-med grags-pa (Abhayakīrti), with his back to the sun, was studying the books on grammar, epistemology, spiritual precepts, and logic, a terrifying shadow fell on them. Looking round he saw behind him an old woman with thirty-seven ugly features: her eyes were red and deep-hollowed; her hair was fox-coloured and dishevelled; her forehead large and protruding; her face had many wrinkles and was shrivelled up; her ears were long and lumpy; her nose was twisted and inflamed; she had a yellow beard streaked with white; her mouth was distorted and gaping; her teeth were turned in and decayed; her tongue made chewing movements and moistened her lips; she made sucking noises and licked her lips; she whistled when she yawned; she was weeping and tears ran down her cheeks; she was shivering and panting for breath; her complexion was darkish blue; her skin rough and thick; her body bent and askew; her neck curved; she was hump-backed; and, being lame, she supported herself on a stick. She said to Nāropa: 'What are you looking into?'

'I study the books on grammar, epistemology, spiritual precepts, and logic', he replied.

'Do you understand them?'

'Yes.'

'Do you understand the words or the sense?'

'The words.'

The old woman was delighted, rocked with laughter, and began to dance waving her stick in the air. Thinking that she might feel still happier, Nāropa added: 'I also understand the sense'. But then the woman began to weep and tremble and she threw her stick down.

'How is it that you were happy when I said that I understood the words, but became miserable when I added that I also understood the sense?'

'I felt happy because you, a great scholar, did not lie and frankly admitted that you only understood the words. But I felt sad when you told a lie by stating that you understood the sense, which you do not.'

'Who, then, understands the sense?'

'My brother.'

'Introduce me to him wherever he may be.'

'Go yourself, pay your respects to him, and beg him that you may come to grasp the sense.'

With these words the old woman disappeared like a rainbow in the sky.

The venerable Nāropa reflected on the vision of the old woman with thirty-seven ugly features, and taking each as an object of inspection[1] he realized that, objectively, Saṁsāra is misery because it contains thirty-seven kinds of dissatisfaction; that, subjectively, the body with its thirty-seven impure substances[2] is impermanent and perishable; and that, mystically, one comes to understand co-emergent awareness[3] through reflecting on the thirty-seven pathways and thirty-seven kinds of creative potentiality.[4] Then he sang:

> Saṁsāra is the tendency to find fault with others,
> An unbearable fire-bowl,
> A dungeon dark,
> A deep swamp of three poisons,[5]
> A fearful wave of evil lives,

[1] *dran-pa, smṛti.* The reasons why this word cannot be translated by 'memory', I have given in my *Jewel Ornament of Liberation*, p. 230.

[2] Here again we have one number more than the ordinary amount of impure substances.

[3] *lhan-cig-skyes-pa'i ye-śes, sahajajñāna.* According to Sphžg 60*a*, one speaks of *lhan-cig-skyes-pa, sahaja* because two features go together, not that the one is *in* the other. The philosophical implication is that there is no unbridgeable gulf between 'appearance' and 'reality', because appearance is reality inasmuch as it is the appearance of the latter. To make a difference between appearance and reality is the working of our bifurcating mind, but in the immediate awareness that reality is co-present with or emerges together with appearance the seemingly abysmal gulf is bridged. This certainly has not the slightest resemblance to the innatism of Descartes. Hence translations of this term by 'innate' are wrong and must be rejected because they create wrong ideas.

[4] *rtsa, nāḍī; rluṅ, vāyu; thig-le, tilaka* (*bindu*). See below p. 46 and Note F, pp. 268 sqq., for a detailed analysis and the reasons for the rejection of the current linguistic translations.

[5] They are the patterns in which man's emotionally unstable nature manifests itself: passion-lust, antipathy, and bewilderment.

'Tis being caught in a spider's web,
Or a bird entangled in a fowler's net.
'Tis like being bound hand to neck by Māra,
Or immersed in a pond of beastliness.
'Tis like a deer chasing a mirage.
It is the net of fate,
A bee that honey sucks,
Milking the cow of life,
And living 'neath the fleeting shadows of old age and birth.
'Tis being caught by the Lord of Death's rough-coated dogs,
A deer trapped in a snare,
A hunter merciless,
Entanglement in bondage,
An unsafe footpath,
A wild beast captured in a pit.
It is a meadow rich for dichotomic play,
A horse of eight contingencies,[1]
A spearhead beating on a drum,
Merriment with sharpened fangs.
It is a fragile water-plant,
The intangible reflection of the moon in water,
A bubble of bewilderment,
Fleeting mist and rippling water,
A snake conquering by touch and sight,
The taste of honey on a razor blade,
It is a tree with poisonous leaves,
Shooting the poisoned arrow of disturbed emotions,
And poisoning those afflicted by defects.
It is a flame flickering in the wind,
Untruth, a dream, bewilderment,
The waterfall of old age and death.
'Tis Kleśamāra,[2] deception's guide.
Verily I must seek out the Guru.

[1] Gain and loss, fame and disgrace, praise and blame, pleasure and pain.

[2] This term has been explained by sKye-med bde-chen in his *Dohākośa-nāma-caryāgīti-arthapradīpa-nāma-ṭikā*, 34*b*: 'Kleśamāra means the following: Emotional reactivity depends for its existence on an organism and is generated in and through the five senses. The emotional reactions which come about after the

With these words he gave up all his belongings and books. When he announced his intention to seek the Guru who would reveal the sense to him, the congregation at Nalanda thought: 'Among the former abbots there was no scholar so profound as our Nāropa. In performing the duties of an abbot he explained the Doctrine in a holier way than others; when he talked about grammar, logic, Sūtras, or Tantras, he gave superworldly explanations; when he performed the rites of the awakening of an enlightened attitude of confirmation, and other initiations, he was unsurpassable in grace; when he instructed those who practised meditation he was especially gifted in explaining the experiences and realizations. If such an abbot were to go to another country we should be like fish on dry land', and they all were plunged in despair. Then the head of the department at the Eastern gate made this request:

Peerless and glorious Abhayakīrti,
The congregation is the root of Dharma,
To renounce them is against the Dharma.
Stay with us for our sake we pray.

But Nāropa declined. Then the head of the department at the Southern gate said:

The companions in the Dharma are its root.
To leave your friends is against the Doctrine.
Stay with us (we pray).

Again Nāropa refused. Then the head of the department at the Western gate entreated him:

The root of the Doctrine is the Dharma's discipline,
Which to give up is action 'gainst the Dharma.
Stay with us (we pray).

This too was of no avail. Then the 500 scholars of Nalanda together with their patron the king and his ministers, unanimously begged him to stay:

Sublime and glorious sage, Abhayakīrti,
We should have no physician, Dharma's embodiment,

five senses have grasped their outer and inner objects, are called Māra, and to live under the sway of emotional re-activity points to its great power'.

'Gainst the diseases of our blindness and ignorance,
So, saint Abhayakīrti, stay for our sake,
And look with mercy on Nalanda.

The glorious Abhayakīrti only said:

Whate'er is born will die, whate'er is joined will part.
How can we find the path of freedom and immortality
In that which only builds up (Karma)?
I know all the scriptures which are like the sea,
All five branches of learning have I mastered
With grammar and epistemology,
Yet without a competent Guru
The fire of my craving will not die.
If my yearning be not stilled
By the Guru's grace which is like
The nectar stream of Tantra essence
Wide as the ocean, despite my attainments,
Virtues and supersensible cognitions,
I have not seen Reality.
Therefore I shall rely on dGyes-pa rdo-rje (Hevajra)[1]
And seek firmly for the true Guru.

'Let this be my answer to the king; let "it must be" be my answer to the Bhikṣus and to the scholars. I am a scholar well versed in the five branches of learning, but since it is a waste of time to try to turn me from the path of those who have the courage of their convictions, I beg my worthy patrons to allow me to go on.' With these words he shouldered his robe, took his alms-bowl by the rim, grasped his staff, and set out towards the East, saying:

I shall rely on dGyes-pa rdo-rje (Hevajra)
And seek for the true Guru.

A voice came from the sky:

To you the Buddha as Guru will be revealed
If you rely on bDe-mchog 'khor-lo (Cakrasaṃvara).

[1] dGyes-pa rdo-rje, the same as Kye-rdo-rje, Hevajra, stands for Helāvajra and thus attempts to convey by its name something of its positive, blissful, and joyful nature.

And Nāropa said jubilantly:

If from today on bDe-mchog 'khor-lo I rely,
What shall I not achieve?

He bowed to the East and, deeply moved, with tears in his eyes, prayed to Tilopa. When he reached Me-tog snam-bu cemetery he built a grass-hut and repeated the seven-syllabled mantra of bDe-mchog[1] for 700,000 times. The earth trembled, light and a sweet fragrance appeared, and from the sky a voice was heard saying:

In the East there lives Tilopa, embodiment
Of the great bliss of non-dual awareness,
Incarnate and lord of all that lives.
Seek him the Guru Buddha.

Trusting in this voice he sought the Guru for a whole month in the East. When he did not find him he exclaimed:

Alas, I sought but have not found the Guru Buddha,
For by Māra have I been deceived.

Again a voice came from the sky:

You will find the Guru Buddha if you seek him
Without paying homage to that devil Laziness.

When therefore he went further East in his search for the Guru, his tutelary deity 'Khor-lo sdom-pa (Cakrasaṃvara) assured him:

Glorious Abhayakīrti,
I have given you my grace so that you
May find the revered Tilopa.
How will you win Buddhahood
If you find not the Guru?
Search for Tilopa in the East,
He is incarnate Buddhahood,
The Guru who will release your spirituality.
Take then no heed of obstacles.

[1] *Oṃ hriḥ hā hā hūṃ hūṃ phaṭ.*

When he had heard these words he sang:

> Tilopa, venerable Guru,
> Without you I cannot win Buddhahood.
> Whether or no I find you, from today
> I shall heed nor life nor body.
> Why, if undeterred by obstacles,
> Should I not find the promised Guru?

And he proceeded onwards in an Eastern direction.

These were the visions he had:

When he had come to a narrow footpath that wound between rocks and a river, he found a leper woman without hands and feet blocking the path.

'Do not block the way, step aside.'

'I cannot move. Go round if you are not in a hurry, but if you are jump over me.'

Although he was full of compassion, he closed his nose in disgust and leaped over her. The leper woman rose in the air in a rainbow halo and said:

> Listen, Abhayakīrti:
> The Ultimate in which all become the same
> Is free of habit-forming thought and limitations.
> How, if still fettered by them,
> Can you hope to find the Guru?

At this the woman, the rocks, and the path all vanished and Nāropa fell into a swoon on a sandy plateau. When he recovered consciousness he thought: 'I did not recognize this to be the Guru, now I shall ask anyone I meet for instruction'. Then he got up and went on his way praying.

On a narrow road he met a stinking bitch crawling with vermin. He closed his nose and jumped over the animal which then appeared in the sky in a rainbow halo and said:

> All living beings by nature are one's parents.
> How will you find the Guru, if
> Without developing compassion
> On the Mahāyāna path

You seek in the wrong direction?
How will you find the Guru to accept you
When you look down on others?

After these words the bitch and the rocks disappeared and Nāropa again swooned on a sandy plateau.

When he came to he resumed his prayers and his journey, and met a man carrying a load.

'Have you seen the venerable Tilopa?'

'I have not seen him. However, you will find behind this mountain a man playing tricks on his parents.[1] Ask him.'

When he had crossed the mountain he found the man, who said:

'I have seen him, but before I tell you help me to turn my parents' head.'

But Abhayakīrti thought: 'Even if I should not find the venerable Tilopa, I cannot associate with a scoundrel, because I am a prince, a Bhikṣu, and a scholar. If I seek the Guru I will do so in a respectable way according to the Dharma.'

Everything happened as before, the man receded into the centre of a rainbow halo and said:

How will you find the Guru, if
In this doctrine of Great Compassion
You do not crack the skull of egotism
With the mallet of non-Pure-Egoness and nothingness?

The man disappeared like a rainbow and Nāropa fell senseless to the ground. When he woke up there was nothing and he walked on praying as he went.

Beyond another mountain he found a man who was tearing the intestines out of a human corpse and cutting them up. Asked whether he had seen Tilopa, he answered:

'Yes, but before I show him to you, help me to cut up the intestines of this decayed corpse.'

[1] *mgo-bo rduṅ-ba*, lit.: 'to knock on the head' always means 'to play a trick on somebody', 'to cheat a person into doing something'. The pun in this passage is inimitable.

Since Nāropa did not do so, the man moved away into the centre of a rainbow-coloured light and said:

> How will you find the Guru, if
> You cut not Saṃsāra's ties
> With the unoriginatedness of the Ultimate
> In its realm of non-reference?

And the man disappeared like a rainbow.

When Nāropa had recovered from his swoon and gone on his way praying, he found on the bank of a river a rascal who had opened the stomach of a live man and was washing it with warm water. When he asked him whether he had seen the venerable Tilopa he replied:

'Yes, but before I show him, help me.'

Again Nāropa refused, and the man appearing in a centre of light in the sky said:

> How will you find the Guru, if
> With the water of profound instruction
> You cleanse not Saṃsāra, which by nature free
> Yet represents the dirt of habit-forming thoughts?

And the man disappeared in the sky.

After having woken from his swoon Nāropa prayed and journeyed on until he came to the city of a great king whom he asked whether he had seen Tilopa. The king replied:

'I have seen him, but marry my daughter before I show him to you.'

Having taken her he seemed to spend a long time. Then the king, not wishing to let him go, took back the girl and the dowry and left the room. Not recognizing this as a magic spell, but thinking that he would have to employ force with the aid of the bDe-mchog rtsa-rgyud (Abhidhāna-uttaratantra) he heard a voice say:

> Are you not deceived by a magic show?
> How then will you find the Guru
> If through desire and dislike you fall
> Into the three forms of evil life?

And the whole kingdom disappeared.

When Nāropa came to, he travelled in prayer until he met a dark man with a pack of hounds, a bow and arrows.

'Have you seen Tilopa?'

'Yes.'

'Show him to me.'

'Take this bow and arrow and kill that deer.'

When Nāropa refused the man said:

A hunter, I have drawn the arrow
Of the phantom body which from desires is free
In the bow, of radiant light the essence:
I shall kill the fleeing deer of this and that,
On the mountain of the body believing in an I.
Tomorrow I go fishing in the lake.

So saying he disappeared.

When Nāropa had recovered he continued prayerfully in search of the Guru and came to the shore of a lake full of fish. Near by two old people were ploughing a field, killing and eating the insects they found in the furrows.

'Have you seen Tilopa?'

'He stayed with us, but before I show him to you—hallo, wife, come and get this Bhikṣu something to eat.'

The old woman took some fish and frogs from her net and cooked them alive. When she invited Nāropa to eat he said: 'Since I am a Bhikṣu I no longer have an evening meal, and besides that I do not eat meat.' Thinking, 'I must have violated the doctrine of the Buddha to be asked to dine by an old woman who cooks fish and frogs alive', he sat there miserably. Then the old man came up with an ox on his shoulders and asked his wife: 'Have you prepared some food for the Bhikṣu?' She replied: 'He seems to be stupid; I cooked some food, but he said that he did not want to eat.'

Then the old man threw the pan into the fire while the fish and frogs flew up into the sky. He said:

Fettered by habit-forming thoughts, 'tis hard to find
the Guru.
How will you find the Guru if you eat not

This fish of habit-forming thoughts, but hanker
After pleasures (which enhance the sense of ego)?
Tomorrow I will kill my parents.

He then disappeared.

After his recovery Nāropa came upon a man who had impaled his father on a stake, put his mother into a dungeon and was about to kill them. They cried loudly: 'Oh son, do not be so cruel.' Although Nāropa revolted at the sight he asked the man whether he had seen Tilopa, and was answered:

'Help me to kill the parents who have brought me misfortune and I will then show you Tilopa.'

But since Nāropa felt compassion for the man's parents he did not make friends with this murderer. Then with the words:

You will find it hard to find the Guru
If you kill not the three poisons that derive
From your parents, the dichotomy of this and that.
Tomorrow I will go and beg.

the man disappeared.

When Nāropa had recovered from his swoon and gone on in prayer he came to a hermitage. One of the inmates recognized him as Abhayakīrti and asked: 'Why have you come? Is it to meet us?'

'I am merely a Ku-su-li-pa,[1] there is no need for a reception.'

The hermit, however, did not heed his words and received him with due honours. Asked for the reason of his coming Nāropa said: 'I seek Tilopa. Have you seen him?'

'You will find that your search has come to an end. Inside is a beggar who claims to be Tilopa.'

Nāropa found him within sitting by the fire and frying live fish.

[1] Although this is the common Tibetan form of the word, according to Ržd 93*b* it is wrong and should be Ku-sa-li. The author says: 'Ku-su-lu is not correct; in Sanskrit it is Kusali. In Tibetan it means a man who has three thoughts. Apart from thinking about eating and drinking, defecation and urination, and sleeping, he has given up all other occupations and is absorbed in meditative concentration. Such a man is nowadays known as a Ku-su-lu-pa. In India, however, there are two types, a superior and an inferior one. In Tibet one calls a person who has come back from death Ku-su-lu-pa. The meaning of Ku-su-lu is actually one who has given up all work and frequents mountain retreats.'

When the hermits saw this they began angrily to beat the beggar, who asked: 'Don't you like what I do?'

'How can we when evil is done in a hermitage?'

The beggar snapped his fingers, said 'Lohivagaja',[1] and the fish returned to the lake. Nāropa, realizing that this man must be Tilopa, folded his hands and begged for instruction. The Guru passed him a handful of lice, saying:

> If you would kill the misery of habit-forming thoughts
> And ingrained tendencies on the endless path
> To the ultimate nature of all beings,
> First you must kill (these lice).

But when Nāropa was unable to do so, the man disappeared with the words:

> You will find it hard to find the Guru
> If you kill not the louse of habit-forming thoughts,
> Self-originated and self-destructive.
> Tomorrow I will visit a freak show.

Dejectedly Nāropa got up and continued his search. Coming to a wide plain, he found many one-eyed people, a blind man with sight and an earless one who could hear, a man without a tongue speaking, a lame man running about, and a corpse gently fanning itself. When Nāropa asked them whether they had seen Tilopa they declared:

'We haven't seen him or anyone else. If you really want to find him do as follows:

> Out of confidence, devotion, and certainty, become
> A worthy vessel, a disciple with the courage of conviction.
> Cling to the spirituality of a Teacher in the spiritual fold,
> Wield the razor of intuitive understanding as the viewpoint,
> Ride the horse of bliss and radiance as the method of attention,
> Free yourself from the bonds of this and that as the way of conduct.
> Then shines the sun of self-lustre which understands

[1] *lohivagaja* seems to be the Tibetan transcription of a Prakrit sentence which in Sanskrit might have been *rohita avagaccha* 'fish go away!'

One-eyedness as the quality of many,
Blindness as seeing without seeing a thing,
Deafness as hearing without hearing a thing,
Muteness as speaking without saying something,
Lameness as moving without being hurried,
Death's immobility as the breeze of the Unoriginated
(like air moved by a fan).

In this way the symbols of Mahāmudrā were pointed out, whereafter everything disappeared.

(*b*)

Nāropa now thought of suicide in the hope of finding the Guru in a subsequent life. He said to himself: 'Although I have met with various manifestations of the venerable Tilopa I have not had the luck to meet him personally. I have failed in my search and am ashamed to return. Since I have been hindered by this body which is the result of former deeds, I shall discard it with the resolve to meet the Guru in some later life.' In his despondency he composed the following verses:

Pursuing a Ḍāka's prophecy, I gave up
The Sangha, the Doctrine's root, and left
My friends well disciplined in Dharma.
I did not heed the words of those who gave advice,
Despite the hardships that I underwent
I did not find the Guru.
I shall throw away this hindrance of a body
To go on seeking in another life.

When he was ready to cut his veins with a razor—

(*c*)

There came a voice from the sky:

If you have not found, how will you find
The Guru if you kill the Buddha?
Is it not me whom your evil thoughts desire?

And there came a dark man dressed in cotton trousers, his hair knotted in a tuft, and with protruding blood-shot eyes. Nāropa weeping with emotion knelt down, folded his hands and said:

How would I think to find the truth by seeking it
In that which is uncertain and passes like a cloud?
Alas, before you did not show compassion,
Henceforth accept me in compassion.

Tilopa said: 'Ever since you met me in the form of the leper woman we have never been apart, but were like a body and its shadow. The various visions you had were the defilements of your evil deeds and so you did not recognize me.' And he added:

You are a worthy vessel, immaculate,
Resplendent, worthy to receive instruction
In Guhyamantra, the Wish-Fulfilling Gem,
The Ḍākinī's hidden home.
Seize the Wish-Fulfilling Gem, your true spirituality,
The Ḍākinī's hidden home.

He then taught Nāropa in full how to rely on the Gurus of the four transmissions[1] and the message of the Ye-śes mkha'-'gro (Jñānaḍāka) of U-rgyan (Swat), accepted him as his disciple and revived his spirits.

(ii)

UNCOVERING THE WISH-FULFILLING GEM

There are two ways of uncovering the Wish-Fulfilling Gem as the path to maturity through the understanding of symbols:

(*a*) By understanding these symbols the moment they are shown. This is for those capable of instantaneous enlightenment, and

(*b*) by understanding the meaning of the four maturing confirmations indicated by the symbols and their explanation and how thereby true spirituality shines forth. This is for those who come gradually to enlightenment.

[1] The four transmissions are discussed in detail in Sphkh *2a* sqq. The importance of Tilopa lies in the fact that he combined in himself all four. The first is the Mahāmudrā teaching, recognizing all Sūtras and Tantras; the second is the teaching of the Mother-Tantras; the third that of the Father-Tantras; and the fourth the Radiant Light doctrine.

(*a*)

Once, when Tilopa was sitting in the posture taught in the rNam-snaṅ (Vairocanābhi-sambodhitantra), Abhayakīrti approached him, circumambulated him with folded hands, offered a maṇḍala,[1] and kneeling down prayed: 'Guru, kindly instruct me.' By way of answer Tilopa showed him thirteen symbols for thirteen days. He began: 'In order to receive instruction it is necessary first to have the confirmations. Therefore bring some glowing embers and a piece of cotton cloth.' When Nāropa had done so, Tilopa spread the cloth evenly on the ground and fastened the four edges with pegs. Telling Nāropa to hold one side, he lit the other. The ashes retained the warp and woof of the cloth that had been burnt completely. Though the pattern was there it could no longer serve as cloth. Then Tilopa asked: 'Nāropa, do you understand what this means?' and the latter answered: 'I understand that the Guru's illumining understanding and instruction, which is like fire, burns the disciple's emotional instability which is like cotton cloth. Thereby the belief in the solid reality of an external object is destroyed, and since this sort of belief about reality is no longer effective there is no return into worldliness.' And he composed the following song about his understanding:

> The meaning and purpose of my initiation, the fire,
> Has consumed my habit-forming thoughts, the cotton cloth;
> Though in the ash the pattern is preserved,
> The cloth can be used no longer.
> Thus it is with the apparitional body
> Which is intangible when it appears.

Tilopa said nothing. When Nāropa again walked round him with folded hands and asked for instruction, Tilopa merely showed him a transparent crystal. Nāropa said that he understood it to mean that the disciple's spirituality (Being-in-itself) must remain unaffected by falsehood and deceit through abiding in pure commitment.

[1] *maṇḍala* means both an elaborate preparation symbolizing the building and ordering of the whole universe to be offered to the Guru, and a certain way of folding one's hands. To build a *maṇḍala* is 'accumulation of merit', to understand the *maṇḍala* as being nothing in itself, is 'acquisition of knowledge.'

Next Tilopa asked Nāropa to bring him a twisted ball of thread and unloosen it. When this had been done, Tilopa simply threw the thread away and went out. Nāropa declared: 'I understand that the net by which Mind[1] is caught in Saṃsāra, the involvement in eight worldly vices,[2] has to be thrown away and left lying in its place, real mind.'

Tilopa then put a rare jewel on his head.

'I understand that the precious jewel which creates Saṃsāra and Nirvāṇa, is the Guru, and that one has to think of him as indivisible from one's crown of the head.'

Then Tilopa looked at the jewel.

'I understand that to see the Ultimate in this life is to have obtained the highest realization, Mahāmudrā, and that with the glance of unswerving devotion the Guru's action and conduct has to be considered as supreme virtue.'

Tilopa next filled a vessel with pure cold water and asked Nāropa to drink it.

'I understand that the heat of emotional instability found in myself and others is alleviated by the cool water of spiritual instruction.'

Tilopa now filled several vessels with water, emptied them into one vessel and then refilled the many from one.

'I understand this filling and refilling as the fact that one value appears in many (forms) and that the many have only one value.'[3]

Tilopa then showed a triangle as the origin of all things.

[1] *raṅ-sems*, also *raṅ-gi sems*, is a term most likely to mislead the linguistic specialist by inducing him to translate the genitive case *raṅ-gi* as such and render the whole term as 'one's mind', taking 'one' as one entity and 'mind' as another. However, the use of *raṅ* is, to our Western thinking, exceedingly ambiguous. Above all it refers to itself so that *raṅ-gi sems* would have to be translated as 'mind pointing to itself', 'mind in itself', 'mind as such' or any such similar circumlocutions. Further, *sems* is not exactly what we understand by 'mind'. It is a readiness to respond which in a certain sense may be said to be my readiness as it is at the root of my being. The translation 'one's mind' would be correct if we did not understand 'mind' in an entitative sense as we usually do. Not being an entity in the ordinary sense of the word, *sems* does not entail the doctrine of solipsism.

[2] See note 1 p. 26.

[3] *ro-gcig, ekarasa*. This term is often translated as 'having one flavour or taste', which is possible, though in most cases wrong. *ro-gcig* is used pre-eminently in the context of ethics which imply values, not flavours. Even when the term is used in connection with meditative contemplation it rather denotes the transition from contemplation to action.

'I understand this as a symbol that the whole of reality serving as the actuality of the three gates to liberation[1] never had an origin.'

Next Tilopa drew the picture of a dot.[2]

'I understand this as a symbol that all things derive from the creative potentiality of Dharmakāya.'

Tilopa touched his breast and nodded his head.

'I understand this as a symbol that Dharmakāya's creative potentiality is just potentiality.'

Tilopa pointed to a snake uncoiling itself.

'I understand this as a symbol that Saṃsāra becomes free through itself.'

Tilopa pretended to be dumb.

'I understand that the experience of intuitive illumining understanding cannot be expressed in words.'

Finally Tilopa showed him a fruit.

'I understand that when the fruit ripens in the individual self-sufficiency and being-for-others will be fulfilled. This is how I understand each symbol.'

When these thirteen symbols[3] had been pointed out to him, he asked for confirmation of his understanding, and Tilopa sang this great song about the intuitive illumining understanding, containing the solution of the symbols as the path towards spiritual maturation:

> I, Tilopa, smile and say: Listen
> You worthy vessel, immaculate, resplendent,
> The instruction burns like blazing coal
> Emotional instability, the cotton cloth.
> One's true spirituality is as a crystal pure.
> Untie the eightfold knot of vice,
> Look with unswerving faith and love
> At the Jewel of a Guru: drink
> The pure water of instruction,
> For water in all vessels is the same.

[1] Nothingness (*śūnyatā*), unbiasedness (*apraṇihita*), and imagelessness (*animitta*).

[2] *thig-le, tilaka, bindu.* A detailed explanation is given below, pp. 167 sqq.

[3] These thirteen symbols are explained in the same way in Dchlsp 47*b* sqq.

Origination is unoriginatedness,
Dharmakāya by itself as creativity abides.
The finger points for that is its nature.
As the snake uncoils, Saṃsāra frees itself.
Muteness is the ineffability of experience,
Fruit symbolizes the maturing of one's own and others'
Truth. Having solved these thirteen symbols
You know them all. With this confirmation
Which matures the immature, in the Wish-Fulfilling Gem
Of the Guhyamantra, the Ḍākinī's hidden home,
Watch the mirror of mind and become mature.

(*b*)

For those who come gradually to enlightenment, the birth of true spirituality through solving the symbols confers the grace of the maturing confirmations according to the general procedure of the Guhyamantra, Thus Tilopa said: 'Understand by the "jar" confirmation[1] that all appearances are deity and mind and you have then realized that appearance is a magic spell. Understand by the "mystery" confirmation[2] that mind is the noetic act and nothing in itself. Understand by the "transcending awareness through discrimination-appreciation" confirmation[3] that this nothing is bliss. Look for the unity of all this after having understood through the "fourth" confirmation that this bliss is indispersable.'

Then Nāropa asked:

How can I watch when blinded
By my dark ignorance?

[1] It is important to note that this confirmation and the following ones are inner experiences, although their presentation suggests the interaction of two persons. See Note D, p. 267.

[2] Man is not only in-the-world, he also communicates with-others. While the preceding confirmation purified his being-in-the-world, this one purifies his communication with-others. In the deepest sense of the word this confirmation is the mystery of communication. This is possible between subjects, not between a subject and an object. Inasmuch as the 'object'-idea is overcome, the philosophical viewpoint is here the mentalistic thesis that sensa are delusive (*sems-tsam rnam-rdzun*).

[3] As a mere literal translation this name hardly conveys any meaning. See Note E, pp. 267 sqq.

The venerable Tilopa answered:

> Watch without watching for something. Look
> From the invisible at what you cannot grasp
> As an entity. To see and yet to see no things
> Is freedom in and through yourself.

Then Nāropa watched the confirmations without watching for something and looked at them without seeing them as something and he became free in a moment in a state that need not be freed. He prayed:

> When I depend upon the ship, the Guru, the precious
> Jewel of the Mind, I am sure of freedom
> From Saṃsāra's ocean. This practice teaches
> That the path towards maturity is bliss.

But Tilopa said:

> You seem still to be attracted by the teaching
> Of the Guru who understands reality as bliss.
> Your emotions still seem to be unstable since you hanker
> After the instruction on the profound meaning of reality
> By the Guru who understands it as bliss in blissfulness.
> Hanker not for this nor for its opposite.

(iii)

THE TWELVE ACTS OF SELF-DENIAL

This chapter dealing with Nāropa's experiences on the path of freedom, as a result of subjecting himself to severe spiritual exercises, has four sections:

(*a*) His twelve great acts of self-denial in order to obtain the instructions in full and so attune his mind to the Guru's spirituality;

(*b*) His exhortation by Tilopa to act by conduct which cannot be expressed in words and thoughts;

(*c*) His understanding of the meaning of 'coincidence' or the instruction in ultimate identity of awareness developing either into Saṃsāra or Nirvāṇa;

(*d*) His acceptance of his mission by being exhorted to work for the benefit of sentient beings through a life of compassion that transcends all attempts to fathom it by meditation.

(*a*)

I. THE ORDINARY WISH-FULFILLING GEM[1]

Tilopa sat for a year motionless and stiff like a log, as if he had lost the power of movement. He was silent like one bereft of speech; and he remained in a state in which no habit-forming thoughts entered, as if his mind had lost its agility. Nāropa made the appropriate gesture, circumambulated with folded hands, and prayed.[2] When once in a while Tilopa turned his head and stared at him, Nāropa asked for instruction. With the words: 'If you want instruction follow me', Tilopa climbed to the top of the temple of Otantra which had a triple Chinese roof, and straddled the wings of one of the ornamental birds. Then he said: 'If I had had a disciple, he would have jumped down from here.' Thinking that these words were meant for him, Nāropa unhesitatingly leaped down, crashed to the ground, and lay there like a corpse, overcome by intolerable pain. Tilopa asked: 'What is wrong with you?' And Nāropa replied:

> This lump of a body fashioned by former deeds
> Is broken like a reed and nearly dead.

Tilopa said:

> Nāropa, your clay pitcher of a body, believing
> In an I, deserves to be broken. Consider
> The Wish-Fulfilling Gem, the mysterious home
> Of Buddhas and Ḍākinīs in the present, past, and future.

Stroking Nāropa with his hand he restored his body to its former state. He then instructed him in the Ordinary Wish-Fulfilling Gem, which he had received personally from Ye-śes mkha'-'gro

[1] A detailed analysis of this subject matter is found in Part II.

[2] 'To pray' (*gsol-ba 'debs-pa*) is essentially an act of contemplation, not of petition, intercession, or adoration.

(Jñānaḍāka) in U-rgyan (Swat), about the method of realizing the 'Mother lHan-cig-skyes-ma',[1] which includes the procedures symbolized by 'the king' as the unchanging and ever-present reality, 'the three ministers' as the executive, and 'the subjects' as the occasion for practising.

(A) In these instructions the preliminary are 'the three ministers' as executive, which means (i) purification from defilement by evil, or meditation on rDo-rje sems-dpa' (Vajrasattva) and the recital of his mantra; (ii) the perfection of the prerequisites and uniting with the Guru(s); and (iii) the spiritual maturation or acquisition of the capacity for meditative absorption.

(B) The substance is 'the king' as the unchanging reality. It is the approach by the Developing Stage called the Ordinary Wish-Fulfilling Gem.

(*a*) 'Developing Stage' is the name for the purificatory practice of the four modes of origination concerning the three existential phenomena by four creative acts. These are the purifications of (i) womb-birth by five intuitive realizations;[2] (ii) egg-birth by a certain mode of recitation;[3] (iii) heat-and-moisture birth by applying the triple method;[4] and (iv) spontaneous birth by the method of momentary complete inspection.[5]

The object of the Developing Stage is to purify the three existential phenomena of birth, death, and intermediary state between death and (re)birth by their appropriate means. The adept, therefore, conceives of himself as Dam-tshig sems-dpa' (Samayasattva)[6] in the form of the god Heruka, who is the Lord of sixty-two gods and goddesses. He is of deep-blue colour, has four faces and sixteen arms and is embraced by his spouse. His right leg is stretched (and his left leg slightly bent); he expresses the nine moods[7] such as

[1] This is another name for Vajrayoginī or Vajravārāhī. Nāropa composed a small text about her realization, the Vajrayoginīsādhana, the Tibetan translation of which by Mar-pa is preserved in the Tibetan bsTan-'gyur.

[2] This highly complicated technique has been described by sGam-po-pa, xxiv. 6*b* and xxxi. 3*b* in a very concise manner. A more detailed account is given by Padma dkar-po in Sphžg 16*a* sq. and Sphkh 6*a*.

[3] Sphžg 75*b*; 76*a*; 77*a*.

[4] Ibid. 75*b*.

[5] Ibid. See also sGam-po-pa, iv. 4*b*; x. 28*b*; xi. 9*a*; xxxi. 21*a*.

[6] Lit.: 'a being who is committed to a certain task.'

[7] According to Dchb 13*a*, the nine moods are: coquetry, dauntlessness, and

coquetry and others; he wears the eight emblems of the cremation ground and is adorned with various ornaments. He stands on a throne formed by a lotus and a sun, and tramples on Bhairava and Kala ratri.

This lotus and sun throne is in the middle of the Great-Bliss centre in a square palace with four arched gates, and is richly decorated with emblems. Within it are the focal points of authentic existence,[1] and it is surrounded by flames and cremation grounds.

'Birth' is purified when the deities (male and female) have put on their respective apparel[2] and when in a general way the adept feels graced by authentic being.

The 'Intermediate state' is purified by summoning Ye-śes sems-dpa' (Jñānasattva),[3] sealing, worshipping, lauding, and muttering the 'heart'-mantras[4] of the male and female deities.

When by the light radiating from one's heart the world as a vessel and the sentient beings as its content, the residents and their residences, have been gathered and dissolved in oneself, and when finally even 'sound' (*nāda*) is resolved into the radiant light, 'death' is purified by one's continuing in this state for a long time.[5]

The firm pride in the appearance of the deities out of the radiant light as being nothing in themselves is said to be the real sign of the experience of the Developing Stage.

(*b*) The essential purification practice, as regards the three existential phenomena of birth, death, and the intermediary stage by him who practises the Fulfilment Stage, is as follows: structure

repulsiveness relating to being-in-the-world (*sku, kāya*); laughter, awe, and dread to being-with-others (*gsuṅ, vāk*); and tenderness, majesticness, and peacefulness to facing and solving situations (*thugs, citta*).

[1] For a further discussion of these points see below Part II.

[2] These are certain mantras, syllables in specific colours which transform themselves into deities during meditation. One has to visualize them in certain parts of the deity's body. See Dchb 16*b*; Khd 8*a*.

[3] Lit.: 'Transcending awareness being.' This phase of the meditative process indicates the shift from the objective content to the subjective awareness. It is effected by rather complicated procedures. It has been dealt with in Dchb 17*b* sq.

[4] Ibid. 20*a*.

[5] This is to say that death is not a passage into nothingness, but a way of existing as an end attained; everything that has prevented authentic being, has 'died'. See also John Wild, op. cit., p. 218.

or pathways,[1] movement or the activeness of motility,[2] and creativity or enlightenment as potentiality, are brought to radiancy. 'Birth is then purified through the kindling of the inner mystic heat, higher awareness is made to spread, when motility becomes the muttering of the Vajramantra (*oṃ āh hūṃ*) and when the noetic act unfolds itself in intentionality and other intellectual operations.

'Death' is purified when by meditation there is no dispersion taking as entities the four visions which occur when motility recedes into, stays, and is dissolved in the central pathway of the structure as well as in the radiant light of nothingness.

The 'intermediate state' is purified when the indivisibility of motility and mentation which is radiant light, separates from the former psycho-somatic constituents. This moment is the rising of the deity adorned with all his or her perfectly radiant attributes in the framework of being the resident in a residence.

The immediate and vivid experience of the kindling of the inner mystic heat and the subsequent spreading of higher awareness is said to be the real essence of the Fulfilment Stage.

Through the Developing and Fulfilment Stages which purify the three existential phenomena of birth, death, and the intermediary one, the Father- and Mother-inspirations become fully known as one wants to experience them either in their concise or detailed aspects.[3]

(C) When one is doing the four types of practice[4] it is of the utmost importance to keep to the seven rules of eating, dressing, bathing, oblation, muttering, deportment, and sleeping.[5]

[1] Usually this term is translated by 'veins' or 'channels', and 'vital air' is supposed to move up and down therein. This is plain fancy. The rtsa (*nāḍī*) are the end product of a structuring process as well as this process itself. That they have nothing to do with 'veins' or 'channels' is plainly stated in Zmnd 38*b*: 'Those who claim that the *rtsa* are hollow bags and the *rluṅ* breath that comes in and out, and the *thig-le* semen and menstrual blood, do not know at all what it is about.'

[2] Note F, pp. 268 sqq.

[3] This distinction refers to the number of gods and goddesses surrounding the principal deity, be this 'Khor-lo sdom-pa (Cakrasaṃvara) or rDo-rje phag-ma (Vajravārāhī). See Dchb 29*b*.

[4] They are the purification practices mentioned on p. 44.

[5] Dchb 29*b* sqq.

2. ONE-VALUENESS[1]

Tilopa again sat motionless and silent for a year, and when Nāropa asked him for instruction he suddenly got up and went away. Nāropa followed and found him sitting near a blazing fire of sandal-wood. When he begged him for instruction Tilopa said: 'If I had had a disciple wanting instruction, he would have jumped into this fire.' Nāropa did so unhesitatingly, and when his whole body was burnt and unbearable pain overcame him, Tilopa merely asked: 'Nāropa, what is wrong with you?' Nāropa's answer was:

> This log of a body fashioned by former deeds
> Is consumed by fire and so I suffer.

Tilopa said:

> This log of your body believing in an I deserves
> To be burnt, Nāropa. Look into the mirror
> Of your mind (wherein lies) equality,
> The mysterious home of the Ḍākinī.

He touched him with his hand and healed him. He then gave him the instructions on one-valueness.

They consist of two parts: (i) attunement and (ii) one-valueness.

(i) The first is sixteenfold: attunement to the four confirmations;[2] to the four freedom paths;[3] to the four commitments one has to keep in connexion with them;[4] and to the four existential norms as the crowning result.[5]

Or, it is twelvefold: attunement to the four joys in a 'descending'

[1] For a fuller discussion see Part II.

[2] See above, pp. 41 and nn. 1–3.

[3] These are the awarenesses within the confirmatory experiences. See also below in Part II.

[4] They, too, are connected with the confirmations so as to keep the vividness of the experiences alive, not to turn them into a dead concept.

[5] They are: authentic being-in-the-world (*sprul-sku, nirmāṇakaya*); authentic being-with-and-for-others (*loṅs-sku, sambhogakāya*); authentic dealing with situations (*chos-sku, dharmakāya*); and the integration and integrity of these existential norms (*ṅo-bo-ñid-kyi sku, svābhāvikakāya*).

manner; to the four stabilized joys in an 'ascending' manner; and to the four joys as goal attainment.[1]

Or, it is ninefold: attunement to the three existential patterns or norms while dying, sleeping, and becoming awake.[2]

Or, it is fivefold: attunement of passion to the inner mystic heat; of aversion to the apparitional body; of bewilderment-errancy to the radiant light; of haughtiness to the Developing Stage; and of envy to pure appearance.

Or, it is threefold: attunement of death to a way of existing as a goal achieved; of the intermediate state (between death and rebirth) to a way of authentic communication; and of birth to a way of being-in-the-world authentically.

The core of experiencing attunement is to understand the being-this-or-that of Being-in-itself in its being-this-or-that[3] and to preserve this awareness which knows no bias in its naturalness[4] and not to let it swerve away from itself.

(ii) One-valueness is a name for conduct. Not the resultant state of confusion after having mixed different things such as good and bad, but comprehending the being-this-or-that of Being-in-itself in its being-this-or-that is attunement or one-valueness, while the

[1] This kind of attunement is intimately related to the Karmamudrā experience and will be discussed in Part II.

[2] This refers to the experience of the Intermediate state (*bar-do, antarābhava*) in particular. See Part II.

[3] The text makes the important distinction between *gnas-lugs* and *yin-lugs*. The former corresponds to the philosophical term Being-in-itself which cannot be grasped by conceptual thought and which is nothing in itself. The most that can be said is that it names the 'blunt fact' of existing; *yin-lugs* refers to the being-there. The whole of empirical reality, including oneself, which is always this or that (*yin-pa*) and to which we then apply the postulate of existence (*yod-pa*) and non-existence (*med-pa*). Being-in-itself or rather the fact of being is our empirical reality in so far as it is in the being-there, all the acts of the former being manifested in the latter. While the postulates of existence and non-existence would make up what Karl Jaspers, *Die geistige Situation der Zeit*, p. 37 calls 'Dasein ohne Existenz' (being-there without being-in-itself) with the difference that Dasein (being-there) is in his philosophy restricted to the human being, while in Tantrism it refers to the whole world; that which is termed *yin-lugs* is a being-there pervaded by Being-in-itself. This enables us to live up to Being-in-itself, to attune ourselves to its possibilities and then from a state of being tuned-in deal authentically with the fleeting character of empirical reality. This problem has been dealt with by sGam-po-pa, v. 21*a* sqq.

[4] *so-ma*. According to sGam-po-pa, vi. 10*a* and xxvi. 4*b* it is threefold: bodily action is performed in the framework of an unbiased perspective, speech becomes unforced vibrations, and mind operates without conceptual scaffolds.

understanding of this being-this-or-that is then to be tuned-in.

Its application may be illustrated by the phenomenon of sight. When one sees an object there is a subjective counterpart which acts and reacts in a pleasant or unpleasant way (i.e. has an emotively toned experience of something). On closer inspection, however, there is the appearance of something without there being anything. When we analyse this phenomenon still more deeply we find that the external object is both appearance and nothing, that the internal process of becoming aware is not a subject (sharply distinguished from and opposed to the object), and that the noetic relation ending in a distinct content with which formal identity is achieved is transcendence. The three contingent factors (of object, subject, and noetic relation) are present simultaneously in appearance.[1] The same holds good for the other senses such as hearing, smelling, tasting, feeling, and mentation. This is sixfold one-valueness. Experiencing these six forms simultaneously makes us lose our pre-occupation with this life and be mindful of death; it makes us think of the suffering of the six kinds of sentient beings; and it makes us renounce the hustle and bustle of the world and gives us mental-spiritual rest by causing us to become devoted to the Guru whose every action we see as good.

To preserve this state, in which there is no external reference, in an undisturbed way, is the real practice of attunement.

[1] As sGam-po-pa, iv. 4*a*; vi. 3*b*; x. 28*a* sqq.; xxiii. 6*b* and elsewhere points out, 'appearance' (*snaṅ-ba*) is not a three-termed relation in which 'the public, colourless, odourless material substances in mathematical space and time are one term, the aesthetic sensed data in their sensed spatial and temporal relations a second term, and the individual observer is the third term' (F. S. C. Northrop, *The Meeting of East and West*, p. 78), but has a field character. One component of this field is the indeterminate or as sGam-po-pa says, 'bliss, lucidity, and non-dividedness'. It is an invariant factor and primary, because any differentiation is always a differentiation of the indeterminate continuum which it requires for its existence. This is termed the 'certain factor in appearance' (*snaṅ-ba-la ṅes-pa*). The second component is the contingency of subject, object, and the noetic relation between the two. This is called the 'contingent factor in appearance' (*snaṅ-ba-la ma-ṅes-pa*). As is well known, Hume and the modern Western positivists neglected the primary and invariant factor and centred attention on the contingent, transitory differentiations. The Buddhist Tantric analysis of appearance reveals the error of the modern Western supposition that the totality of immediately apprehended fact can be accounted for by the mere aggregation of impermanent differentiations. For a trenchant critique see F. S. C. Northrop, op. cit., pp. 395 sqq. and his *The Logic of the Sciences and the Humanities*, pp. 95 sqq.

3. COMMITMENT[1]

Tilopa spent one year in a dense forest. He constantly wanted food to be given to him as alms. One day, on the occasion of the consecration of a funeral monument (Stūpa), a fair was held in a city nearby. Nāropa happened to go there and when his alms bowl was full he offered the food to his Guru. Eating noisily Tilopa said: 'Nāropa, this is delicious.' Nāropa thought: 'Formerly he never said a word; he seems to be in a good mood today', and so he asked him whether he should bring him some more food. Tilopa replied: 'Yes, do so', and giving him a pitcher full of water and a wooden sword, he added: 'If they do not give voluntarily, pour water on the food; if they pursue you draw the symbol for water in the dust, and if they do not turn back brandish your wooden sword.'

In this country it was the custom that if anyone came to a house for a second time he would not be given alms again. When therefore people said, 'you have had something before', and were unwilling to give him alms again Nāropa poured water on the food. Hearing the shouting 'this man spoils the rice' some men ran after him. When they were about to seize him he drew the symbol of water in the dust and a lake appeared which the pursuers could not cross. Then an old woman advised them 'Drain the lake'. They started digging and soon were able to pursue him. Then Nāropa brandished his sword. It became an iron hut and Nāropa found himself sitting inside. The old woman said to the men 'Bring coals and a pair of bellows and kindle a fire', which they did. When Nāropa could not stay inside any longer because of the heat he rushed out and fled. He had almost come to Tilopa when they caught him and beat him half-dead with sticks and stones. Tilopa approached and asked: 'Nāropa, what is wrong with you?' And Nāropa answered:

> Thrashed like rice and like sesame crushed
> My head is splitting and I suffer.

Then Tilopa said:

> This twisted copper kettle of Saṃsāra
> Deserves to be smashed, Nāropa. Look

[1] For a fuller discussion see Part II.

Into the mirror of your mind which is commitment,
The mysterious home of the Ḍākinī.

He touched him with his hand and healed him. Then he gave him the instruction on the Wish-Fulfilling Gem of Commitment.

This instruction consists of two parts: (i) trust and (ii) observation.

(i) Generally speaking there is commitment if one does not counteract that which one has taken upon oneself to do, be it only observing the rite of taking refuge. In particular, however, commitment plays a role in the mantra-teaching and especially in the unsurpassable discipline when after having obtained the 'jar'-confirmation one does not fail in one's commitment to look upon the world as a divine mansion and upon the sentient beings therein as gods and goddesses.

Here, the experience of the 'jar'-confirmation which is the basis of the commitment to be authentically in the world and called 'Extent' is the Ordinary Wish-Fulfilling Gem.

The experience of the 'mystery'-confirmation which is the foundation of the commitment to authentic communication and is termed 'Non-Duality', is found in the Six Liberation Practices which go under the name of 'The Upper Gate'.[1]

The experience of the 'transcending awareness through discrimination-appreciation'-confirmation which is the basis for the commitment to deal with situations authentically and is called 'Profoundness', is the mystic association with the Ḍāka (transcending awareness of) Eternal Delight[1] and is known as 'The Lower Gate'.

The experience of the 'fourth' confirmation which is the commitment of the indivisibility of the various aspects of authentic being and named 'Utter Profoundness' is the illumination of Mahāmudrā awareness.[2] In its application one has to try to live in such a way that this unitary experience does not fall to pieces, that one never becomes separated from service and attention, that one partakes of this spiritual nourishment, that one retains its mystic character, and that one guards this authentic being.

The commitment named 'Extent' is threefold: (*a*) a meditative

[1] So also Tshk 3*b*.

[2] Ibid. 4*a*. A fuller account is given ibid. 7*b*–8*b*. See also Part II.

absorption into the ground (of one's being) or preserving authentic situationality through co-emergent awareness;[1] (*b*) a meditative absorption into great bliss as its experience or preserving authentic communication through intuitive understanding; and (*c*) a meditative absorption into a feeling of fellowship or preserving authentic being-in-the-world through recognizing (this spiritual nature of every sentient being).

The commitment named 'Non-Duality' is also threefold: (*a*) to recognize the nature (of one's being); (*b*) to experience the traversing of the path; and (*c*) to confess one's failure to reach the goal.

(*a*) While mind as the non-duality of the noetic act and nothingness cannot be grasped as anything, there is incessant appearance as merriment of this very mind. Therefore appearance is mind; mind is the ultimate and, since this is not separate from Dharmakāya, it cannot be thought of as being something and somewhere.

(*b*) Having recognized the necessity to preserve the Wish-Fulfilling Gem of commitment while the contents of mind come and go, is to have experienced it.

(*c*) Since one is guilty of a grave offence when one fails in one's commitment to authentic being which is the Guru, one has to confess this in the following way: if one's Guru is alive one has to ask him for confirmation after one has practised the meditation on Vajrasattva until the special features of this meditation have become realized. If he is no longer alive one has to ask someone who is in his spiritual line for the confirmation seven or three times or as often as the case may require.

Similarly if one has committed an offence by having become angry with one's companions in the Dharma one has to confess in front of the shrine.

But if one has committed an offence by doing evil or violating the precepts one has to make a detailed confession and to start again from the beginning.

If one takes care not to fail in one's commitment to authentic being which is the Guru himself, all commitments will be kept. By applying the technique in which the Guru and the tutelary deity in its Father–Mother aspect are inseparable, the Guru

[1] See note 3, p. 25 for this term.

reveals himself as this deity and the Mother becomes rDo-rje rnal-'byor-ma (Vajrayoginī). The Three Jewels also coincide with authentic being, the Guru. That is, the Guru's being-in-the-world is the holy congregation, and since the Dakas, the Protectors of the Doctrine, and the companions in the Dharma are the holy congregation they form the Guru's being-in-the-world. Communication is the Noble Doctrine, and authentic solutions of one's situations are Buddhahood.

(ii) Observation is to guard the commitments to authentic being or the Guru in a state of stability where one commitment leads to the other and integrates with it.

Briefly, it is gladdening confidence in which no sense of self-reproach and guilt can enter, because good is realized in the knowledge of good, however small the cause may be, and because evil is shunned in the knowledge of evil, however small its cause may be.

4. THE MYSTIC HEAT[1]

Tilopa again sat motionless and silent for a year in a border country. When Nāropa had made the appropriate gesture, circumambulated him with folded hands, and asked for instruction, Tilopa said, 'Follow me', and went away. Then sitting near a dark and deep pool, full of leeches, he said to Nāropa: 'If I had had a disciple he would have built a bridge over this pool.' Taking these words literally Nāropa began building a bridge. When he was waist-deep in the water, he slipped and went under. Since the water had been disturbed, leeches and other vermin came in swarms and bored into his body. The loss of blood gave him the sensation of being dissolved, and the water flowing into this emptiness made him feel frozen. Tilopa asked: 'Nāropa, what is wrong with you?' And Nāropa answered:

> I dissolve, I freeze, through the bites of leeches,
> I am not master of myself and so I suffer.

Tilopa said:

> This pool of your body fashioned by former deeds
> Deserves to be turned into ice, Nāropa.

[1] A detailed analysis of this subject-matter is given in Part II.

Look into the mirror of your mind which is the mystic heat,
The mysterious home of the Ḍākinī.

When he had healed him by touching him with his hand he gave him the instruction on the mystic heat in which eternal delight and warmth are self-glowing.

This instruction is twofold, consisting of (A) how to trust in the possibility of experiencing this heat through imagining it vividly, and (B) how to use it as a means.

The first (A) is threefold: (*a*) (The mystic heat has to be imagined as) Being-in-itself accessible through body-mind (or being-oneself), through spirituality, and being something common to both; (*b*) the modes of experiencing this mystic heat are the path (that leads to) (*c*) the goal or the realization of authentic being which is eternal delight and nothingness.

As regards this division the great scholar Nāropa has said:

Being and the Path
And the Stages in the realization of the goal.[1]

The first section (*a*) has three divisions: (i) Being viewed as a psycho-organism, (ii) as spirituality, and (iii) as something common to both.[2]

The first division (i) again has three subdivisions: (1) the pathways[3] or the static, (2) motility[4] or the dynamic, and (3) enlightenment-potentiality or the creative. As Nāropa stated:

The pathways are static, motility is dynamic
And enlightenment is creative.

[1] Although lHa'i btsun-pa Rin-chen rnam-rgyal ascribes this verse to Nāropa, it actually goes back to Tilopa himself. He gives these lines in his *Āhapramāṇasamyak-nāma-ḍākinī-upadeśa*, 1*a*. The authoritative Tibetan text of the bKa'-brgyud-pas varies in the arrangement of the subject-matter from the one preserved in the bsTan-'gyur. In this translation the term Being (*dṅos-po'i gnas-lugs*) is a short form for the more exact, though lengthy, 'being-there as possible Being-in-itself'.

[2] This classification differs from the one given by Tilopa. The term *thun-moṅ* 'common', 'general' signifies being-oneself, the self-conscious individual who is aware of Being-in-itself or the transcendent totality of truth through his being-himself. It thus belongs to the psycho-organism, rather than to the all-encompassing spirituality (*sems*). As such it is commented upon by Padma dkar-po in his Sphžg 12*a*.

[3] See above note 1, p. 46 for the translation of this term.

[4] See Note F, pp. 268 sqq., for this translation.

The first of these (1) has three sections: (i) the coarse, (ii) the subtle, and (iii) the very subtle.

(i) In the middle of the indestructible psycho-organism, which is like a stūpa, there is a central pathway which is the axle of this system. It enters the fontanelle above and ends in the perineum below and has four properties.[1] To the right the *ro-ma* (*rasanā*), which is white and red with a preponderance of white, branches off four inches below the navel and leads to the right nostril. At the same spot but to the left the *rkyaṅ-ma* (*lalanā*), which is red and white with a preponderance of red, branches off and leads to the left nostril. Both have many branches. Then two thick ones enter the central pathway at the region between the eyebrows, forming the white part of the head. Many others branch off from here, two thick ones entering both eyes and nostrils and functioning there. All except the two thigh branches are multiple.

In the central pathway, in the head region, there is the 'head' focal point of eternal delight, like a lotus with thirty-two petals. It is multicoloured or white, represents the cohesive force, and is turned slightly downwards. In the throat region we find the 'throat' focal point of communication, a lotus with sixteen petals. It is red, represents temperature, and is turned upwards. Between the two breasts or in the heart there is the 'heart' focal point of situationality dealings, a lotus with eight petals. It is black and represents movement and is turned downwards. In the navel region we have the 'navel' focal point of structure, a lotus with sixty-four petals. It is yellow, stands for the solidifying force, and is turned upwards. The total number of these coarse structure ways is 120.

(ii) Each point of the eight petals of the 'heart' focal point branches off into three pathways. These connect the twenty-four parts of the organism. Each of the latter has three branches so that there are seventy-two lotus-seated ways. These again branch off until their final total is 72,000.

(iii) There are as many very subtle pathways as there are hairs on the body.

(2) Motility or the dynamic is twofold: (i) actuality and (ii) differentiation.

1 They are: redness, lustrousness, straightness, and hollowness. See Sphkh 12*a*.

(i) That which makes a body animated by a mind and serving as the basis of all activity, expand, and move, is here considered as the actuality of motility.

(ii) Differentiation is based on the five types of motility developing into vibrations along the pathways.

(*a*) The 'Downwards-Moving One' is Amoghasiddhi, the vibration in movement; it is green and localized in the pubic region. It serves to eliminate or retain faeces and urine.

(*b*) The 'One like Fire' is Ratnasambhava, the vibration of solidification. It is yellow, has its station in the navel region, and is responsible for digestion.

(*c*) The 'life-holder' is Akṣobhya, the vibration of cohesion. It is blue, stays in the heart region, and is responsible for respiration.

(*d*) The 'Upwards-Moving One' is Amitābha, the vibration of temperature. It is red, stays in the throat region, and is responsible for the flow of saliva and other fluids.

(*e*) The 'Encompasser' is Vairocana, the vibration of spaciousness. It is white, found in the head and limbs, and is responsible for bodily movements and postures.

There is another division according to the secondary forms of these five primary types:

(*a*) A branch of the 'One like Fire' is called 'Moving One'. It is found in the eyes, is shaped like a full-blossomed sesame flower, and is responsible for sight.

(*b*) A branch of the 'Life-holder' is the 'Really Moving One'. It is a groove in the ears and is responsible for hearing.

(*c*) A branch of the 'Upwards-Moving One' is the 'Obviously Moving One'. It is like a copper needle in the nose and is responsible for smelling.

(*d*) A branch of the 'Downwards-Moving One' is the 'Speedily Moving One'. It is in the tongue in the shape of a half-moon and is responsible for tasting.

(*e*) A branch of the 'Encompasser' is the 'Very Rapidly Moving One'. It is found throughout the body like feathers on a bird. In particular it is found in the skin and the sex organs and is responsible for sensitivity.

Another differentiation is by function. This is twofold: (i) action-motility, and (ii) awareness-motility.[1]

Still another differentiation is according to the sensations during meditation. It is threefold and called (*a*) male, (*b*) female, and (*c*) neutral.[2] Each of these is again subdivided into three aspects (male–male, male–female, male–neutral; female–male, female–female, female–neutral; neutral–male, neutral–female, neutral–neutral).

Finally there is the differentiation by the vibratory rate. In the case of a full-grown man who is healthy and resting, though not from fatigue, the rate of breathing comprising exhalation, inhalation, and the intermediate state between these two, reckoned as one unit, is for one full day and night (twenty-four hours) 21,600 times. This rate belongs to the central pathway. Similarly by dividing day and night into two equal halves the rate becomes 10,800 times in each case. This rate belongs to the right and left pathways. By further dividing this period into four 'thun-chen' (360 minutes each) the rate becomes 5,400 times. This belongs to the focal point of sexuality. A further division into eight 'thun-phran' (180 minutes each) gives the rate of 2,700. This belongs to the 'heart' focal point. The following division into sixteen 'pho-ba'' (ninety minutes each) results in the rate of 1,350. This belongs to the 'throat' focal point. Another division into thirty-two 'chu-tshod' (forty-five minutes each) gives a rate of 675. This belongs to the 'head' focal point of eternal delight. A last division into sixty-four 'dbyug-gu' (twenty-two and a half minutes each) has the rate of 337½. This belongs to the 'navel' focal point.

In relation to the zodiacal signs the vibratory rate is 1,800 each. This rate belongs to the four focal points. Moreover, in the twelve-petalled lotus of the focal point of variable delight in the sex region the vibratory rate of the zodiacal signs is 1,800 each. Each petal branches off into five points with a total of sixty in which the rate is 360 each. During the transit periods there enters a vibratory rate from awareness-motility[3] from the central pathway,

[1] See Note F, pp. 268 sqq.

[2] This distinction is found in Tilopa, op. cit., 2*b*. 'Male' refers to the ordinary motor act, 'female' to the incipient detachment from the external reference of the sensory motor act, and 'neutral' to the successful detachment. See also Sphžg 96*a*; Sphkh 16*b* sq.

[3] See Note F, pp. 268 sqq.

which is eleven and a quarter. In the houses of the twelve-petalled lotus the rate is fifty-six and a quarter. Altogether the vibratory rate of the awareness-motility from the central pathway is for the period of one day and night 675. This vibration is hardly perceptible.

Motility, as the motor act of the five sense organs, is coarse. As the eighty self-contained reaction patterns,[1] it is subtle; and as awareness-motility operating in three reaction potentialities,[2] it is very subtle.

(3) Enlightenment-potentiality or the creative is threefold: (*a*) The coarse is designated A-Haṃ (i.e. 'I'); (*b*) The subtle is the being-oneself as possible Being-in-itself, indestructible and infinitely open to new possibilities, reaching into my being-there through the heart;[3] (*c*) The very subtle is the affinity of the materiality-producing forces in beginningless Being, symbolized by the colours white and red.[4]

(ii) Being viewed as spirituality-(mentality) is threefold: (*a*) as the five sense perceptions it is coarse; (*b*) as the eighty self-contained reaction patterns it is subtle; and (*c*) as the three reaction potentialities it is very subtle.

(iii) Being as common to both the psycho-organism and spirituality means that motility in its subtle aspect[5] and spirituality-(mentality)

[1] The reaction patterns evolve out of the reaction possibilities and potentialities. The former determine overt behaviour, but are themselves preconscious. Thirty-three patterns have their root in the potentiality to aversion, forty in that of passion-lust, and seven in that of bewilderment. These patterns are more like empty forms which are filled with a determinate content in conscious experience. See Barb 3*b*; 8*b* seq.; Bargd 12*b* sqq.; Sphžg 10*b* sqq.; Tsoṅ-kha-pa, vi. 3, 15*a* sq.; vii. 1, 143*b*, 203*a* sq., 205*b* sqq.

[2] They are: 'aversion', 'passion-lust', and 'bewilderment-errancy'. These names, however, are slightly misleading. They are not determinate emotions, but potentialities which gradually develop into concrete emotive experiences through and within the reaction patterns referred to before. See also below, p. 170. I have made use of the rare 'errancy' in order to indicate the straying away from the real.

[3] This is a paraphrase rather than a translation of the original *mi-śigs-pa'i thig-le*. The attribute *mi-śigs-pa* means 'indestructible' and names my very self, both as Being-in-itself and being-oneself. *thig-le* designates 'creative potentiality' and thus shows that Being is not a well-defined entity but something that is open to infinite possibilities. The same idea is discussed at length in Zmnd 34*a* sqq.

[4] So also Ržd 153*a*. See also below p. 65 for an analysis of this idea.

[5] i.e. the eighty reactions patterns. The text could be paraphrased in modern language: the indivisibility of motility and mentation is the cradle of conscious emotive behaviour.

as the reaction potentialities have been indivisible from time immemorial, like water poured into water, and thus fully perform what is called Saṃsāra and Nirvāṇa. So it is said in the rDo-rje 'phreṅ-ba (Vajramālā).

(B) The modes of experiencing the mystic heat as the path (to goal achievement) are:

(*a*) The meaning of the word *gtum-mo*. The syllable *gtum* ('fierce') signifies the direct overcoming of all that is not conducive to enlightenment, that is, all that has to be given up; the syllable *mo* ('mother') indicates motherhood as producing spontaneously all the good in virtues, that is, all that has to be attained.

(*b*) Its actuality is the awareness of eternal delight and nothingness that has come about by the spreading of a self-kindled glow.

(*c*) Differentiation is into an external, internal, mystic, and ultimate heat.

(*d*) Its comparability is that the external one is like fire, the internal one like a medicinal drug, the mystic one like a lion, and the ultimate one like a mirror.

(*e*) Its function is as follows. The external one overcomes the 80,000 obstacles and produces a feeling of warmth in the sentient organism.

The internal one makes the eighty-four diseases subside and produces a sense of delight.

The mystic one conquers the 84,000 instinctive forces and produces the awareness of eternal delight and nothingness in the sentient organism.

The ultimate one is *gtum-mo* in the true sense of the word. It is *gtum* because it dispels the darkness of unawareness and *mo* because it is the mother who bears (her child) awareness as the noetic act.

(*f*) Its efficacy. The external one makes the body-structure[1] glow in a vermilion-like light; the internal one lets radiation[2] spread straight like the tense string of a bow; the mystic one lets motility[3]

[1] *lus-kyi gnad*. Outwardly this term refers to the postures one adopts during meditation. Essentially it is the triadic structure of the pathways, one in the middle and one to the right and left of it.

[2] *dmigs-pa'i gnad*. This term refers to the five-coloured light that one sees and experiences to emanate from and to return to one's body. See Sphkh 12*a*.

[3] *rluṅ-gi gnad*. This term designates the removal of all hindrances that make the sensation of vibrations difficult to perceive. Ibid.

develop forcefully like a skilled archer shooting an arrow; and the ultimate one preserves spirituality as diligently as one would a light in a gale.

(*g*) The mode of its glowing, upwards, by flaring up into self-existing awareness it illumines the 'Upper Gate'[1] pathway; downwards, radiating into undefinable eternal delight it illumines the essence of the 'Lower Gate'[1] pathway; and intermediately, glowing in the continuity of Saṃsāra it shows the limitation of the pathways and of motility along them.[2]

(*h*) Its effectiveness. That of the external one is that even if the technique related to the control of vibrations is sometimes weak bodily warmth will not get lost. That of the internal one is that no chance diseases will occur. That of the mystic one is that the working of action-motility[3] can be stopped, and that of the ultimate one is that discursive thought and man's dividedness against himself turns into transcending and unitary awareness.

(*i*) Its ten signs. There are (1) five general signs connected with the control over the materiality-producing forces, and (2) five special ones in connexion with the control having been fully established.

(1) The former are as follows. When the vibration of solidification comes under control one has the experience of seeing smoke; when that of cohesion there comes a glittering before one's eyes; when that of temperature there is a glow like that of a glow-worm; when that of movement there is the light of a flame; and when that of spaciousness one has the feeling-vision of a cloudless sky. Hence Tilopa said: 'When the vibrations of the five materiality-producing forces come under control one has the vision of smoke, a glittering before one's eyes, a glow-worm, a flame and a cloudless sky.'

(2) When the control of the vibration of solidification has been fully established and this vibration remains stable, the body-mind

[1] See Part II.

[2] Attention to the pathways of the structuring process and the motility in connexion with the process is only one step in the process of emptying the mind from all concepts. As long as they dominate the picture mind is still fettered. After all the diagram of the 'body' in Tantrism is only a means, not an end.

[3] See note F, pp. 268 sqq.

feels settled and one has the vision of sun-rays; when the same happens with cohesion the body perspires and feels cold and there is the vision of moon-rays; in the case of temperature the body feels very hot and there is a flash of lightning; in that of movement the body is very powerful and quick-moving and there is the vision of a rainbow; and in that of spaciousness the body feels wide and full of delight without, however, having an idea of its existence, and one has the vision of sun and moon fusing into each other. The higher types experience this as if it happened in nature, the mediocre ones in a sort of feeling-sentiment, and the lower ones as if in a dream. Therefore Tilopa said: 'The five signs of stabilization which one sees directly, are sun-rays, moon-rays, lightning, rainbow, and the fusion of sun and moon.'

(*j*) The eight qualities. There are (1) four common ones of attraction, and (2) four sublime ones.

(1) The four former mean that, through the pathways one acquires wealth, through motility people, through creative potentiality authenticness, and by the presence of all three factors in equal perfection life and beauty in the three worlds.[1]

(2) The other four are that by gaining control over the 'Downwards-Moving One' and the 'Upwards-Moving One'[2] one cannot be harmed by the all-consuming fire that starts when the world comes to an end and which destroys a thousand suns and moons. By the control over the 'Life-holder'[2] one can make a powerful stream flow upwards; and by that over the 'Encompasser' one can walk, sit, and fly in mid-air.

5. APPARITION[3]

Tilopa sat motionless and silent for another year. Nāropa made the appropriate gesture, circumambulated him with folded hands,

[1] The pathways which signify a live structure in the narrower sense of the word and man's authentic being in a wider context, are thus symbolic of the richness of life. Man's being-in-the-world is no longer a sordid affair. Similarly motility which develops into the motor act and into speech as the readiest means of communication, enables him to communicate with other people as individuals rather than as objects for the will of power or the impulse to destroy. And being open to infinite possibilities one does not become petrified into the rigid banality of a particularity and objectivity.

[2] See Part II.

[3] A fuller account is given in Part II.

and, when Tilopa glanced at him, asked for instruction. Tilopa said: 'If you want instruction, bring fire, some reeds and fat.' When Nāropa had brought these things Tilopa split and sharpened the reeds with a knife. Then he dipped the ends into the fat that had been heated on the fire and held them against Nāropa's body. When the pain became intolerable, Tilopa merely asked: 'Nāropa, what is wrong with you?' And Nāropa answered:

> This noose wherein the essence lies
> Of Buddhahood tortures me. I suffer.

Tilopa said:

> This noose of your body believing in an I
> Deserves to be cut, Nāropa. Look into the mirror
> Of your mind where rises the phantom body,
> The mysterious home of the Ḍākinī.

He healed him by touching him with his hand and then gave him the instruction on apparition which is free in itself from the eight worldly concerns.[1]

This instruction has two parts: (i) The illusion recognized by all schools of thought and (ii) the experience of an apparition as a magic spell as taught and practised in Vajrayāna.

(i) A magician mutters a spell over stones and pieces of wood and produces the illusion of men, women, horses, oxen, asses, mules, rooms, houses, and many other illusory appearances which although they do not exist in reality seem to do so. People who have been blinded by the magician's performance then believe what they see to be true and hanker after these things; the magician, however, is not attracted to what seems to be houses and oxen and so on. A man who is not affected by this atmosphere of magic has no such erroneous visions of houses and oxen, which for him are but stones and pieces of wood. Similarly all phenomena appear to the common man as being true and in his hankering after them he accumulates Karma and will have to suffer its effect. Pratyekabuddhas and Bodhisattvas who have an intuitive grasp of nothingness see the same phenomena as true but do not hanker

[1] See above note 1, p. 26.

after them. Only for the Buddhas is there no bewildering phenomenality and no hankering after it; there is only pure appearance. Phenomenality can be illustrated by Nāropa's twelve similes:

> A magic spell, a dream, a gleam before the eyes,
> A reflection, lightning, an echo, a rainbow,
> Moonlight upon water, cloud-land, dimness
> Before the eyes, fog and apparitions,
> These are the twelve similes of the phenomenal.

In brief, having learned that Saṃsāra is a conflict-situation one becomes aware that death is uncertain and one leaves everything as it appears to the senses as it is; one continually says to oneself that all is a dream and a magic spell, and in thought one attunes oneself to last night's dream in all its translucency. So one constantly strives to get a better understanding of the magic spell by an inspection of it and by not letting the three gates of action (by body, speech, and mind) become disordered.[1]

In particular, this deals with the mystic apparitional body. That is, the psycho-organism of every ordinary being is twofold: (*a*) ephemeral, and (*b*) real.

(*a*) The former is the organism built up by the materiality-producing forces and clothed in the experientially initiated potentialities of experience and taking birth in any of the six forms of life.

(*b*) The real one is mere motility and mentality-spirituality. This real one does not leave or become separated from the ephemeral one.

Even if the coarse body is discarded this does not mean that the sentient beings no longer have an ephemeral body. The 'mind body'[2] endowed with all sense faculties in the intermediate state

[1] i.e. in overcoming the belief in physical limitation as making up the whole of reality, a more authentic being-in-the-world is achieved, and in this connexion also the barriers to communication, which a careful analysis of everybody's speech reveals, are removed, and lastly in not falling into the false opinions and beliefs that have intercepted man's relation to himself and to others one can deal with situations authentically.

[2] The term 'mind' must not be allowed to mislead us. The original word *yid* (*manas*), though currently translated by 'mind', always refers to something before there is a mind as we understand the word. The technical term *yid-kyi*

between death and rebirth is the ephemeral body. But this 'mind body' is not the real one. Its nature is rather like water and its warmth. The real body, consisting of mere motility and mentality-spirituality, may be compared as to its nature with water and its moistness. As long as the coarse body, formed by the materializing forces as their product, is present, the ephemeral one is like a guest-house and the real one like the guest therein. Therefore the subtle and real 'body', motility-mentality, is the basis for attaining apparitional existence as a being-there pervaded by Being-in-itself.[1]

(ii) The essence of the experience stages. The foundation is laid by the excitation and perception of sensations through deep breathing (imagined to move) upwards, downwards, and to the middle (of the mystic diagram of the body), or the kindling of the mystic inner heat. After that a different kind of breathing, being the vibrations of the three syllables (*oṃ āḥ hūṃ*), takes the lead. Absorption then is achieved through two meditative processes, dissolution[2] and evaporation.[3] When one feels how gradually all

lus might be rendered more adequately as 'the human constant', in so far as that which is designated by this term underlies all human activity. Yet it must not be assumed that this 'constant' is an invariable. It has been group-patterned by the carry-over of traces of former experiences and according to their varying degrees of intensity this constant itself may be variously charged. For a further detailed analysis see Part II.

[1] *rten daṅ brten-par bcas-pa*. According to Sphžg 7*b rten* is synonymous with *lus* 'body-mind' and *brten-pa* with *sems* 'spirituality'. In Sphkh 4*b* 'spirituality' is said to be 'action-born' (*thabs-byuṅ*). This means that spirituality is evolved in the course of one's endeavours. It is not a negligible by-product. Hence the Tantric conception cannot be equated with epiphenomenalism. Nor does the statement imply any causal theory. There is a 'forward reference' from body-mind or being-there and being-oneself to spirituality or Being-in-itself, but this has nothing to do with the metaphysical principle of teleological causation, rather there is here a kind of natural teleology which coincides with the progressive enhancement of values in the growth of man. In Sphžg 14*a brten-pa* = *sems* = *sems dṅos-po'i gnas-lugs* is defined as 'value' (*yon-tan*).

[2] The existentiality of Buddhahood formed out of motility and mentality into a white shape with three faces and six hands is possible communication. But since this does not act for sentient beings it must turn into the Buddha Akṣobhya of white colour with three faces and six hands. In his heart is the letter *hūṃ*. Its light dissolves the whole body from head to foot and absorbs it in the *hūṃ*. The letter *hūṃ* then dissolves gradually from the bottom into the half-moon over it, the dot above it, into sound which also is allowed to fade into nothing. Or, just as a snow-flake turns into water, so also this phenomenon becomes smaller and smaller and finally dissolves. This is dissolution.' Sphžg 179*a*.

[3] 'This is similar to the contemplation of the *hūm* in the heart region of Ak-

the sensitive parts of the body are affected thereby and the central pathway is illumined by the lustre of the partner's vibrations,[1] through the power of concentration the movement of action-motility is stopped and all vibrations enter, stay, and fade in the central pathway. The sign of vibration entering upon the central pathway is an even movement, that of its stay thereon is the immobility of the abdomen and that of its fading are the four signs associated with the dissolution of solidity in cohesion, of the latter in temperature, of this in vibration, and of this in noetic capacity: a glittering before one's eyes, smoke, a glow, and lamp-light respectively. When these four signs have passed and when awareness as a soft glow (like that of the moon) by the descent of a stream of nectar from the *haṃ*-polarity[2] to the heart region, and awareness as a spread of light (like that of the sun) by the flare of a red fire from the *A*-polarity[3] to the heart region, and the darkness that comes about by the extinction of sun and moon, have been passed through, the radiant light which is complete nothingness, Dharmakāya, shines in all its nakedness. Then, when motility begins to stir in this light of complete nothingness, and in reverse order darkness has set in, this indivisibility of motility and mentality, the vehicle of the primordial radiant light, separates from its former psycho-somatic elements and, being adorned with all the major and minor auspicious marks in highest perfection,

ṣobhya. From this *hūṃ* light shines forth dissolving all the worlds and the sentient beings therein into light. After that this light is allowed to fade into nothingness, like breath disappearing on a mirror.' Ibid.

[1] *phyag-rgya, mudrā.* This term is ambiguous because it may be interpreted as *las-kyi phyag-rgya, karmamudrā* or *ye-śes-kyi phyag-rgya, jñānamudrā.* The former is a real woman and through her one comes to the experience described. The latter refers to the inner experience or awareness, symbolized as a female.

[2] The materializing forces which are responsible for the rigidity of our ordinary 'I' (*ahaṃ*), a tensional pattern produced by the fertilizing powers of father and mother, divide into poles after an initial unity. The one deriving from the father ascends to the 'head' region and terminates in the *haṃ*. It is thought of as being white and, physiologically, it produces the lustre of the body. The other deriving from the mother descends to the 'navel' region or even below this and terminates in the *a*. This is red and produces biological warmth. Through the practice of kindling the inner mystic heat the tension between the two polarities is resolved. The disruptiveness of the 'I', on which ordinary life is based, is gradually mended and one finds oneself; in more philosophical language, a shift from the being-there and the being-oneself to the Being-in-itself is aimed at. See also Tsoṅ-kha-pa, vi. 3, 23*b* sq.

[3] See the preceding note. Ržd 153*a* sqq.

participating in five similar and five special features,[1] this motility becomes an apparition of brilliantly white light in a being-there pervaded by Being-in-itself[2] with distinct features of a body, a face, and other limbs. This at first is merely an idea, later an existential fact. After that appearance (being always the appearance of) the basic noetic capacity becomes an awareness which is bliss and nothingness and is present as the magic of the being-there pervaded by Being-in-itself. To feel one with it, unswervingly and without any sense of duality, is the essence of this experience. This genuinely divine figure in its environmental setting recedes into one's self in the same way as (in the Developing Stage) Ye-śes sems-dpa' (Jñānasattva, awareness-being) fades into Dam-tshig sems-dpa' (Samayasattva, commitment-being) or the old psycho-somatic elements, and in this process the visionary signs appear in reverse order. When it comes to a glittering before one's eyes, everything is realized as nothing and this, in turn, is eternal delight, the merriment of gods and goddesses.

(iii) The result or the realization of coincidence: such an apparition can unite with as many partners of experience as there are atoms in the mythical mount Meru. And by the power of its repeated entrance into the primordial radiant light, internally, awareness is purified from every stain and becomes aware of everything possible; externally, since the limits of the knowable now no longer exist, awareness knowing the most subtle spreads far and wide. In the formal identity between the indeterminate relational form of the noetic act and the object by which the empty form is terminated[3] the radiant light as path and goal form

[1] The five similar features are what would ordinarily be called the five psycho-somatic elements: shape, feeling, sensation, motivation, and consciousness. The five special features are: life in the heavenly sphere Akaṇiṣṭha, manifestation as rDo-rje-'chaṅ, the entourage of male and female Bodhisattvas of the ten spiritual levels, the effulgence of the primordial radiant light, and time (as time rather than an event in time).

[2] See above note 1, p. 64. Dnz 13*a*.

[3] This is a term which linguistic translations leave untranslated. It is clearly explained by sGam-po-pa, x. 31*b* as 'the absolutely specific characteristics of all the entities of Saṃsāra and Nirvāṇa'. At the same place he defines *ye-śes* as 'spirituality pure in itself from its very beginning and radiant'. See also xxxi. 27*b*; v. 23*a*, 26*a*, 27*a*, 30*b*, 45*a*; vi. 11*a*, where the text has to be corrected on the basis of the preceding passages.

a unit. This is the realization of fullest communication, Sambhogakāya, characterized by seven features.[1]

6. DREAM[2]

Tilopa sat silent and motionless for another year. Nāropa made the appropriate gesture, circumambulated him with folded hands and, when Tilopa glanced at him, asked for instruction. 'If you want instruction follow me', said Tilopa and went away. When in the middle of a wide plain a man appeared carrying a load, Tilopa said: 'Pursue him!' Nāropa tried to do so, but the man kept receding into the distance like a mirage and Nāropa was unable to catch him. Urged on to pursue this vision he did so and when he could not stir from exhaustion, Tilopa came and asked: 'Nāropa, what is wrong with you?' And Nāropa answered:

> As when a deer chases a mirage, something false
> Appeared and passed away. And so I suffer.

Tilopa said:

> This rope of the three worlds, Saṃsāra,
> Should be cut, Nāropa. Look
> Into the mirror of your mind, the place of dreams,
> The mysterious home of the Ḍākinī.

He healed him with his hand and gave him the instruction on dreams or the self-abrogation of bewilderment.

This instruction is in two parts: grasping a dream (i) by waiting for it to come, and (ii) by attending to vibrations.

(i) Both Sūtras and Mantra-texts assert that the whole of entitative reality is like a dream. By heeding this the mistaken belief in a Pure Ego is undermined. Moreover, in dreamless sleep one treads the path of death; in dream one passes through the intermediate world between death and (re)birth;[3] and when one awakens one is in the world of concrete patterns. Therefore for undermining the belief in the exclusive reality of what appears

[1] See Part II.
[2] A fuller discussion is found in Part II.
[3] So also sGam-po-pa, x. 43*a*.

during daytime, the fact of dreaming is the most excellent index from among the twelve similes[1] as to the illusory-hallucinatory nature of our world.[2]

The practice is as follows: when a man who has given up his preoccupation with this life and can hold steady the vision of his apparitional existence, falls asleep at night or any other time, all his attention and sensitivity becoming focused on the centre of the 'throat' focal point, the indication of sleep comes, a tiny, quick-moving, soft glow which in the 'heart' focal point becomes a strong, but non-effulgent light, difficult to apprehend. (From there) immediately after motility has stirred in the primordial radiant light, a dream will appear at the 'throat' focal point and one must concentrate on holding whatever appears as a perceptual display for the five senses as long as possible. Having succeeded in this practice one must next multiply (this perceptual content), transform the unfolding drama into something auspicious, and use it to counteract fear. When one has practised this wondrous creativity of a dream process in which one may see Buddha-realms and other things, the bewilderment which consists in taking for truth all that appears in daytime in the waking state, is annihilated.

(ii) A yogi who is well versed in kindling the mystic inner heat and its spreading a sensation of heightened vitality[3] as well as in attending to the vibrations of the three mystic syllables (*ōṃ āḥ hūṃ*) carries out the same practice when he goes to sleep at night or at any other time. However, when a dream appears, his dream-life is particularly blissful and he concentrates as long as possible on the vision of himself as Heruka in his divine setting. When he has done so he multiplies the scope of his vision by ten and more, transforms the unfolding drama into pure Buddha-realms and

[1] See above p. 63.

[2] So also sGam-po-pa, x. 8*b*: 'When one wakes up after a dream one should think: "What is the difference between last night's dream and what appears now?"—There is no difference.'

[3] *gtum-mo 'bar-'dzag*. This is explained in the texts in the following way. Through the heat rising towards the 'head' region the 'white bodhicitta' is made to descend. In a less symbolic language this means that by allowing the 'warmer' feelings to become expressed the 'cold' rigidity of the ego is melted and freed from its isolation. sGam-po-pa, xxxii. 21*b* sq. also speaks of a 'blazing mystic inner heat' (*'bar-ba'i gtum-mo*).

the like, and creates various enhancing situations. In some cases he will purify his former Karma, accumulated in the six forms of life; in others he will enter, stay in, and emerge from a great variety of meditative absorptions; or he will listen to the Dharma under the Buddhas of many and various realms. By practising this dream-state the bewilderment of holding as true what appears as an outer object in the waking life will be annihilated and internally the rigid interconnexions of the pathways will be resolved.

7. THE RADIANT LIGHT[1]

Tilopa again sat motionless and silent for a year. Nāropa made the appropriate gesture, circumambulated him with folded hands, spoke his prayers and, when once Tilopa glanced at him, asked for instruction. 'If you want the Dharma, follow me', said Tilopa and went away. When they met a minister conducting his bride home on an elephant, Tilopa said: 'If I had had a disciple he would have pulled them down and dragged them about.' Nāropa did so, but the minister and his attendants beat Nāropa thoroughly and when he was unable to move with pain Tilopa came and asked: 'Nāropa, what is wrong with you?' Nāropa answered:

> You cannot play with this craftsman of a minister,
> In a jest he ground me to a powder, and so I suffer.

Tilopa said:

> This rock of your body believing in an I
> Must be ground to powder, Nāropa.
> Look into the mirror of your mind, the radiant light.
> The mysterious home of the Dākinī.

When he had healed him with his hand he gave him the instruction on the radiant light, the inexistence of the darkness of unknowing.

This instruction has three sections: (i) the ground or Being-in-itself (as indicated by) the synonyms of 'radiant light'; (ii) the path or the experience of (going along it or through) the stages in

[1] For a detailed analysis see Part II.

the semblant light; and (iii) the goal or the realization of the ultimately real light.

(i) The synonyms are: (*a*) basic, (*b*) ultimately real, (*c*) semblant, (*d*) intuitive, (*e*) effulgent, (*d*) non-effulgent, and (*g*) experiential light.

(*a*) This is the luminosity and indestructibility of the noetic act presently experiencing the bliss and misery of Nirvāṇa and Saṃsāra respectively.[1]

(*b*) This is a name for the transcending awareness which is bliss and nothingness together that come after and above the realization of the high-grade one-valueness in one's being.[2]

(*c*) This is the name for the transcending awareness of composure, when it extends from the high-grade unitary experience[2] to the low-grade one-valueness.

(*d*) This is recognized to be the transcending awareness of composure coming about after a low-grade non-concretization of things or non-diffusion is becoming active in one's being.

(*e*) This is the awareness of liberation following on the experience of the high-grade non-concretization of things.[3]

(*f*) This is said to be a meditative absorption which extends from the unitary experience to the medium-grade non-concretization.

(*g*) This is generally said to be the meditative absorption of the low-, medium-, and high-grade unitary experience.

(ii) A man who walks the path lets the radiant light shine forth either by mediative concentration during daytime, or forces it to do

[1] Saṃsāra and Nirvāṇa are interpretations, not entities. It is possible to give them an independent status on the basis of a realistic and intentional logic. However, one should be cautious in applying the Western categories.

[2] The current translation of this term by 'one-pointedness of mind' is correct for the Sūtras and the Abhidharma. In these works emphasis is laid on the content. In the Tantras the experiential character is stressed. Using the word 'mind' in a non-specific sense, one might say that it has a 'field character', part of which is indeterminate, primary and persistent, and part of which is determinately variable. In the experience termed *rtse-gcig* the 'field character' has been realized and 'the gulf between the variable and the invariable has been bridged'. See Phntm 4*b*.

[3] This is a state which is beyond every formulation by concept and speech. Epistemologically speaking, the subject-object dichotomy has subsided. Yet it is not nihilism. Whatever appears is at once recognized as what it is, and in this experience bewilderment, the tendency to reduce everything to a concept or label, is overcome and the gulf between 'bewilderment and freedom' has been bridged. Ibid. 4*b*.

so by controlling sleep at night. In this context the latter technique is intended.[1]

When an individual, built up by the six materializing forces,[2] as is the case with man of this world-sphere, falls asleep, the non-effulgent light shines when four materiality functions[3] have dissolved one into the other and when thereafter mentality resides in the 'heart' focal point. When one recognizes this peculiar moment through the help of the 'profound' instruction, the bewilderment of what appears in waking life turns into meditative-concentrative absorption. This is the essence of loosening the entanglement of the pathways in the 'heart' focal point. In possession of the four confirmations, keeping the commitments, experiencing the Developing and Fulfilment Stages, knowing the nature of misery, and being capable of unswervingly inspecting a given subject-matter, such a yogi will have to avoid the four kinds of getting food[4] and in solitude, heeding only the biological functions,[5] he will have to be absorbed in his existential self for full six months.

(iii) By observing day and night the patterns of concretization, non-concretization, and utter non-concretization,[6] like fire melting ice, one disentangles the pathways and straightens them out in the central pathway; action-motility is totally stopped and the instinctive forces[7] become transcending awareness. The 'red' and 'white' materiality producing forces become the unitary creative potentiality. Physically the organism becomes a transfigured body and mentally-spiritually radiant light, bliss, and nothingness —Dharmakāya.

[1] sGam-po-pa, xv. 11*b*; xxxi. 8*b*.

[2] Solidification, cohesion, temperature, motion, noetic capacity, and spatiality.

[3] Solidification, cohesion, temperature, and motion.

[4] Feast for the dead, feast for the living, stealing and robbery.

[5] *b(h)u-su-ku*: eating and drinking, sleeping, and defecation and urination. See Sphžg 148*ab*.

[6] The former two types refer to the experience with the Karmamudrā, the latter to those with the Jñānamudrā. See Part II for a detailed discussion, and Sphžg 118*a*; 146*b*.

[7] *ñon-moṅs, kleśa*. They are the three reaction potentialities named after their manifestation as 'passion-lust', 'aversion', and 'bewilderment'. They are the matrix of the 'eighty reaction patterns' which illustrate man's 'normal' emotional instability.

8. TRANSFERENCE[1]

Tilopa again sat silent and motionless for a year, and when Nāropa as before had made a maṇḍala and spoken his prayers, Tilopa went away with the words: 'If you want instruction follow me.' When they met a king with his queen and their retinue Tilopa said: 'If I had had a disciple, he would have thrown the queen down and dragged her about.' Nāropa did so and the king and his followers beat Nāropa until hardly any breath was left in him. While he was suffering Tilopa came and asked: 'Nāropa, what is wrong with you?' And Nāropa answered:

> The happiness of the king, master of the bow,
> Has flown like an arrow, and so I suffer.

Tilopa said:

> This propensity of your body believing in an I
> Must be got rid of, Nāropa.
> Look into the mirror of your mind, transference,
> The mysterious home of the Ḍākinī.

When he had healed him with his hand he gave him the instruction on transference.

This instruction contains as the ground of the existential self the recognition of the capability of its transference; as the path the stages in the experience of transference; and as goal the realization of the confines of transference.

(i) Transference is recognized in all Sūtras and Mantra-texts. However, in the three lower Tantra sections[2] and in the Sūtras it is said to be the behaviour corresponding to one's status after rebirth in a pure realm by having sent up one's spirituality-mentality through the fontanel opening, by means of the mystic syllable *HIK*, from one's present life which is believed to be something base.

He who practises the Developing Stage which is part of the highest Tantra section[3], lets the radiancy of the deity together with

[1] See Part II for a detailed discussion.
[2] The Kriyā-, Caryā-, and Yoga-tantras.
[3] The Anuttarayogantras such as the Guhyasamājatantra, Hevajratantra, Kālacakratantra, and others.

its mansion (on which he meditates) unite with the radiant light in the 'heart' focal point and with the help of motility (*rluṅ*) sends the mystic letter *HŪṂ* standing for the five types of transcending awareness[1] (and symbolizing his basic noetic capacity) up through the fontanel opening. After having been reborn either in the Akaniṣṭha heaven or in U-rgyan (Swat) he is said to follow a life that behoves the mantra-fold.

He who practises the Fulfilment Stage and is highly intelligent realizes the 'rainbow body' (authentic existence) during his lifetime and becomes (spiritually) immortal. He who is of medium intelligence recognizes and holds to the radiant light at the moment of death and does not pass through the experiences of the intermediate state between death and rebirth. The lowest type of those who practice the Fulfilment Stage has the experience of this intermediate state in such a way that, if he is intelligent, immediately after the light of the intermediate state has begun to shine, he absorbs it in the radiant light by means of the two types of concentration[2] and rises as a god or, at the time of the 'little death' during the first week (after the physical death), recognizes the radiant light and attains authentic existence. When he has come to a stage where the possibilities of taking birth in various forms

[1] They are: (i) *dharmadhātujñāna*, (ii) *pratyavekṣaṇajñāna*, (iii) *kṛtyānusthānajñāna*, (iv) *ādarśajñāna, and* (v) *samatājñāna*. They have been explained variously by various schools of Buddhism. sGam-po-pa, viii. 13*b* sq. uses *thamal-gyi śes-pa* 'original awareness' instead of *dharmadhātujñāna* and explains the others as follows: 'The intuitive awareness in which there is no division into subject and object is immediate apprehension (*so-sor-rtog-pa'i ye-śes, pratyavekṣaṇajñāna*); the fulfilment of everything in an instant without travelling the five paths and passing through the various levels of spirituality is accomplishment-awareness (*bya-ba grub-pa'i ye-śes, kṛtyānusthānajñāna*); the understanding that the entities of commonsense reality are like images in a mirror is mirror-like awareness (*me-loṅ-gi ye-śes, ādarśajñāna*); the fact that Saṃsāra and Nirvāṇa as terminal contents of the noetic act are the same is identity-awareness (*mñam-pa-ñid-kyi ye-śes, samatājñāna*)'. Zmnd 193*b* explains as follows: 'The relationship between cause and effect, after the knowable and the knower have been apprehended from an unbiased viewpoint, is immediate apprehension awareness; the nothingness in itself is mirror-like awareness; the miraculous unfolding is accomplishment awareness; the intuition of the sameness of all entities is identity awareness; and the fact that these forms of awareness have never moved away from the ultimate nature of awareness is ultimate awareness.'

[2] 'Dissolution' and 'evaporation'. See above notes 2 and 3, p. 64.

dawn upon him and when he sees his prospective parents engaging in coitus and feels hatred towards his father and love for his mother (provided he should be a male, while in the case of a female it would be the other way about) he transforms his mother's womb into (what is called) Samayasattva residing in his mansion, and himself enters there as Jñānasattva from his father's mouth, nose, or other part of the body. Conceiving the human body as a particularly well-suited foundation for the mantra-behaviour, he attains authentic existence after having been reborn.

If he is of low intelligence he becomes frightened at the idea of staying in a womb when he sees his prospective parents engaging in cohabitation, and transferring himself to the Akaṇiṣṭha heaven or to U-rgyan (Swat) follows the behaviour of the mantra-fold there.[1]

For him who does not understand the being-oneself of Being-in-itself in its being-oneself, there is bewilderment, Saṃsāra, unknowing; with reference to him the instructions which explain the being-oneself by means of the four confirmations, the Developing and Fulfilment Stages and other techniques, are called 'transference'. Moreover, those who understand the being-oneself of Being-in-itself in the being-oneself, have the status of being transferred to authentic being. To declare that evil has been abandoned and good which formerly was not has been attained as something new, or that evil has been turned into good, has nothing to do with, and is to fail to understand, the being of Being.

(ii) The experience is briefly: a man who is capable of immediate realization serves his Guru for a long period and then solely for the purpose of realization stays in solitude far away from all disquieting elements, and then he can look at whatever appears as it is without being upset by it; he sees whatever appears as the profound nature of transference.

A man who gradually comes to realization first prepares himself as does an expert archer, then he shoots the powerful arrow of his noetic capacity at the desired target, and lastly having hit the mark he fuses with the three existential norms.

[1] The highly intelligent or positive mystic is not afraid to live in the world, but it is the negative mystic who is afraid and tries to run away. Heaven or paradise is an escapist notion.

9. RESURRECTION[1]

Tilopa again sat silent and motionless for a year. As before Nāropa made a maṇḍala and venerated his Guru with folded hands. When Tilopa's glance fell on Nāropa the latter requested him for instruction. With the words 'If you want instruction follow me' Tilopa went away. When they met a royal prince, freshly bathed, richly adorned with jewels, surrounded by an army, and riding in a chariot, Tilopa said: 'If I had had a disciple he would have dragged this prince from the chariot and pushed him around.' Nāropa did so, but the army beat him almost to death with arrows, spears, swords, and stones. After the army had passed by Tilopa came and asked: 'Nāropa, what is wrong with you?' And Nāropa answered:

> Like deer without a shelter
> I suffer with no refuge and my pleasure flies.

Tilopa said:

> This deer of your body believing in an I
> Deserves to be killed, Nāropa.
> Look into the mirror of your mind which is resurrection,
> The mysterious home of the Ḍākinī.

When he had healed him with his hand he gave him the instruction on resurrection.

The instruction on resurrection is of two types: (i) a common, and (ii) a superior one.

(i) The former again is twofold: (*a*) having recourse to certain ingredients and (*b*) to making use of powerful mantras.

(*a*) This is practised in India by all people who know how to do so: either a certain ointment is applied to the corpse, or one eats a certain drug. In both cases consecrated water is used in order to achieve the desired result.

(*b*) This involves the use of evil spells which go against Truth.

(ii) The superior type is by means of meditation and is subdivided according to (*a*) the Developing, and (*b*) the Fulfilment, Stages.

[1] See Part II for a fuller discussion.

(*a*) He who practises the Developing Stage, after having attained the tactile and visual marks (of his visualized deity) to a certain degree, is resurrected (as the deity) by the power of deep absorption which is a means to become purified from his evil and to achieve the special intuitive understanding of the Fulfilment Stage.

(*b*) He who practises the Fulfilment Stage is capable of letting all vibrations enter, stay and dissolve on the central pathway and when the four signs connected with this process[1] appear is resurrected for the benefit of others by virtue of his power of motility and mentality.

While there are thus many types of resurrection, in this context only the experience of resurrection (or more properly of transference) for the benefit of others by means of the Developing and Fulfilment Stages, the 'profound' paths, is shown.

The experience is (i) instantaneous or (ii) gradual.

(i) This is the utmost profound technique of rising in the shape of a deity in its mansion. He who with unflagging devotion and reverence for the Guru understands and realizes authentic existence ('rainbow body') by experiencing the glow and flow of the inner mystic heat, during daytime is concerned with his apparitional existence, while at night he does the same with his dream life.

(ii) The gradual experience is related to the time, the object (in which resurrection takes place), the material as to the time at which resurrection takes place in the next existence and as to the capacity of keeping this new lease on life, and the association with consciously experiencing this new life.

10. ETERNAL DELIGHT[2]

Tilopa again acted as before for one year, and when Nāropa, after having made a maṇḍala and paid reverence with folded hands, asked for instruction, Tilopa said: 'Get a girl.' When Nāropa associated with a girl who was healthy and very faithful, for some time he felt very pleased, but afterwards he did not listen to what the girl said, nor she to him. He became lean, his skin grew

[1] See p. 65.

[2] A fuller explanation is given in Part II.

rough, and he took service with a smith. When he was suffering from this unaccustomed change, Tilopa came and asked: 'Nāropa, are you happy?' Nāropa answered:

> I suffer by being constantly engaged
> With my self-dividedness in an apparent dual world.

Tilopa said:

> Nāropa, you should strive
> For Saṃsāra and Nirvāṇa's unity.
> Look into the mirror of your mind, which is delight eternal,
> The mysterious home of the Ḍākinī.

Then he gave him the instruction on eternal delight, 'the Lower Gate', which is the most excellent way of the Vajrayāna discipline. This instruction is threefold: (i) the nature of the female consorts to be taken as the starting-point; (ii) the order of experience of the four types of delight as the path; and (iii) the realization of eternal delight as the result.

(i) There are four types of girls: Padminī (*padma*), Hastinī (*glaṅ-po*), Mṛginī (*ri-dvags*), and Citriṇī (*sna-tshogs-can*)[1]. The best among them comes from the Brahmin caste, is endowed with the relevant signs of the three behaviour levels in their overt, covert, and mystic aspects, and free from the four defects of the padma[2] (genital organs): not having the menstrual flow, not smelling foul, not being diseased, and when inebriated by sexual desire not knowing any shame or restraint with the yogic partner. Her age must range from sixteen to twenty-five.

(ii) He who practises the Fulfilment Stage, which is one of the two methods of developing spirituality in the unsurpassable Mantrayāna, is eager to realize the authentic being ('rainbow body') in his lifetime when he becomes aware of the signs that accompany the fading of all vibrations on the central pathway.

[1] There is no agreement as to the type names or the typification of females. Tilopa, op. cit. 4*a* uses the terms *padma-can*, *duṅ-can-ma* (Śankhinī), *ri-mo-can*, and *ri-dags-can*. Padma dkar-po follows the nomenclature of Tilopa in Sphžg 149*a* and says that *glaṅ-po-can* is another name for *ri-dags-can*. Ras-chun-pa in his Dchog 3*a* recognizes only the *padma-can*, *ri-mo-can*, and *duṅ-can-ma*.

[2] According to Ras-chuṅ-pa, op. cit. 4*a*, the four defects are dryness, wetness, closedness, and coolness.

Such a man endeavours to experience the meaning of his own or his partner's being. The first is experienced by stimulating one's sexual power and vitality, not allowing it to decrease; the second by absorbing the partner's equivalent, so producing a constant feeling of bliss and nothingness.[1]

The essence of this experience is to learn to become well versed in four techniques:

(*a*) 'Downward motion'; like a smith hammering a metal mirror, making the four types of delight[2] descend slowly like a tortoise from the head to the sex region) and so realizing them in their natural order.

(*b*) 'Retention': to hold, like a lamp in a storm, constant in one's inner vision the reality of co-emergence delight.[3]

(*c*) 'Backward motion': like an elephant drinking water, to make the four delights ascend (to the head region) and to keep them stable.

(*d*) 'Saturation': like a farmer watering his crops carefully to saturate every pore and experience the delight as consummation.

(iii) This is the realization of authentic being ('rainbow body') without any external reference, when the whole of reality as presented to the six types of perceptiveness rises in the continuity of unsullied eternal delight.[4]

When a few days had passed Tilopa came and said: 'Nāropa, how is it that you who have renounced the world according to the teaching of the Buddha, as a Bhikṣu are living with a girl? This is not a proper thing, punish yourself.' Nāropa said: 'This is not

[1] The two techniques are discussed at length in Sphžg 148*a* and 152*b* sqq.; Sphyd 98*ab*.

[2] They are: 'joyous excitement' (*dga'-ba, ānanda*),
'ecstatic delight' (*mchog-dga', paramānanda*),
'absence of excitement' (*dga'-bral, vilakṣaṇa*), also sometimes termed 'special delight' (*khyad-dga'*), and
'co-emergence delight' (*lhan-cig-skyes-pa'i dga'-ba, sahajānanda*).
The former three have a determinate character, while the last one is indeterminate and encompassing the other with which it is always present, even if unnoticed. This again stresses the conception of a 'field character'. The problem has been very clearly discussed by Padma dkar-po in his Sphžg 156*b*–157*a*.

[3] This is a name for the noetic act that cognizes everything as being of the nature of bliss. It is thus cognition and feeling together in its purest and most intense form.

[4] The six types of perceptiveness are those of the five senses and of 'mind'.

my fault, but that of this', and he hit his erected penis with a stone. When through excessive pain he was near death, Tilopa asked: 'Nāropa, is something wrong with you?' And Nāropa answered:

I suffer from having hit my penis
In answer to desire which is the root of evil.

Tilopa said:

Listen to my words, listen, Vimala (prabha).
You should beat yourself, Nāropa,
To realize that pain and pleasure are the same.
Look into the mirror of your mind where values are as one,
The mysterious home of the Ḍākinī.

He then touched him with his hand so that he could at least urinate again, gave him the name Nāropa, and instructed him in the sixfold sameness of value.

This instruction is that all the entities of the world of appearance are but the motion of original awareness. But although they remain the creative play of the co-emergence of bliss and nothingness, internally this awareness, defiled by its own obscurating power, becomes co-emergent ignorance,[1] and externally this ignorance, postulating a duality of the world of appearance (as subject and object and object and object), by taking this duality as final becomes ignorance mistaken about cause and effect. As a result of this one rises (from the primordial light) as a ghost, the result of one's former tendencies, and interpreted according to the twelve topics of the Law of Interdependent Origination (Pratītya-samutpāda) such as motivation and others. Then as a result of the three poisons[2] one becomes oppressed by misery in the same state of bewilderment-errancy as the six kinds of sentient beings. One will only understand through oral instruction by a competent Guru that this bewilderment causes a certain form of life.

[1] This is the transition, as it were, from Being-in-itself to being-oneself, the self consisting of the three reaction potentialities (*snaṅ-ba gsum*), developing into the reaction patterns underlying all conscious behaviour. See Sphyd 49*a*. sGam-po-pa, viii. 13*a*.

[2] They are the three reaction potentialities——'passion-lust', 'aversion', and 'bewilderment'.

By understanding how transcending awareness, which is the noetic act, enters into one's life again, and by preserving it so as not to become alienated from it (by taking it for something which it is not), the whole of reality, all that appears to the six forms of perceptiveness, remains the play of co-emergence delight. In brief, just like a feather drifting in the wind, one roams among things without becoming attached to them. The experience of the three conditions (for existence),[1] being of a subtle, coarse, and opaque type, as having the same value, is the profound essence of this instruction.

11. MAHĀMUDRĀ[2]

Again Tilopa acted for one year as before. When Nāropa made his maṇḍala and venerated him with folded hands, Tilopa glanced once at him. Nāropa prayed and asked for instruction. 'If you want instruction, give me your girl!' When Nāropa did so, the girl turned her back to Tilopa, looked at Nāropa, smiled and cast sidelong glances at him. Tilopa beat her and said: 'You do not care for me, you only care for Nāropa.' Nāropa did not lose faith in the propriety of his Guru's action, and when he sat there happily without the girl, Tilopa asked him: 'Are you happy, Nāropa?' And Nāropa answered:

> Bliss is to offer the Mudrā[3] as fee
> To the Guru who is Buddha himself, unhesitatingly.

Tilopa said:

> You are worthy of bliss eternal, Nāropa,
> On the path of infinite Reality.
> Look into the mirror of your mind, which is Mahāmudrā,
> The mysterious home of the Ḍākinī.

And he gave him the instruction on the illumining Mahāmudrā transcending awareness.

This instruction is threefold: (i) through mystic illumination to determine the unoriginatedness or the ground (Being-in-itself)

[1] They are motility-mentality as the primary condition, the fertilizing power of both father and mother as the organizatory condition, and the materiality developing process as the concomitant condition. Sphžg 16*b*.

[2] For further particulars see Part II.

[3] See Note G, p. 270.

Mahāmudrā; (ii) through subsequent presentational knowledge to recognize the unceasing or the path Mahāmudrā; and (iii) through the relation of coincidence to realize the ineffable or the goal Mahāmudrā.[1]

(i) Original knowledge, genuine and transcendent, is in itself nothing, but may under conditions become anything. In itself it is ultimately beyond truth, conventionally in its working it is not falsehood. It does not originate as the extreme of existence, nor does it vanish into the extreme of non-existence, nor does it remain in differentiatedness. Free from the eight possible extremes,[2] beyond the three pitfalls of bewilderment-errancy,[3] nothingness (and yet) having all causal characteristics it is directly realized in mystic illumination which recognizes spirituality as it is in itself.

(ii) In nothingness which is present unceasingly there arises pure sensation. In its manifestation as unceasing pure sensation, individual mind affected by the emotions, clings, inwardly looking, to an ego and, looking outward through the five senses, it particularizes. This bewilderment of dual appearance of subject and object which is called Nirvāṇa and Saṃsāra respectively, has never appeared as true appearance, and is only pointed out by similes applying to bewilderment in dreams. This presentational knowledge is realized (as what it is) when (its contents) come up like an apparition or as nothing (solid).

(iii) This pure sensation which is ineffable even if one tries to express it in words, which is radiant and yet nothing, which is devoid of the three conditions (of concretization),[4] beyond the four types of delight, even more superb than the radiant light, utterly transcendent, rises as nothingness, having the intrinsic character of compassion for the benefit of sentient beings. It is realized when one has reached the stage of great one-valueness or coincidence.[5]

[1] See Note H, pp. 270 sq.

[2] They are: origination, annihilation, eternalism, nihilism, singularity, plurality, coming, and going.

[3] They are the three reaction potentialities. This passage again suggests a field character, one factor or part of which is beyond all determination, while the other is determinate or, as the texts say, 'having all causal characteristics'.

[4] They are appearance, symbols (gestures and language), and possibilities of experience.

[5] See p. 70.

Its mode of experience is such that when at rest one sees that which rests face to face; it is a brilliant sensation which is nothing in itself, devoid of and beyond all words and thought, like the expanse of a bright sky. When it appears as the objects of the five senses one sees that which appears face to face; it is eternal delight which also like an apparition is nothing in itself, in the one-valueness of all that appears and that apart from it is held to be absolutely true. When moving one sees that which moves face to face; this light of the intuitive understanding through mystic illumination, which is not concerned with a determinate object and yet is compassion for the benefit of bewildered beings, is realized after the lower stage of the realization that there is nothing to be meditated upon.[1] This is the profound mode of seeing that which rests and moves face to face.

Although the state that there is nothing to be meditated upon is for ever mystic illumination, it is not contradictory to the manifestation of presentational knowledge as compassion or the way leading beyond this world. In the sDud-pa (Ārya-Prajñāpāramitāsaṃcayagāthā, fol. 23*a*) it is stated that:

> (A Bodhisattva living a life of enlightenment)[2]
> Knows that all is nothing and unborn since time without beginning.
> He is compassionate to those who have not yet attained mystic illumination,
> And so he parts not with the Buddha's teaching.

12. THE INTERMEDIATE STATE[3]

Again Tilopa acted as before for a year, and when Nāropa had made a maṇḍala, venerated him with folded hands, and spoken his prayer, the venerable Tilopa said: 'If you want instruction, follow me.' He went into a large desert, but although he proceeded leisurely, Nāropa, no matter how much he hurried, could not catch up with him and sat down exhausted. When he begged Tilopa that

[1] See p. 70.

[2] This line is missing in the text and has been translated from the text in which it is said to be found.

[3] Further details are to be found in Part II.

he might care to reveal something which would indicate that now, as the result of his labours, he had realized the significance of the ultimate, Tilopa said: 'If you want instruction, make a maṇḍala.' Since he had no grain he made the maṇḍala out of sand and when he declared that, having sought everywhere, he could not find any water for sprinkling, Tilopa asked: 'Has your body no blood?' Nāropa let the blood gush from the arteries, and when he let his eyes roam, not finding any flowers, Tilopa chided him: 'Have you no limbs? Cut off your head and put it in the middle of the maṇḍala; take your arms and legs and arrange them round it.' When Nāropa had done so and offered this maṇḍala to his Guru, he fainted from loss of blood. When he had regained consciousness, Tilopa asked: 'Nāropa, are you happy?' And Nāropa answered:

Happiness is to offer to the Guru
This maṇḍala of one's own flesh and blood.

Tilopa then said:

Nāropa, this body with its sullied pleasures has no reality,
Yet it should be a source of delight eternal.
Look into the mirror of your mind, the intermediate state,
The mysterious home of the Ḍākinī.

Then he touched him with his hand, healed him, and gave him the instruction on the intermediate state.

This instruction is fivefold: (i) that which has to be purified or the recognition of the intermediate state of one's physical existence; (ii) the ground on which the process of purification is performed and the place whither one comes by this process, the intermediate state having the characteristic of the ultimate, or the pointing out of the reality of the radiant light as 'mother'; (iii) that which has to be purified or the intermediate state of the ultimate and its impure manifestations; (iv) the purifying process or the means of making the radiant light as 'child' shine forth by the instruction on attunement or the path; and (v) the realization of the goal.

(i) The intermediate state between birth and death is this our body consisting of flesh and blood as the result (of former actions); the dream state (as the intermediate state between sleep and wakefulness, *rmi-lam bar-do*) is the subtle body consisting of the indivisibility of motility and mentality; the intermediate state of possibilities (between death and rebirth) is the 'mind-body', called Gandharva.

(ii) When people of the human world die their four materiality functions gradually fade one into the other; after the soft light the intense spread of light and the inner glow have ceased to shine, the radiant light which is complete nothingness and, like the pure morning sky in autumn, bursts forth for all sentient beings. This radiant light is the 'mother'.

(iii) The intermediate state of the ultimate as having determinate manifestations is the static and the moving. The static possessing the impurity of bewilderment-errancy is the cause of animal life. The moving having the impurity of passion and aversion is the cause of life among spirits and in hell respectively. This impurity split up into three poisons has to be purified.

(iv) When in an individual who practises the Path, all vibrations converge, stay, and dissolve on the central pathway, and thereby the four signs of the three types of nothingness[1] have appeared, and when finally the radiant light which is complete nothingness shines forth, this light is called the 'child'. The task is to attune it to the existential modes of birth, death, and the intermediate state.

(v) In the case of a person who practises the Fulfilment Stage, one has to distinguish between a man of keen perception and one of dull senses. The former is such a man that when the four signs and the three types of nothingness have appeared and passed, immediately after motility has again become active in the sphere of radiant light, this indivisibility of motility and mentality becomes a pattern which has five features similar to the five specific ones of the Buddha-level.[2] He then awakens to Buddhahood from the Sambhogakāya state.

A man of dull senses, immediately after motility stirs in the radiant light, experiences an intermediate state which has six determinate and indeterminate features.[3] By virtue of his capabi-

[1] See p. 171.

[2] They are the individuality of the Buddha, his realm, his listeners, the time of his discourse, and his teaching.

[3] They are mentioned in Bargd 21*ab*. The six determinate features are that 'while he formerly was hindered by walls and other solid things he is not now

lity of entering the radiant light again and again from this status which is characterized by seven qualities,[1] he acquires authentic being ('rainbow body') when motility stirs in the radiant light of the second week after death. From this situation he awakens to Buddhahood. If he is unable to do so, as a being of the human world he sees his prospective parents engaged in coitus and considering them as an especially suitable occasion for conduct, he enters his mother's womb. From here he can realize authentic being.

When Nāropa had received all these instructions in full, he came to the monastery of Śrī-Kamala. There he defeated the pandits who were preaching their doctrines. Tilopa was displeased and said: 'Nāropa, what the books have to say are mere words, as bad as the adulterated milk you buy in the bazaar.' When Nāropa, however, questioning the advantage of having thus become immaculate through the power of spiritual sustenance, asked Tilopa whether he should meditate in the East, in the cremation ground of Kāmarūpa (Assam), Tilopa gave him a skull filled to the brim with an impure and stinking mess and said: 'Eat this.' When dejectedly, but powerless, he swallowed the contents, the uneatable mess turned out to be delicious. Then Nāropa thought: 'Now, when there is spiritual sustenance, this mess has the eight types of flavour,[2] but when there is no spiritual sustenance it seems to be vile. Similarly, if one does not meditate, emotivity seems to be the cause of Saṃsāra, but if one meditates it is the bliss of Nirvāṇa. Therefore (my Guru) wanted to say that

so; while formerly others heard what he said this is not now so; while he formerly could see the sun, the moon, and the stars he cannot do so now; while formerly his steps left traces they do not do so now; while formerly he cast a shadow he does not do so now; and while he formerly had no supersensible cognitions he has them now', and the indeterminate features are that 'his stay is uncertain and he may go any moment anywhere; his food is uncertain; his dress is uncertain since anything may appear; his friends are uncertain because he may associate with anyone; his conduct is uncertain because he may have various visions of what is to be done and what not; his mentality-formation is uncertain because it may have this or that reference and is tossed about like a feather in the wind'.

[1] See p. 182.

[2] Ordinarily only six types of flavour are mentioned. See *Abhidharmakośa*, i. 10. Here the eight flavours associated with Nirvāṇa seem to be implied. They are: permanence, peace, no growing old, no death, purity, transcendence, unperturbedness, and bliss.

I should meditate for the benefit of myself and all others.' Tilopa said: 'It is just as you thought', and he gave him the instruction in the removal of obstacles in general and those for transforming the various ways of conduct into ultimately valid norms.[1] Thus Tilopa and Nāropa became one in mind.

(*b*)

NĀROPA IS ADVISED BY TILOPA TO ACT IN A WAY WHICH IS BEYOND WORDS AND THOUGHTS

Once Tilopa said to Nāropa:

> The blind do not see by tarrying
> And the deaf hear not,
> The dumb do not understand the meaning
> And the lame walk not.
> A tree does not grow roots
> And Mahāmudrā is not understood.

Nāropa thought that these words implied he should act so that benefit might accrue. He put on cotton trousers, took a skull in his hand, and set out as a mendicant, muttering the word '*vaidūrya*'. This is a symbol for being able to digest whatever one eats. When he met some children, one of them understood the symbol, handed him a razor, and asked him to eat it. Nāropa took it by the handle and put the blade into his mouth. When it melted like butter all were greatly astonished. In course of time the rumour of this feat reached the ears of the king. Not coming to the right decision as to what to do the king had swords attached to the tusks of one of the elephants in his army and let the beast attack Nāropa. Nāropa looked fixedly at the elephant and the animal died. Afraid that the smell of the dead carcass might infect the city the inhabitants were plunged into distress. The king, too, was grieved that his elephant had died and he chided his ministers: 'This is your fault. You must provide me with another elephant.' They tried to shift

[1] The removal of obstacles and the living up to ultimately real norms consists essentially in not relapsing into objectifying thought. Among others this removal also relates to the technique of avoiding unfavourable forms of birth. See Tshk 9*b* sq.

the responsibility and finally came down to the parents of the child (who had given Nāropa the razor). When these were on the brink of tears an old woman came and said: 'You should ask the yogi himself.' They did so by folding their hands and venerating him. By the power of his concentration he removed the carcass, relieving the misery of the inhabitants. Then by the power of his spiritual sustenance he brought life back to the elephant and restored it. The king and the child's parents were freed from their grief. The king became very devoted to Nāropa, invited him to his palace, showed him great honours and gave him his daughter, the princess Ye-śes sgron-ma (Jñānadīpī), as consort. After she had received the initiations and instructions, the teacher (Nāropa) was seen by others in his male–female aspect hunting deer with a pack of hounds. They were shocked. In particular the king's officiating priests and courtiers told him about it all. They said: 'Dismiss this evil-doer, or if you do not listen to our advice, he will corrupt the households.' When the king had with his own eyes seen what was going on he counselled the teacher and said: 'Don't do such things.' When Nāropa continued hunting, the courtiers declared: 'Your Majesty, either you banish this scoundrel or we leave you.' The king thought: 'If I let my courtiers go there will be evil talk that I have not upheld the religious tradition of my forefathers. Might it not be a good thing to have him killed while he is still here?' And forthwith he consulted with the Śrāvakas. Then he ordered the teacher to come. The king with his retinue and the other courtiers shouted at him as he and his consort were being led away: 'You do what must not be done; you destroy the religion of the Buddha.' They bound him tightly, beat him with clubs and swords, and lastly burnt him in a blazing fire of sandalwood.

The following day, a courtier and a man from the king's retinue intending to throw the ashes into the river, approached the place of execution and saw the teacher in his male–female aspect dancing in the middle of the fire which was still alive, and standing in a dazzling light. Frightened they returned and reported the matter to the king. All the people said:' this is impossible' and went to see for themselves. Everything was as had been reported. When the king asked: 'Is the teacher not dead after having been executed?', Nāropa answered:

The harsh words, abuse and swords
Helped to raise the shield of patience, be it e'er so small;
The fetters of Karma causing my agonies
Helped to free me from the poisons three;[1]
This fire of sandal-wood helped me
To burn the stump of belief in an ego;
The sharp swords helped
And cut Saṃsāra's ties;
The clubs of the ruler's judgement helped
To crush the evil demon of belief in an ego;
Killing others[2] without premeditation,
Not violating the three disciplines[3] and
Therefore not falling into evil forms of life,
Helped me, Nāropa, to act properly.

(Then he added):

Not inquiring into my motives
You had me, Nāropa, man and woman, burnt
Owing to your courtiers' jealousy.
To burn me was no real burning.
Not avoiding Karma with its cause and its effect,
How will you fare when you are reborn in evil forms of life?
Better would it have been had you appreciated me.

Then and there the king and his followers were overcome with grief, and in a dream they saw the earth opening and themselves suffering for aeons in hell, just as is related in the Aśokarājasūtra. When they woke up they were utterly contrite and unanimously they prayed:

Nāro, not inquiring into your motives
In passion and hatred have we accumulated Karma.

[1] Passion-lust, aversion, bewilderment.

[2] 'Killing others' is a metaphorical term for overcoming the naïve belief in the concrete existence of things. It relates to the experience of the apparitional character of everything we perceive. Lzzl 40*b*.

[3] See note 2, p. 21.

We have seen ourselves reborn in hell
As the result of this.
In contrition we offer our apologies,
Deign to forbear the Karma we have massed!
From the bow of the eight wordly concerns[1]
The arrow, like a Guru's word, has been shot and hit
the mark:
We have dreamed of our rebirth
In three evil forms of life.
Deign to forgive our error!
In flames for many aeons
Burn the faulty teaching,
And by burning our belief in this and that
Deign to forgive the evil we did not want to do,
In accordance with the Aśokarājasūtra.

Nāropa said: 'Your Majesty, if you and the others really want to atone, mere words will not suffice. Heed the following:

Listen, kings and patrons:
The knot of the eight worldly concerns has been loosened;
The three poisons of Saṃsāra's swamp have dried;
Ignorance, the weapon of darkness, has been repelled;
Contrition, the great fire of supreme awareness, has been
kindled:
Confess in the sphere of the unoriginated.[2]

The king and the patrons were purified from their evil and accepted again. When the Hīnayāna had become the Mahāyāna all patrons had won liberation.

Then Nāropa went to another country. He acted like a small child, playing, laughing, and weeping with the children.[3]

[1] See note 1, p. 26.

[2] The constantly valid type of moral conduct to which man must be true under all circumstances is rooted in the indeterminate field factor of human nature. Moral codes that lay down determinate lines of conduct are transitory, they can never be expected to hold under all circumstances. This problem has been pointed out clearly by F. S. C. Northrop, op. cit., pp. 344 sq.

[3] The symbol of the child for conduct is frequently met with in Tantric literature. It indicates the spontaneousness, open-mindedness and disinclination to force oneself upon other people's attention, and suggests the cultivation of an intuitive fellow-feeling for all that lives. Of course, the symbol is appropriate as long as one does not associate the idea of the problem child with it.

(*c*)

NĀROPA UNDERSTANDS THE MEANING OF COINCIDENCE

The way in which he realized the intuitive understanding of the relation of coincidence or one-valueness is fivefold:

(1) The statement as to the fact of being deceived by all that is created by mind;

(2) The request to be relieved of the fear that bewilderment might encroach on transcendence;

(3) The statement as to the rejection of attachment to the appearance of Saṃsāra and Nirvāṇa as either bad or good;

(4) The request to be enabled to cut off all imputations by giving up attachment; and

(5) The statement as to transcendence pointing to itself by itself.

I

Once Tilopa, surrounded by a host of spiritual heroes and spiritual powers, appeared in the sky and sang:

Ah, Nāropa,
Without the permission of the Guru, the Ḍāka,
Without inner experience and intuitive understanding,
And while still not free from spontaneous attachment,
Do not act, Nāropa.

Nāropa thought: 'Does this mean that I should listen to the Dharma?' As an answer came the words:

To listen to the Dharma is like drinking salt water;
(It means that) you still crave, Nāropa.

Nāropa reflected: 'Since I am a great scholar, does it mean that I must teach?' Again the answer was:

By extending the limits of words
The meaning is not understood, Nāropa.

'Then, does it mean that I should meditate?'

When spontaneous craving becomes free in itself,
Do not meditate on this experience, Nāropa.

'Or, does it mean that I should act?'

Where the subject-object realm has been transcended
Action is not possible, Nāropa.

'Does it mean that I shall look at my being-oneself in Being-in-itself?'

Since transcendence is not a content of mind,
You cannot see Being, Nāropa.

'Does it mean that the result, the goal, will be reached by itself?'

Where there is no longer wishful thinking nor despair
No result need be effected, Nāropa.

'If there is nothing to be done, then the desire to do something must be bewilderment. I shall ask the Guru to resolve my doubts.'

2

Nāropa asked:

If a myriad forms
Exist in the unoriginated,
Action is possible;
If not, what is this wish to act?

If this capacity for thought, radiant and self-aware,
Is attainable in Voidness which is nought,
Desire is possible;
If not, why do we desire it?

Spirituality, light, and nothingness
Are neither positive nor negative,
If entities, they can be experienced,
If not, what is this experience?

If in great bliss, sufficient in itself,
There be merit and defect, happiness and misery
Are possible; but
If all be equal
What do doing good and shunning evil mean?

3

Tilopa answered:

Listen, great pandit Nāropa:
Until you understand that (all)
Appearance due to interdependent factors has never come about,
Do not fail
To accumulate merit and knowledge, which are like the two wheels of a carriage.

Towards the teacher who points out the unoriginated
Let appearance rising red and white, and the capacity
For thought, fly like a crow from off a ship.[1]
Enjoy the goods of earth, Nāropa.

[1] This is an allusion to one of Saraha's similes. In his *Dohākośa-nāma-mahāmudrā-upadeśa*, 123*a* he says:

Just as the pilot-crow which has flown from the ship,
After roaming in all directions returns and settles on the ship,
So also mind original returns to its originality
Though it may have followed the paths shown by desirous mind.

With slight variations this verse is found in Saraha's Dohākośa, verse 72. In his commentary thereon gÑis-med, Avadhūti says: 'Just as merchants who want to cross the ocean put a pilot-crow on their ship, so also the yogis who want to cross the ocean of existence let the pilot-crow of memory [as a power, not as an act, *dran-pa, smṛti*] fly. As has been said by Saraha: "Just as the pilot-crow which has flown from the ship...." In the same way as the pilot-crow settles again on the ship because it did not find any land to settle on, so also the crow of memory settles in non-memory (*dran-med, vismaraṇa*) unoriginatedness (*skye-med, ajāta, anutpāda*), and transcendence (*blo-las 'das-pa, matyatīta*), [because it cannot find any "object"], as Saraha implies: "Having roamed about settles on the ship again"' (*Dohākośahṛdaya-arthagīti-ṭīkā*, 90*b*). The intention of the verse here is that appearance in its polarity of subject and object ultimately refers back to the indeterminate field factor. Although the goods of earth are no solid basis for conduct, they are not to be despised but to be enjoyed in utter detachment.

Until you understand that spirituality, self-aware and radiant,
Is the same as the spontaneous rising of appearance,
By experiencing it with attachment
You fetter yourself, Nāropa.

While all that is without and is within
From the start has never been and is beyond both thought and words,
Knowing that remembered experiences are but accidental
And untrue, act as you will, Nāropa.

The various ideas on this and that
Which cause birth in Saṃsāra,
Cut them as they arise, Nāropa,
With the sharp knife of intuitive understanding.

When attachment grows
For earthly goods with form and sound,
It's like a bee attached to honey.
Dismiss then this attachment, Nāropa.

4

Nāropa said:

It is my fault that habit-forming thoughts spread like the blemishes of the moon
And through attachment cling like a bee attached to honey,
That desire is freshened through the rain (of objects),
That the three poisons,[1] the swamp of Saṃsāra, become deeper and deeper,
That uninterruptedly the bond of Karma is tightened
And that ignorance grows thicker and thicker in darkness
So that the experience of the real is scarce like the hairs of a tortoise,
And intuitive understanding as non-existent as a flower of heaven.
How am I to give up desire in my blindness?

[1] See note 1, p. 88.

5

Tilopa sang this song of his oral instructions in which the meaning of supreme goal-realization is condensed:

Nāropa, you are a worthy vessel:
In the lamasery of Pullahari
In the spacious sphere of radiant light, ineffable,
The little bird of mind as transference has risen high
By its wings of coincidence.
Dismiss the craving of belief in an ego.

In the lamasery of non-dual transcending awareness,
In the offering pit of the apparitional body
By the fire of awareness deriving from the bliss and heat of mystic warmth
The fuel of evil tendencies of normal forms
Of body, speech, and mind has been consumed;
The fuel of dream tendencies has been burnt up.
Dismiss the craving for the duality of this and that.

In the lamasery of the ineffable,
The sharp knife of intuitive understanding
Of Great Bliss, of Mahāmudrā,
Has cut the rope of jealousy in the intermediate state.
Dismiss the craving that causes all attachment.

Walk the hidden path of the Wish-Fulfilling Gem
Leading to the realm of the heavenly tree, the changeless.
Untie the tongues of mutes.
Stop the stream of Saṃsāra, of belief in an ego.
Recognize your very nature as a mother knows her child.

This is transcendent awareness cognizant in itself,
Beyond the path of speech, the object of no thought.
I, Tilopa, have nothing at which to point.
Know this as pointing in itself to itself.

Do not imagine, think, deliberate,
Meditate, act, but be at rest.[1]
With an object do not be concerned.
Spirituality, self-existing, radiant,
In which there is no memory to upset you
Cannot be called a thing.

Nāropa then said that action which is free from all bias had been fully understood.

Nāropa had imbibed all the qualities that were to be found in the treasure-house of Tilopa's mind. He had realized the twelfth spiritual level[2] and he expressed his intuitive understanding in the words:

One need not ask when one has seen the actuality,
The mind beyond all thought, ineffable, unveiled;
This yoga, immaculate and self-risen, in itself is free.
Through the Guru's grace highest realization has been won,
One's own and others' interests fulfilled. Thus it is.

(*d*)

NĀROPA IS EXHORTED TO ACT

The advice to act for the benefit of others in compassion is not a sentimentality to be pondered about, it is as follows.

Tilopa said:

In the lamasery of Pullahari
Dispel the darkness of Mati's ignorance
With the sunlight of supreme awareness, ever free.
Bathe him in the light thereof.

Having thus made a reference to Mar-pa, Tilopa went to the monastery of gTsug-gi nor-bu (Śiromaṇi).

1 These are the famous six topics of Tilopa. They have been commented upon by sGam-po-pa, xxxi. 2*a*, 5*b*; and by Padma dkar-po in Sphžg 61*b*.

2 The ordinary conception is of ten spiritual levels. According to Sphyd 29*a* sqq., they are up to fifteen levels. The twelfth level is characterized by the perfection of Buddha-activity and a step beyond the sphere in which experientially initiated potentialities of experience can be activated (32*a*). It is the level of a Sceptre-Holder (*rdo-rje-'dzin*) (33*a*).

The great scholar Nāropa had removed the blemishes of his being-in-the-world by the first three acts of self-denial, and as a result of the jar confirmation he had realized the lower grade of one-valueness and the qualities of the sixth spiritual level—Nirmāṇakāya (authentic being-in-the-world). By the subsequent three acts of self-denial he had removed the blemishes of his being-with-others and as a result of the mystery confirmation he had realized the medium grade of one-valueness and the qualities of the eighth spiritual level—Sambhogakāya (authentic being-with-others). By the following three acts of self-denial he had removed the blemishes clinging to his dealing with situations, and as a result of the transcending-awareness-through-discrimination-appreciation confirmation he had realized the superior grade of one-valueness and the qualities of the tenth spiritual level—Dharmakāya (authentic situationality). By the last three acts of self-denial he had removed the blemishes of the three patterns together and, as a result of the fourth confirmation, he had realized both the lower and mediocre grades of non-meditation and the qualities of the twelfth spiritual level—Svābhāvikakāya (authentic being as such). When thus all knots had been untangled, acting free from all bias, he went to a country which was as yet unsettled (i.e. non-Buddhist).

At that time Riripa and Kasoripa came to the monastery of gTsug-gi nor-bu, greeted Tilopa with folded hands and venerated him. When they did not find Nāropa there they asked where he had gone. Tilopa answered. 'He has attained the highest realization, Mahāmudrā, and with the words that nothing remained to be asked whether I or rDo-rje-'chaṅ were there, he went to unknown countries. I gave him this admonition: in Tibet, the land of spiritual darkness, there lives Mar-pa Mati, capable of kindling the lamp of the Noble Doctrine. Burn away the darkness of his ignorance, and when the light of transcending awareness shines on the beings there, go yourself to the realm beyond thought. I have no news of where he is now.' Riripa and Kasoripa both said: 'We three were brothers in spirit. But he is like a second Buddha and without equals. He is capable of acting for the benefit of sentient beings, and so he should be exhorted to this effect.' When Tilopa suggested that they should call him, they asked: 'What if he does not come though we ask him?' Tilopa replied: 'Tell him my message to come.'

The two set out and though for a long time they searched for him in all regions they did not find him. When in their despondency they had spoken their prayer, they soon found him, sitting in a valley. The two circumambulated him with folded hands and inquired how he was. They said: 'Most venerable Nāropa, since you are like a second Buddha and without equal, it is absolutely wrong that you, not acting for the benefit of sentient beings, are staying in a sphere which is beyond thought. Tilopa said that you should start acting.' When they asked him to come, he said: 'If the venerable Tilopa says that I should go, in truth I must go.' The three set out and, when they had come to Tilopa, the latter said: 'You three have come quickly, that's very good.' Then Tilopa addressed Nāropa: 'Nāropa, since I have given you all my instructions, act for the benefit of sentient beings.' Finally, he summed up his instructions together with their injunctions:

> Listen to this order, great pandit Nāropa:
> With rain from the cloud of the Noble Doctrine
> In the sky of self-awareness, radiant in itself
> And not to be born as some content of mind,
> Ripen the crop of those who should be taught.

Then Riripa prayed:

> Reject the attitude of the Śrāvakas and Pratyekabuddhas
> Concerned only with their own peace and happiness;
> And with the lamp of Dharma
> Dispel the darkness of sentient beings, Nāropa.

And Kasoripa:

> Nāro, as the physician of the Dharma
> By using the medicine of the Noble Doctrine
> Alleviate the suffering from emotionality,
> The disease which strikes sentient beings.

Nāropa folded his hands and said:

> According to the order of the Guru, The Buddha,
> And the prayers of the brothers in spirit
> I will make the essence of the Sūtras and the Tantras
> Renowned in the land which is as yet unsettled.

When he had spoken thus, Tilopa became invisible.

(iv)

NĀROPA SETS THOSE WHO MAY BE TAUGHT ON THE PATHS OF MATURITY AND FREEDOM

Nāropa spent some time in his glory in the western part of India, and then, having proceeded towards the 'Gold Mountain Monastery' at Pullahari in the vicinity of the 'Flower Ornament Valley', he taught the Buddhist religion. Once his tutelary deity 'Khor-lo bde-mchog (Cakrasaṃvara-Mahāsukha) revealed his face to him and praised him:

> Washing away the stains of emotional instability
> With the nectar of speech, which is not normal speech,
> From the pure stream of the instruction
> By the Guru, like the tree of paradise,
> Nāropa speaks, but not with normal words.
>
> Dispelling the spiritual darkness of sentient beings
> With the sun of transcending awareness, light as when clouds in the sky have disappeared,
> Nāropa this non-dual spirituality enjoys.

Later, one morning, in a sphere of brilliant light he had the vision that the best of his spiritual sons, the interpreter Mar-pa, had come to India and stayed with the novice Prajñāsinha, to whom he sent an instructor with the message: 'A Bhante from Tibet is staying with you, bring him to me.' The novice and the interpreter Mar-pa came together to Pullahari. The novice made the introduction, and when the venerable Mar-pa had met

Nāropa, greeted him with folded hands again and again, and presented him with a lavish present of gold, Nāropa said:

My son, predicted by my Guru,
Worthy Mar-pa blo-gros,
It is good that you have come from beyond the snowland
In order to take over the kingdom of the spirit.

And he was most happy.

The venerable Mar-pa came thrice to India. The first time he was initiated into the dGyes-pa rdo-rje (Hevajra) by Nāropa, and when he had heard all the instructions, explanations, and liberations and further had studied under his predicted Guru the great Yoga texts such as the gSaṅ-ba 'dus-pa (Guhyasamāja), the gDan-bži (Śrī-Catuḥpīṭhamahāyoginītantrarāja) and the essence of all, Mahāmudrā, he returned to Tibet. As he had lost his books in a river he returned to India and, after having spent a huge amount of gold on his Gurus in order to evoke their kindness, he spent twelve years and a half in particular with Nāropa. When he had heard all that which belongs to the unsurpassable Guhyamantra, and when he had been given permission, he went back to Tibet and spread the Dharma.

Nāropa had seven famous disciples who were like him in explaining the Sūtras and Mantras. They were: Lord Maitripa, Śrī-Śāntibhadra, the mahāsiddha Ḍombhipa, the great pandit Śāntipa, sPyi-ther-ba from Nepal, the novice Prajñāsinha, and Ākarasiddhi from Kashmir. He had many hundreds of pandit disciples, Buddhist and non-Buddhist, such as the great sage Smṛti, the pandit Śāntivarman, Jñānākāra, Sumatikīrti, Devacandra, Nāgakīrti, and others. He further had 800 siddha disciples, both Buddhist and non-Buddhist, such as Pham-thiṅ-pa and others. Then he had fifty-four yogis who observed certain vows, such as Ben-da-pa (Paiṇḍapātika from Nepal) and others, and he also had 100 yoginīs who all had the signs of spiritual attainment. All of them he brought to spiritual maturity. In Tibet the famous Father-Tantra lineage derives from Nāropa.[1]

[1] The most important Tantra belonging to the 'Father' line is the Guhyasamājatantra. It has been the favourite Tantra of Tsoṅ-kha-pa. As to the disciples of Nāropa see also George Roerich, op. cit.

(v)

NĀROPA'S DEATH

The efficacy of his being-in-the-world, communicating-with-others, and situationality arriving-at-a-solution expressed itself in inconceivable activity, and by the miraculous conquest of the limitations set by the four constitutive elements of physical existence he matured and liberated infinite beings, visible and invisible. In order to end his life in the Fulfilment Stage, in the excellent hermitage of Pullahari he passed away in the Iron-Male-Dragon year (A.D. 1100) on the eighth day of the first month at the age of eighty-five. To those beings with pure vision his authentic ('rainbow') Vajrakāya, resplendent in a fivefold light, endowed with all the major and minor marks in highest perfection, surrounded by music and perfume, became more and more subtle and was completed as Dharmakāya which is ultimate fulfilment, unoriginatedness, the indestructible sound *A*[1], radiant light, and nothingness. To those beings who had various visions of reality he seemed to have attained eternal life and to pass from sight like a water-bubble, or to have attained the authentic Vajrakāya and to continue existing in it. To those who were not yet purified of their Karma, and as an object of devotion and reverence for the beings still to come, he seemed to pass into Nirvāṇa, his physical body being left behind. When it was cremated it is claimed that countless relics were found.

(vi)

THE VENERABLE MAR-PA OBTAINS THE ORAL TRANSMISSION AND SPREADS THE DOCTRINE IN TIBET

When Mar-pa was about to leave once more for India and had collected money for the journey, three girls in heavenly robes

[1] The letter *A* is a symbol of the intermingling of being-as-such and being-oneself, indestructible and the starting-point of every development into determinate aspects. See in particular Sphžg 9*b*; Sphkh 6*a*; Zmnd 69*a*.

appeared to him in a vision.[1] To give his enterprise a good start and to fulfil the intention of Nāropa's prophecy they said:

The sky-flower, the Ḍāka riding on the foal
Of a barren mare, the Oral Transmission,
Has scattered the hairs of a tortoise, the ineffable,
And with the stick of a hare's horn, the unoriginated,
Roused Tilopa in the depth of ultimate reality.

Through the mute Tilopa, the ineffable resisting all attempts at communication,
The blind Nāropa became free in seeing Truth which is no seeing.
On the mountain of the Dharmakāya which is the ultimate, the deaf Nāropa,
The lame Mati (Mar-pa) ran in a radiant light, which neither comes nor goes.
The sun and moon and dGyes-pa rdo-rje—
Their dancing is one-valueness in many.

The conch-shell has proclaimed its fame in all directions,
It has called out to the strenuous, who are worthy vessels for instruction.
The focal points, Cakrasaṃvara—the world
Is the wheel of the Oral Transmission:
Turn it, dear child, without attachment.[2]

After these words they faded like a rainbow.

As a result of this vision Mar-pa went to Gro-bo-luṅ, and since a few days were still available, a Ḍāka appeared to the venerable Mi-la-ras-pa and said: 'Through long meditation you have attained Mahāmudrā, the awakening to Buddhahood and the Six

[1] Lit.: Where sleep and light mingle.

[2] This is a typical example of the symbolic language of the Tantric instructions. Without a competent Guru it remains unintelligible. In this verse 'sun' and 'moon' are symbols for the structural pathways to the right and left of the central one, referred to by dGyes-pa rdo-rje. The dancing, or the vibrations that pass along the pathways, is ultimately nothing and hence has at every stage the same value. The focal points of possible experience, cakras, are held together by Cakrasaṃvara. These focal points collect the whole world and become intelligible by, as well as interpret, the world through the Oral Transmission. This is the 'turning of the wheel of Dharma'.

Doctrines, but you do not possess the instruction on transference and resurrection, which is the special means of awakening to Buddhahood by a short meditation.'[1] The venerable Mi-la-ras-pa went to Mar-pa and asked to be taught resurrection. Then Mar-pa said that such a method existed but that he did not seem to have learned it; teacher and disciple went through all the books. Although they found many references to transference, there was not one single text on resurrection. The Mar-pa said: 'This vision of yours points to this purpose, I must depart quickly.'

When he arrived in India he met the novice Prajñāsinha who told him: 'You have come late, on last year's new moon he (Nāropa) passed away.[2] He said many praiseworthy things about you and, convinced that you would come, he left his Vajra and bell and this painted scroll for you. The Vajra and the bell were stolen. But he (Nāropa) is still alive.' With these words he gave him the painted scroll of Hevajra. Although Mar-pa got this visible sign, in his yearning for his Guru he shed many tears of grief. Like a person who is denied meeting his Guru or whose merits are not up to the mark, he asked the novice whether he had any Oral Transmission instructions. The latter replied: 'I have not even heard the word "Oral Transmission". But since your devotion is equal to the compassion of the venerable one who sees with the eyes of the Dharma, you will certainly meet him, but you should make offerings with all the gold you have with you.' So Mar-pa made an offering each month in the presence of Lord Maitripa, Śrī-Śāntibhadra, the Ḍākinī Rus-pa'i rgyan-can (Kaṅkhalī-bhūṣaṇā), the novice Prajñāsinha, and Nāropa's former co-students Riripa and Kasoripa. The first prophecy he received was:

> The dream that the jewel has been placed on the
>   royal banner
> While a dancing girl gazed askance into a mirror,
> A bird rose and settled on the royal
> Banner and a captain steered his ship,
> Means that you will meet Nāropa.

[1] Here the forcible method is implied. See p. 199.

[2] Meditation is often compared with death, obviously because in proper meditation man is 'dead to the world'.

The second:

The dream that the revered Nāropa
With elephantine glance
Spread light o'er Tibet
From his eyes, the sun and moon,
Means that you will meet Nāropa.

The third:

The dream that a conch-shell blown upon three mountains
Guided beings from the lower valleys,
And that the light glowing in a lantern
Filled the whole human world
Means that you will meet Nāropa.

The fourth:

The dream that the blind have been led
From the desert of the misery of an I,
So that the eyes of ignorance have been opened
And the mirror of mind is seen
Means that you will meet Nāropa.

The fifth:

The certain fulfilment of the prayer
Imbued with the power of good
By the spiritual Dharmarāja
Means that you will meet Nāropa.

The sixth:

In steadfast Pullahari
(Like) the disk of the full moon
Nāropa will display the mirror
Of the Dharmakāya which is spirituality.

Exuberant with joy at these assurances and travelling through jungles and cities in search of his Guru, Mar-pa encountered countless difficulties. For instance he was imprisoned for three months by a tyrannical king. Released from prison he continued his search for another eight months, in the first of which he heard a voice saying:

Are you not deceived by the bewildering dream
Of two women catching hold of you
While riding on a lion, dancing and singing
On top of the sun and moon?

In the second month another voice said:

If you spur not on the horse in incessant confidence
And devotion with the whip of strenuousness
Will you not roam in Saṁsāra with its duality
Like a deer caught in the hunter's snare?

In the third month:

If you know not that his tracks are as hard
To trace as a bird's passage through the sky,
Will you not fall into abysmal senselessness
Like a dog pouncing on the shadow of a bird?

In the fourth:

If by that which never was
The snake's coil of doubt is never loosened
In the spiritual Dharmakāya, which is ultimate reality,
Your endeavour is as useless as a needle with two points.

In the fifth month, when he had the vision of meeting his Guru, a voice said:

If you know not that his being
Void of desires, is subtle as a rainbow,
How, like a blind man in a circus,
Will you cognize what it means?

In the sixth month, when he again had the vision of meeting his Guru and offering him a gold maṇḍala, he heard a voice saying:

Since all that is is pure from the beginning,
Unless you offer a maṇḍala of ultimate reality

Will not costly maṇḍalas [offered] with desire
Unite in friendship with all worldly interests?

In the seventh month he saw in a vision his Guru sitting in a ravine and eating the brain of a dead man. When he refused in disgust to eat his share from a bone ladle a voice said:

Since the enjoyment of great bliss has but one value
In the vessel of Great Bliss,
If you partake not of it as great bliss
Great Bliss you will ne'er enjoy.

In the eighth month when he was sitting exhausted after vainly pursuing the vision of his Guru, a voice said:

If the horse of non-action, radiant light, the ultimate,
Does not race and neither comes nor goes,
Why, in the desert void of sense do you run
Like a deer chasing a mirage?

Praying in despair and saddened by memories of the great scholar Nāropa, in his search he came to the jungle Ri-mun-bcan. He offered some gold to a shepherd and asked him about Nāropa. When he was shown a foot-print by a block of quartz his joy that he would now meet the venerable one was immeasurable. He prayed fervently and said: 'At last father and son will meet.' When he saw his Guru he felt as happy as when he attained the first spiritual level,[1] and he began to talk incoherently. He placed his Guru's feet on his head, embraced him, fainted, and when he had come to, he made all his gold into a maṇḍala and offered it to Nāropa. Although he was told 'I do not want it', he pressed it on his Guru and was saddened when Nāropa was about to throw it into the jungle, saying: 'May it be an offering to the true Jewel of a Guru.' However, the venerable Nāropa handed the gold back and said: 'I do not need it; all that is here is gold', and touching the ground with his big toe turned it all into gold.

When Nāropa was asked about the instruction on resurrection

[1] The name of the first spiritual level is 'The Joyful One' (*rab-tu dga'-ba, pramuditā*).

and the Oral Transmission, he said: 'You have been brought here by the grace of Tilopa. These promised instructions are in Pullahari.' When asked about the prophecy, he answered:

In the lamasery of Pullahari
Dispel the darkness of Mati's ignorance
With the sunlight of supreme awareness, ever free.
Bathe him in the light thereof.

Then he said: 'Come' (and both went away).

Mar-pa, terrified at the thought that his Guru must in time depart, and afraid of Tilopa's anger at their meeting, circumambulated Nāropa and begged for his protection. Nāropa prayed:

O Guru, deign to dispel all obstacles
Sent by Māra's daughters to afflict
The son promised me by you:
The worthy Mar-pa blo-gros.

In answer to this prayer Tilopa with a host of wrathful deities, carrying various frightful weapons, removed all obstacles. The Ḍākas folded their hands in terror and said:

We take refuge in the great terrifying
Body armed with fearful weapons,
In that Body and with terrifying
Speech we will do no harm.

When the moon has risen in full splendour twice
Let him ride the horse of the great carriage.
Venerable Nāropa, since the prophecy
Has beeen fulfilled, live among spiritual beings.

With these words they all disappeared. It is said that at this time Mar-pa himself saw half of Tilopa in the clouds.

Then Nāropa and Mar-pa went to Pullahari. When Mar-pa asked for the Oral Transmission and in particular for the teaching on transference and resurrection, Nāropa asked him: 'Did you remember to ask for resurrection, or did you receive a revelation?' Mar-pa replied: 'I did not receive a revelation, nor did I remember it myself; I have a disciple named Thos-pa dga', he had a revelation by a Ḍāka.'[1] Then Nāropa said: 'How wonderful, in the dark country of Tibet there is a being, bright like the sun rising over the snow.' He then lifted his folded hands to his head and with the words

> Salutation to the being
> Thos-pa dga',
> Like the sun rising o'er the snow
> In the dread darkness of the North,

he closed his eyes and nodded thrice towards Tibet. It is said that also the hills and trees of Pullahari nodded thrice towards Tibet and that they all lean that way.

Nearly two months later when he had received the symbolic initiations and instructions in the Oral Transmission, Nāropa appeared to him in the sky in the shape of the deity Hevajra with eight goddesses,[2] and asked him whether he made obeisance to him or to the tutelary deity. Mar-pa answered: 'To the tutelary deity.' Nāropa said:

> There where there is no Guru
> Not even the name of Buddha is heard.
> The Buddhas of a thousand aeons
> Depend on the Guru for their appearance.

'The fact is that they are His manifestations.' The tutelary deity then disappeared in the Guru Nāropa who declared: 'Because of this your interpretation your human line will not last long. Yet it is of an auspicious nature for sentient beings. Be happy that the line of the Dharma will continue as long as the Buddhist teaching lasts.' In a thanksgiving ceremony Nāropa laid his hand on Mar-pa's head and sang this revealing song:

> The bird of the Five Buddhas[3] has risen
> In the vastness of the ultimate,
> It holds the jewel of a universal monarch.
> The human line has faded like a flower,

[1] Thos-pa dga' was Mi-la-ras-pa's first name.
[2] Gaurimā, Caurimā, Vaitālī, Ghasmarī, Pukkasī, Śabarī, Caṇḍāli, Ḍombinī.
[3] Vairocana, Ratnasambhava, Amitābha, Amoghasiddhi, Akṣobhya.

The Dharma has become a river.
Saṃsāra's wave, that dazzling picture
Of desire, of its own has passed away.

Understanding this Mar-pa made obeisance to Nāropa who was immediately drawn by a Ḍāka to the spiritual realm.

Mar-pa hurried back to Tibet and handed the instructions in the Oral Transmission, together with the injunctions, to his spiritual son Mi-la-ras-pa. The latter gave to Ras-chuṅ-pa and Ṅan-rdzoṅ-pa the instructions and maturing confirmations, and to Dags-po rin-po-che (sGam-po-pa) the 'Liberation Path', known as the Six Topics of Nāropa. Thus he kindled the lamp of the Buddhist doctrine in the snowland of Tibet.

Such was the wondrous life of Nāropa, a second Buddha.
By the power of his former resolutions he attained the best form of existence,
The world renounced, he embodied the three disciplines on the path to liberation.
He was an outstanding sage, explaining, discussing, and composing Sūtra and Tantra texts,
In Pullahari he spread the teaching of the first Piṭaka (Vinaya),
In Nalanda, after the defeat of his opponents, he was asked to act as abbot.
He taught the Sūtras and the Abhidharma after overthrowing many Tīrthikas,
Inspired by twelve minor visions of the Ḍāka's prophecies, he sought the Guru,
He met and obeyed Tilopa through twelve acts of self-denial, he attained
The highest realization, the experience, and intuitive understanding
Of attunement by experiencing the four confirmations
Of the 'Oral Transmission', of resurrection, and of other practices.
All has been recorded faithfully according to the siddha-king's transmission,
And is endowed with the oral instructions which contain the meaning and the purpose
Of the teaching in a nutshell, so that they may easily be understood.

In Jambudvīpa, unexcelled, where in the Golden Age thousands of Buddhas appeared,
In the Snowland (of Tibet) where in this degenerate age the Sūtras and Tantras are widely taught,
In Brag-dkar where the obstacles of the central path were removed by the venerable Mi-la-ras-pa,
This is the place where spiritual heroes and Ḍākas meet and where meditation prospers,
Hallowed by the noble saints of the past and future,
Like the outspread wings of the Garuḍa bird, which span at least a mile,
Near the palace of rDzoṅ-dkar oft visited by Avalokiteśvara,
The place where Lord Atīśa stayed and part of mÑa-ris bskor-gsum,
I, lHa'i btsun-pa Rin-(chen) rnam-(rgyal), have written this story of his life as it occurred.

Indeed,
By the power of good in my intention to write this book
May there be prosperity and peace in the land where once
Lived Khu and dbOn,[1] father and son, and may
All sentient beings who as mothers are related to each other,
Incarnate come into contact with the Guhyamantra teaching,
And may they be accepted by the siddha-gurus.
Through the power derived from penetrating the outer and inner conditions
By means of the pathways, motility and
Creative potentiality that in itself is indestructible
May they realize the Three Norms that have been since time without beginning.

Also through this book may the essence of the teaching contained in the Sūtras and
Tantras spread and flourish and last for a long time.

May good increase!

[1] Khu-ston brTson-'grus g'yuṅ-druṅ (A.D. 1011–75) and dbOn-po 'byuṅ-gnas rgyal-mtshan. The latter became abbot when the former died, hence the 'father-son' relationship.

PART II

THE PHILOSOPHY

WHAT IS TANTRA?

THE line of thought which Nāropa represents is named Mantranaya or Mantrayāna. It is an aspect of Mahāyāna Buddhism,[1] the product of an intensely philosophical spirit inspired by an insatiable ambition to know reality directly, not by rumour or description. It relies on the 'inner light' rather than on the mere rationality of philosophy with which it is nevertheless well acquainted. By its very name it claims to be the expression of the Real or the spirituality of Buddhahood.[2] But since the immediate experience of the Real is an unusual and privileged state of being, it is also said to be 'secret'.[3] The philosophical significance of Mantrayāna has been much obscured by irresponsibly applying to it the name 'Tantrism', probably one of the haziest notions and misconceptions the Western mind has evolved. Hence before using this, now common, term, it may be profitable to find out what Tantra and Tantrism are.

It is customary in certain Western circles and among those in the East who have come under Western philosophical and Christian influence, or who are anxious to commend the East to the West by establishing an identity between Eastern and Western doctrines, to consider Tantrism as a medley of ritual acts, yoga techniques, and other practices, mostly of an 'objectionable' type, and therefore as a degenerative lapse into a world of superstition and magic. The reasons are not far to seek. Buddhism became

[1] In the *Tattvaratnāvalī*, a small text contained in *Advayavajrasaṃgraha*, p. 14, Mahāyāna is said to consist of Pāramitāyāna and Mantrayāna. The same distinction is found in sGam-po-pa, v. 26*a*, and Tsoṅ-kha-pa, ii. 2, 63*a*.

[2] *sṅags*, *mantra* is according to sGam-po-pa, x. 45*b* 'the spirituality of Buddhahood because it is not something which becomes an entity'. Its function is said to be 'the protection of mind' (*yid skyob-pa*, *manastrāṇa*) so that it may not become dissipated in the objects of its desires and its basic spiritual value may remain unimpaired. This interpretation goes back to *Guhyasamājatantra, p.* 156, and has been commented upon by Nāropa. *Sekoddeśaṭikā*, p. 33 and Tsoṅ-kha-pa, vi. 4, *10a.* Mantra is commonly associated with more or less intelligible syllables or word-series. This is actually one of its most insignificant aspects. Essentially *mantra* is a name for symbolic transformation-processes and their experience, in which language partakes, being, as it were, its final shape. Inseparable from mind, *mantra* is its activity as such.

[3] See note 1, p.6.

known to the Western world at a rather critical period, when the West expected scientific thought and rational argument to further morality and religious contentment. It accepted the Christian code, whether practised or not, as the norm of moral action, the Christian religion as a way of salvation, and reduced philosophy to a purely academic pursuit. The possibility that philosophy itself might provide guidance in conduct, and that as a way of life and quest for meaning it might involve the whole of man and not merely his brain, was overlooked. This parochialism was fortified by repression and puritanism; and the assurance with which the prejudices against everything that did not agree with this pattern were voiced greatly assisted the habit of identifying human with Western nature. Consequently that which is labelled 'Tantra', which speaks in symbols charged with multiple meanings, was put into an unfavourable light. In the development of Buddhist thought through the ages, Tantrism was conceived to be a late product and to deviate shockingly from an imagined or *a priori* postulated innocence.[1] Although this theory appears to be self-consistent, it is a conglomerate of loosely assorted beliefs and wishes. It starts from the mistake of judging texts, studied improperly, by an arbitrary scale of values; it labours under the unwarranted assumption that, because the Tantras were the last texts to become known to the West, they must be the last phase of Buddhist literary activity; and it even seems to contain some pious reminiscences of the story of The Fall of Man in Genesis.

Nothing of what is thus fancied about Tantrism is borne out by the original texts. Although this crude and yet highly cherished

[1] The main charge levelled against Tantrism is that it makes use of sex. As is well known, sexual imagery is excluded from religious symbolism in the West, while erotic forms are freely used in the East for conveying religious feelings. Sex has no evil associations for a follower of the Tantras. But this does not imply licentiousness. To be unaware of the difference between East and West, and on the basis of such ignorance to outline a development of Buddhist thought, can hardly be said to do justice to Buddhism. The various histories of Buddhist thought that have been written, all bear the stamp of the second half of the nineteenth century. The so-called Higher Criticism which often is insane arbitrariness, is in the field of Buddhist studies an inverted form of popular Darwinism, an attempt to understand everything in terms of evolution and—degeneration. On the unsound methods of this Higher Criticism see Walter Kaufmann, *Critique of Religion and Philosophy*, pp. 269 sq.

dogma has been challenged recently,[1] the question 'what does Tantra mean?' has remained unanswered. Tantra is dealt with as a literary document, which actually is only the communicatory aspect of Tantra as such. What then does Tantra mean? The Guhyasamājatantra, one of the oldest Buddhist Tantric literary documents, defines the word as follows:[2]

> '"Tantra" is continuity, and this is threefold:
> Ground, Actuality, and Inalienableness.
> "Actuality" is immanent causality, "Inalienableness" is
> the effect,
> "Ground" is the process.'

Commenting on this cryptic aphorism, Tsoṅ-kha-pa declares:[3] 'The meaning of the term "Tantra" (*rgyud*) is continuity, and Nāropa has explained this as meaning that "actuality" is the experimenter, an individual likened to a precious jewel as an individual as such, or continuity as immanent causality; "ground" is the four techniques communion and realization by means of the two Stages (Developing Stage and Fulfilment Stage) or continuity as an operational process; and "inalienableness" is the unlocalized Nirvāṇa, rDo-rje-'chaṅ (Vajradhara), the pattern of identity, or continuity as effect.'

At first sight this commentary does not seem to be very enlightening, because it makes use of too many terms which need clarification. Thus 'actuality' is a particular individuality which, in its own peculiar fashion, is what it is and which cannot be described or referred to otherwise than being itself. Actualized in a human being it is its own unique contribution to the 'particular concrete occasion'—as A. N. Whitehead would say[4]—which is this particular human being. Although identical in so far as being

[1] Thus D. L. Snellgrove, *The Hevajra Tantra*, is quite explicit that the old dogma of Tantrism being a degeneration is nonsense. However, he, too, does not say what Tantra means and deals with it as a literary document.

[2] *Guhyasamājatantra*, p. 153. The translation given here is based on the Tibetan version of this verse according to which the *ākṛter* of the printed text has to be corrected into *ākṛtir*.

[3] Tsoṅ-kha-pa, iv. 2*b*.

[4] A. N. Whitehead, *Science and the Modern World*, chapter Abstraction.

itself, it varies from one occasion to another according to the difference of its actualization on that occasion. Thus there is a gradation in actuality, because there are other occasions or human individuals. The reference to an individual who is like a precious jewel is meant to point to the actuality in its fullest and unrestricted actualization.[1] In other words, every actual occasion is defined as to its character by how this 'actuality' is actualized for that occasion. However, since this actualization is determined as it goes along by causes which are intrinsic to the actualizing process itself, we can speak of 'actuality' as immanent causality. Being continuous it is not linear and dotted like the traditional causal sequence, in which every event is linked to the preceding and succeeding event with rigid unalterability. The causal situation here is rather a fluid one, and within it new patterns of performance are possible at any moment. The idea of immanent causality indicates the presence of an active agency which is within the process itself, or rather is the process.

This at once leads to the second characteristic: continuity as process. Figuratively it is the 'ground' on which we move along in the process and by which it is sustained. The operations here, summarized by the contemplative technique of the Developing and Fulfilment Stages, are not uncaused, but their causality cannot be formulated in terms of linear temporal sequence. They are determined at the moment of their exercise in accordance with the nature of the 'actuality' of the total causal situation. In this respect they are the excercise of freedom which is never a thing to be approached or to be missed, but a way of existing. Freedom is the opposite of compulsion, not of causal determination.[2] It is therefore well to note that when we say that the cause controls or determines its effect, this is rather an inexact and ambiguous use of words

[1] In Sphžg 4*b*, Padma dkar-po explains five classes of beings: (i) he who is like a precious jewel will immediately realize the ultimate, but those who are like (ii) a blue, (iii) white, or (iv) red lotus flower, or like (v) sandal-wood, must be led gradually. So also Tsoṅ-kha-pa, iv. 13*ab*. This distinction between an immediately capable and a gradually capable type of man is already found in Tilopa, op. cit. 1, where Tilopa adds that what is good for one type is not necessarily good for another.

[2] See John Hospers, *An Introduction to Philosophical Analysis*, p. 270; Judson C. Herrick, op. cit., p. 213.

which should be specified. The control and with it the determination are there, but they are exercised within the event, not upon it.

This consideration brings us to the third characteristic: continuity as effect or 'inalienableness'. We have seen that in a causal situation the cause is not an external agent acting upon something inert, but is this situation itself, and that the control or directive operation is intrinsic to the situation as a whole. This implies that the effect also is not something extraneous, but is rather an emergent arising within the process as such. Although such an emergent implies a 'forward reference', it would again be wrong to describe the process as 'a pursuit of an end'. This would contradict all that has been established so far. Moreover, an end not yet reached has no significance in the total situation. It now becomes evident that, although such terms as 'cause' and 'effect' are employed, the primary concern is not with temporal or spatial sequence. The teleology involved here is rather the recognition that in a causal situation, as is the individual human existence, every directive process, such as the subjectively experienced Developing and Fulfilment Stages, 'has a restricted finalistic character defined by the end-state toward which it is directed and actually implemented not by the end-state but by the existing trend toward that end'.[1] This genuine teleology is most easily recognized in human action and conduct, but this does not imply teleological causation with its assumption of an action upon a natural process by an external causal agent in the manner of a *deus ex machina*. To have an idea of the future is a present act.

The unbrokenness of the cause-process-effect situation, when objectively examined, usually appears to be set in a frame of perceptual space and time as a linear succession of events, but subjectively the frame of reference is radically different. Here the integrity remains unimpaired by the analytic process employed in its investigation. This unitary character is referred to by the 'pattern of identity' which means that reality is one and undivided and identical with itself; hence the same reality is found in the cause and in the effect, or rather is both together.[2] Wherever we

[1] C. Judson Herrick, op cit., p. 153.

[2] *zuṅ-'jug, yuganaddha.* This term has quite a long history. In the Abhidharma

may look, forward or backward, within or without, in either case we find the same, not merely alike in kind but identically the same, reality: the extremes coincide.

An essentially similar, but more detailed explanation of 'Tantra' is given by Padma dkar-po who links it more clearly with man's existence or actuality, a proper knowledge of which will make all the difference to his actual status. In order to understand the full philosophical importance of Padma dkar-po's account a few introductory remarks will be necessary.

Padma dkar-po sets out to illumine the idea of Being which is both Being-in-itself, the transcendent totality of man, and being-oneself, the self-conscious existence of the individual. In its former sense it has an affinity to the existentialist term *Existenz*. For Padma dkar-po, as for Karl Jaspers, Being-in-itself cannot be known as an object, nor can it be grasped as a subject behind the phenomena. It is its very own and so far as I am concerned it is my very self. It is nothing determinate and hence infinitely open to new possibilities. It cannot be defined or characterized in any way. But it seems (or is felt) to be a vast continuum, out of which all entities are somehow shaped, and which surrounds and pervades the worlds. In this respect Padma dkar-po's account comprises what Jaspers calls *Existenz* and *das Umgreifende* (all-encompassing). Against this there is my being-there or, as Jaspers calls it, *Dasein*. A better term would be being-this-or-that, because it has specific traits and characters. It is determined. It is this or that. Even so it is possible to say that Being-in-itself is in my being-oneself and my being-this-or-that, in so far as I am all this. This double (or triple) nature allows me either to give priority to my being-this-or-that and become lost in the objects of its desires (Saṃsāra), or to give priority to my Being-in-itself-*cum*-being-oneself and in so doing become a Buddha (Nirvāṇa) while still in my being-this-or-that. Finally, like Jaspers, Padma dkar-po rejects any ontology or theory of being. Although there is a considerable similarity between Buddhist Tantrism and Western existentialist thought, it

literature it is still taken literally as 'juxtaposition'. In Tantrism it is exclusively used as the relation of coincidence; since this relation has the properties of symmetry, transitiveness, and reflexiveness it is of the formal nature of identity. In this sense the term is already used in *Pañcakrama*, chapter vi.

must not be assumed that the two lines of thought can therefore be equated. As F. S. C. Northrop has pointed out, for the Western existentialist there is no exit, whereas there is an exit for the Buddhist.[1]

Padma dkar-po's words are as follows:[2]

'The concrete fact of Being we term the Being-itself continuity, because it continues existing like the serene sky [whether clouds appear in it or not] (encompassing everything), beginning with sentient beings and ending with Buddhas. Since this Being-itself is not tainted by experientially initiated possibilities of experience[3] and exists as an ultimate inner light,[4] it is referred to by many names like 'Suchness', 'Cause-Sceptre-Bearer', 'Primordial Buddha', 'Ground-Mahāmudrā', 'Being-itself-Co-emergence', 'Tathāgatagarbha', and others.[5] If it were not of the nature of light it

[1] See in particular F. S. C. Northrop, *The Logic of the Sciences and the Humanities*, chapter Logic and Civilization.

[2] Sphžg 5*b*–7*a*.

[3] I owe this term to C. D. Broad, *Religion, Philosophy and Psychical Research*, p. 66.

[4] 'Light' (*'od-gsal, prabhāsvara*) is a purely operational term. As sGam-po-pa, xvii. 3*b* points out, for practical reasons one distinguishes between light as noetic performance (*rig-pa 'od-gsal*) and light as Being-itself (*raṅ-bžin-gyi 'od-gsal*). The former is not like the noetic light of the Vijñānavādins (mentalist-idealists) entitatively absolute, it is rather an encased light, but through its light character related to the light as Being-itself which does not depend on anything but itself for its illumining operations. As such it is also determined as bliss, but this does not mean that it is a feeling-judgement of the type an ordinary man makes when he has a pleasant feeling, or of the Hīnayāna quietism. It is not conceptual but the experienceable feeling-tone of transcending awareness in which the opposites have been resolved. Therefore also it is nothing (*stoṅ-pa, śūnya*). This again does not mean that it is a sort of subsistent nothingness. The term is only an index so as to point out that to speak of light as Being-itself is to say too much. All this goes to show that 'light' is a term which enables us to regard ourselves or our human existence in two different ways which reveal two distinct but inseparable phases of our being. In the above quotation 'exists as an ultimate inner light' the verb 'exists' (*gnas-pa*) has the meaning of the technical term *Existenz*, the fact of being, rather than existence (*yod-pa*). Unfortunately no Western language is capable of expressing adequately the subtleties of the classical Tibetan language.

[5] Padma dkar-po is quite explicit that these terms are mere names and not things. Hence to conclude from the term 'Primordial Buddha' (*daṅ-po'i saṅs-rgyas, ādibuddha*) that Mahāyāna Buddhism is theistic is to misunderstand the situation completely. The term 'Cause-Sceptre-Bearer' is also highly significant. In Sanskrit it is Vajradhara, which is rendered in Tibetan as *rdo-rje-'dzin* and *rdo-rje-'chaṅ*. The former refers to Reality from the viewpoint of human striving and accomplishments, the latter to Reality from the viewpoint of Reality. Here,

could never become translucent, just as coals will not become white by washing. Byams-pa (Maitreya) there said:

'Instability of thought and of emotion
Does not inhere in sentient beings,
Their Being from beginning pure
In themselves has always been maintained.'

'Although never parting from its Being-itself, it is infinitely open to new possibilities as the appearance of things (animate and inanimate) which have traits and characters. Thus it becomes the causal situation for the psycho-physical constituents, materiality producing forces, interactional fields, and other phenomena belonging to impure Saṃsāra; but it also becomes the causal situation for the inexhaustible patterning (of one's life) by a Buddha's existential, communicable and spiritual significance,[1] when it is purified of the former stains. In this aspect it is spoken of as "class" "all-traitness", or "all-controllingness". As is stated in the brTag-gñis (Hevajratantraraja):

"Neither Buddha, nor sentient being,
Not even an ontological one."

'In the Chos-kyi dbyiṅs-su bstod-pa (Dharmadhātustotra):

"That which has become the cause of Saṃsāra,
Purified by a process of purification
Is Nirvāṇa:
Dharmakāya."

as so often, the Tibetan wording is more exact than the Sanskrit prototype. 'Being-itself-Co-emergence' (*raṅ-bžin lhan-cig-skyes-pa*, *svabhāvasahaja*): emergence being what it is, is another index of the intimate relation between Being-in-itself and being-this-or-that. That which is here under discussion has nothing to do with the innatism of Descartes, hence to translate this term by 'the Innate' is to misrepresent the philosophical situation of Buddhist Tantrism.

[1] *sku*, *gsuṅ*, *thugs*. These terms correspond to Sanskrit *kāya*, *vāk*, *citta* which are usually translated by body, speech, and mind. However, what we ordinarily understand by them is in Tibetan *lus*, *ṅag*, *yid*. The Tibetan terms *sku*, *gsuṅ*, *thugs* never refer to concrete phenomena, but rather to their significance. Genetically speaking, *sku*, *gsuṅ*, *thugs* are present even before there is a body, speech, or a mind in the conventional sense of these words. On the other hand, they are no Platonic ideas either. Hence whenever philosophical exactness becomes necessary the ordinary linguistic translations will not do and must be replaced by others.

'And in the rDo-rje rtse-mo (Vajraśekhara-mahāguyayogatantra):

> " 'Tantra' is continuity:
> Saṃsāra is considered as Tantra.
> 'Later' means beyond:
> Nirvāṇa is the Later Tantra."

' "Class" has been explained by the author of the rNam-'grel (Pramāṇavarttikā) in his own commentary to it by "similarity", because again and again it is stated that the similarity between different things is "class". So also an ordinary man in the street says that this or that belongs to this or that class, because in this or that respect there is similarity and thus to this or that class he gives the name of "shell" or "bone".[1] Since this (Being-itself) is also the causal factor in Buddhahood, the mahāsiddha Lavapa's words that the cause continuity is an individual which is rarely met with,[2] must be understood to mean that this (Being-in-itself-*cum*-being-oneself) is the individual's subtle self. And when Nāropa speaks of an individual like a precious jewel, this must mean that inasmuch as one calls such an individual a person who is determined by class to be a great philosopher, the subtle self must be determined by class from the very beginning. The coarse individual is a coarse self; and since he believes in a perceiving self when he sees his psycho-physical constituents, it has been stated in the dbU-ma 'jug (Madhyamakāvatāra vi. 124) that

' "No self is found apart from the psycho-physical constituents", because there is nothing to be held to be as a self apart from the psycho-physical constituents and their being perceived. There is nothing that could hold a self and the psycho-physical constituents to be different. Since the idea of a self emerges in the perceiving act, a self is said to depend on the psycho-physical

[1] Padma dkar-po combines the ideas of classes being in nature and being man-made. See John Hospers, op. cit., p. 21: 'Classes are in nature in the sense that the common characteristics can be found in nature, waiting (as it were) to be made the basis for a classification. On the other hand, classes are man-made in the sense that the act of classifying is the work of human beings, depending on their interests and needs.'

[2] He is capable of immediate realization, because he has not succumbed to worldly desires. Indeed, few can be said to be not involved in purely worldly considerations. See sGam-po-pa, vi. 13*b*; x. 33*a*.

constituents. In the work just mentioned it is stated (vi. 138–9):

> "Śākyamuni therefore has shown that a self
> Depends on the six forces: solidification, cohesion, temperature,
> Motion, spatiality, and cognition, and on the
> Six bases: the visual and other senses,
> And has spoken of mind and mental events."

'The coarse self is called the inferior person, the subtle self the great man. In speaking of a subtle self one must not assume that this is identical with what the Hindus say. Although this subtle self is referred to by the name "self", its immediate experience is the strongest argument against a Self. Thogs-med (Asanga) says in his Theg-bsdus (Mahāyānasangraha) that on the level of an ordinary person one does not see one's source, but only when one has attained a certain spiritual level. And so the statement in the bZaṅ-skyoṅ-gis žus-pa that by not having seen truth one does not understand the noetic performance, must mean that one does not see the openness to new possibilities because of the apparitional flow of one's chance-producing acts, because the openness is the field of those who have attained the level of a saint. Similarly it is said in the rDo-rje 'phreṅ-ba (Vajramālā):

> "There is nothing in the three worlds by my life
> That has become the essence of my being.
> By the flow of apparitions the three worlds
> Are made to seem like visions in a dream."

'Since one has to go in and to this pure Being-in-itself, by relying on the instrumental experiences of maturation and liberation, one speaks of a path, and inasmuch as this continues from the preparatory level up to the Vajra-level,[1] there is a gradation and one also speaks of stages on the path. Since this going is the ground on which all virtues grow and on which they rest, one speaks of a ground continuity and, since it is also the concomitant factor in the attainment of enlightenment, one speaks also of an operational

[1] *rdo-rje-'dzin*, see above note 5, p. 118.

process continuity. The attainmentof a Sceptre-Bearer's level is the source of all being-for-others[1] not tainted by spurious impulses to do good, out of the causal situation and its process character, or the effect; and since the enlightening will continue as long as there are sentient beings as infinite as the sky, there is a stage of emergence, and this is the stage of the effect being born on the effect continuity. Since its absolutely specific characteristic is that its being-for-others does not wane, as is the case with those who think that the obstacles created by the experientially initiated possibilities of experience must be removed and dumped somewhere, or who have passed into a Nirvāṇa in which the stream of the noetic enterprise has been cut off, it is inalienable continuity.'

The above definition of 'Tantra' as continuity in Being-itself, in its directive process and its emergent effect, is the one adopted by all who follow the discipline of Tantrism. This definition shows that Tantra is the affirmation of the absolute unity of reality and of its being known directly. This it has in common with mysticism.[2] The important point to note is that it reveals our being in the world where two ways are open: either to give oneself over to one's being-there in one's capacity of being-this-or-that, in which case we become untrue to ourselves; or to give oneself over to the infinite openness of being-oneself-*cum*-Being-in-itself and thereby become

[1] *gžan-don, parārtha.* This term is sometimes translated by 'altruism'. However, we usually understand altruism as the opposite of egotism. Such an opposition is not implied here. The term refers to an immediacy of otherness and thus indicates the solution of the dilemma of realism and idealism. Of course, realism and idealism have to be understood in a general way, not in any specific one. Our 'phenomena' are not opposed to the 'real', but on the basis of this view acquire the immediate objectivity they seem to have. In addition this term indicates that which William Ernest Hocking, *The Coming World Civilization*, p. 28, calls 'a veritable consubjectivity'.

[2] Although the common usage of 'mysticism' is what would better be described as mystification, the contribution of mysticism to philosophy is tremendous. This is commonly recognized by philosophers and historians of philosophy. But because of its derogatory usage in common speech it is necessary to recall the words of William Ernest Hocking, *Types of Philosophy*, p. 255: 'as a form of philosophy, mysticism is not to be associated with occultism or superstition, nor with psychical research, nor with an application of the fourth dimension to psychology, nor with a cult of vagueness, nor with a special love of the mysterious for its own sake.' In the history of human thought it has always been the mystic who opened new vistas. See also Walter Kaufmann, op. cit., pp. 229 sqq.

true to ourselves. But the attainment of this privileged status does not come about by chance or by constructing conceptual systems. It is the result of a hard training—the way of how we go about making ourselves—and this also is 'Tantra'.[1] The training follows a definite plan, so that the frozenness of our being-this-or-that is dissolved and wider and wider horizons of reality are revealed to the student. Only a few will submit to such training in full. But here and there in the vast flux of human history we find someone who has grown up to Being and who can arouse us to our own Being. Nāropa is an instance of such a personality. And what is more, with him the whole course of training is available as laid down in his biography and transmitted to others.

[1] According to whether preference is given to 'action' (*thabs*, *upāya*) or 'discrimination-appreciation' (*śes-rab*, *prajñā*) or to their unity (*gñis-med*, *advaya*) one distinguishes between 'Father-Tantras' (*pha-rgyud*), 'Mother-Tantras' (*ma-rgyud*), and 'Non-dual Tantras' (*gñis-med rgyud*). All of them are forms of the exercise of the highest philosophical acumen (*bla-na-med-pa'i rnal-'byor*, *anuttarayoga*). The subdivisions are based on the difference of the symbolism employed. See Dchzr 1. According to sGam-po-pa, x. 20*a*, 'action', which in the narrower sense of the word is the practice of the Developing and Fulfilment Stages, belongs to the period where mind has not yet risen to an unrestricted perspective.

THE PROBLEM OF TRANSLATING TANTRIC TEXTS

TANTRIC texts, of which the biography of Nāropa and the essence of his teachings is an instance, tax a translator's capacity to the utmost. The difficulties of rendering Eastern philosophical terms into a Western language are not entirely related to the linguistic intricacies, although these must not be underestimated; they are much more linked up with the differences in thinking. Of the latter the linguistic specialist is usually unaware; with a few exceptions, he probably lacks, and may even scorn, a philosophical or psychological training. The result is that he begins his work from a natural, though mistaken, assumption. People who speak a given language (English, Tibetan) frequently use a certain specific sound (*dog*, *khyi*) with the same reference and so come to think of the *sound* as the word. Similarly the written *mark*, which may appear on the pages of a dictionary, is taken for the word, and this leads to the popular phrase 'to look up the meaning of the word in the dictionary'. But this natural diction is exceedingly inappropriate, because meaning does not attach to any one term of the triadic relation 'means' or 'symbolizes'. Meaning attaches to the sound or mark (1) as used by someone (2) to refer to something (3). Failing to note this subtlety and being forced to select terms which already have a fixed common usage, and negligent of ascertaining beforehand whether the term in question has the identical usage in both languages, linguistic specialists very often produce translations which are philosophically irrelevant, if not wrong and misleading, however self-consistent their presentation may be. Thus for instance *lus* is given as 'body' in a dictionary. But while we habitually use the word 'body' in opposition to 'mind' this does not hold good with *lus*, which is always used as 'the body lived in by the subject', i.e. body-mind. And the usage of *lus* 'body-mind', is again different from *sku*, which is also given as 'body' in a dictionary, but which apart from other non-body meanings implies man's existential significance, his being in an environment, the pattern of his existence. Many more such instances could easily be adduced.

Philosophers, on the other hand, who are aware of the difference in thinking, instinctively feel the inadequacy of linguistic translations, but are themselves unable to point them out, because they usually do not know any Oriental language. The result is that they either do not bother about Eastern philosophies or simply fit the information they derive from linguistic translations into their preconceived (Western) systems.

There is a marked difference between Eastern and Western philosophies. Although there is no unanimous agreement as to what one has to understand by philosophy, the tendency in the West is to conceive of philosophy as the creation of such imposing systems as those of Descartes, Hume, Berkeley, Kant, Hegel, Bradley, Royce, and many others, and above all, there is the conviction that all knowledge must be expressible in concepts. The pivot of Western thought is the object which, as William S. Haas points out, 'must not therefore be taken in a material, and still less in a materialistic significance. It indicates the form of mind which deals with any kind of data in an objective way, and attempts to determine them by concepts which are the expressions of reflective thought, and then to organize the various spheres of existence according to the principle of unity in variety. Thus, if the physical world should vanish from sight, the Western mind could and would still continue to express itself adequately in the formation of the immaterial world. This is precisely what it did in the days when theology shaped the transcendental realm as an objective world on which man depended but which in no way depended on man. The same thing is true of the main metaphysical systems of Western philosophy where the absolute, whatever be its determination and its relation to the human mind, does not depend upon the latter.'[1]

This objectifying tendency applies to philosophy as such. It is most natural for a Westerner to ask 'What is philosophy?'

In vain one seeks for something similar in the East. Here the pivot is the subject which remains the subject and never is absolutized and thereby objectified. While the ideal of Western

[1] William S. Haas, *The Destiny of the Mind*, p. 115.

philosophy would be the complete objectivation of the objectifying mind, the subject itself having undergone the process of objectivation, in the East subject and object are not in opposition, the one to be swallowed up by the other, but in juxtaposition, engulfed by something which is neither subject nor object. The insistence on the primacy of the subject is essentially the recognition of the fact that the subject determines the reality of its world. William S. Haas remarks in this connexion: 'Determination does not mean creation. It means . . . that a strict correspondence exists between certain fundamental forms of subject and their worlds.'[1] Even so it must not be assumed that the subject is something invariable or absolute, existing apart from the objects which it devours. The subject is something that is active everywhere, it may grow and expand or shrivel. From such a point of view philosophy is not an objective phenomenon. It is embedded in the subject and in this way a function of the subject's status or being. When there is a change in the being of the subject there is a corresponding change in the nature and amount of knowing. One has but to remember the different classes that were discussed in the analysis of the word 'Tantra' above. The Easterner therefore will not ask 'What is philosophy', but will say 'By philosophy I will discover and strive to live in and with the Real'.

This difference in thinking may be stated in still another way. The East tends to concern itself with the immediately apprehended factor in the nature of things, be they natural objects or inspected selves, whereas the West concentrates on the doctrinally designated factor. In developing their respective presentations the East uses concepts by intuition, the West concepts by postulation. F. S. C. Northrop makes the following valuable distinction: 'A concept by intuition, therefore, is one the complete meaning of which is given by something immediately apprehendable',[2] while 'a concept by postulation is one, therefore, designating some factor in man or nature which, in whole or in part, is not directly observed, the meaning of which may be proposed for it postulationally in some specific deductively formulated theory'.[3] However, since one and

[1] William S. Haas, *The Destiny of the Mind*, p. 117.

[2] F. S. C. Northrop, *The Meeting of East and West*, p. 447.

[3] Ibid.

the same word, for instance 'red', may be used in the sense of a concept by intuition when referring to a sensed colour, and as a concept by postulation when referring to a certain wave-length of light, we are faced with a systematic ambiguity which may, and often has, become a harmful ambiguity. Matters are not improved when Northrop points out another important difference between concepts by intuition and concepts by postulation. The former, he says, are 'mere names for particulars. That this is the case is shown by the fact that no amount of syntactical discourse can convey what such a concept means unless one has immediately apprehended and experienced that to which it refers',[1] and 'concepts by postulation, on the other hand, are universals. This is shown negatively by the fact that what they mean is not to be found denotatively in any particular aesthetic intuition or experience. It is shown positively by the fact that they gain meaning only syntactically by virtue of the logical and grammatical relations in which they stand to each other in the postulates of some deductively formulated theory. Such postulates are always general propositions referring to all instances.'[1] This distinction is valid only when the experiential character of that to which the concept refers is emphasized; it is wrong when in the traditional way universals and particulars are given an ontological status. A concept, whether by intuition or postulation, is always universal, only the experience is particular or individual. In any occasion of cognition, that which is known is an actual occasion of experience which exhibits itself as a process. As A. N. Whitehead remarks: 'In so disclosing itself, it places itself as one among a multiplicity of other occasions, without which it could not be itself. It also defines itself as a particular individual achievement, focusing in its limited way an unbounded realm of eternal objects.'[2] That is to say, in being brought before the mind in a concept, the particular experience becomes universal and predicable of many. However, we are here not primarily concerned with the nature of the concept. The important fact to note is that the West uses the concept for arriving

[1] F. S. C. Northrop, p. 448.

[2] A. N. Whitehead, *Science and the Modern World*, p. 176. 'Eternal object' is Whitehead's substitute for the traditional 'universal'. The very choice of words emphasizes the Western emphasis on the object.

at formally and doctrinally expressed, logically developed, and deductively formulated treatises of a scientific or philosophical character. The East uses the concept as a stimulus to retrieve the experience from which it has been abstracted.

This insistence on immediate experience must not lead us to overlook the important distinction between practical or existential awareness, manifested in deliberations about concrete situations and in our moods and feelings, and of theoretical awareness. Both types have not been adequately dealt with in Western philosophies for certain reasons. Indeed, the former has been seriously neglected in modern philosophy, and the latter has been restricted to abstract scientific theorizing which is held to be the only source of valid knowledge. The East, on the other hand, has held practical and theoretical awareness together. It is convinced that practice itself requires theory. (This is acknowledged in the West in the technological branches of knowledge but nowhere else.) As is well known, Kant and many existentialist thinkers defended the supremacy of the practical over the theoretical, because it is from practical awareness that we gain our first and most direct knowledge of existence. But without the clarifying influence of theoretical awareness all practice becomes vague and confused. If we want to know what something is in itself, we must turn to theory. We must gain detachment from practical concerns and situations. This is achieved in what is called a point of view. In most cases practical presuppositions still remain, though in a less subjective and restricted way. The ideal is the attainment of an unrestricted perspective from which a sound direction of human action will at least be possible. Therefore, the Tantras claim that pure theory must precede action, both of which are then reinforcing each other. The unrestrictedness of perspective and the cognitive indeterminacy which underlies the whole noetic enterprise is ever and again insisted upon.

This difference in thinking makes all our philosophical terms inadequate. They are tainted by certain presuppositions, since none of them can claim to have been born from the unrestricted vision which is the starting-point of Tantric philosophy. Therefore, in order to grasp the philosophical premises of the East correctly, we must be extremely cautious and careful so as not to read Western notions into Eastern statements because of the fixed common usage of our philosophical terms. The safest way would be to develop a completely new terminology of a most abstract and sophisticated type. This I have attempted in certain instances (knowing full well that thereby I am likely to incur the wrath of the linguistic specialist). Another way, no less safe, is to resort to the technique of multiple definition, 'accompanying any definition or distinction we make use of with a set of rival definitions in the background of the mind. Only so can we protect ourselves from the coercive suggestion of any one interpretation which seems for the moment to fit. It is not enough simply to resolve that we will regard our logical schema as hypothetical. By itself this is only a rechristening of tradition. New hypothesis is but old dogma writ large. Unless we do actually and constantly sketch out alternative definitions using different logical machinery we shall not gain the ability to experiment in interpretation which comparative studies require.'[1] In practice this amounts to rendering one technical term of Eastern philosophies by many in English.[2] This has the advantage that the reader who is interested in philosophical problems of the East, is not baffled by a revolutionary new and (sometimes) obscure concept, and yet is constantly reminded of the fact that his habitual mode of thinking (realist, idealist, positivist, Marxist, and so on) does not hold good and that he will do well to exercise his imagination. In this respect I have derived unending benefit from a study of sGam-po-pa's works. They abound in multiple definition. In the notes I have therefore

[1] I. A. Richards, *Mencius on the Mind*, p. 90.

[2] This, too, will find little favour with the linguistic specialist. He will claim that one term has to be consistently translated by one and the same in English. But in view of the multiple meaning content of any Eastern terms and of what sGam-po-pa, for whom philosophizing was of primary concern, does, this claim is exceedingly funny. In sGam-po-pa, x. 31*b*—we find the triad: *chos—chos-can—chos-ñid* and on 18*b* the triad: *chos—chos-ñid—blo*. Both contain the word *chos* which corresponds to Sanskrit *dharma*, but in the first instance he defines it as 'the objective reference of a perceptual situation in ordinary consciousness', in the latter as 'the enlightenment mind as the noetic act in itself'. Similarly, in the former the term *chos-ñid* (*dharmatā*) is defined as 'limpidity which is not an *ens*' and in the latter as 'self-rising transcending awareness which from beginning to end is not dependent on causes and conditions, originally limpid and not a concrete awareness content'.

constantly referred to sGam-po-pa, to whom the teachings of Nāropa were entrusted. Of similar importance is Padma dkar-po who, besides many other works, wrote profound commentaries on the teachings of his predecessors, in particular on those of Tilopa, the teacher of Nāropa. Lastly, the 'Oral Transmission' texts of gTsaṅ-pa He-ru-ka and other indigenous Tibetan works are invaluable for understanding the intrinsic meaning of Nāropa's message. However, I am far from claiming to have exhausted or fathomed their profundity.

THE THEORETICAL CONTENT OF NĀROPA'S TRAINING

In the following the attempt shall be made to give a more comprehensive account of what is merely outlined in the body of the text of Nāropa's biography. Although much belongs to practice which can only be learned from a competent Guru, the practice itself remains unintelligible and meaningless if its theoretical background is not grasped.

I. THE WISH-FULFILLING GEM

These practices are still followed today. The preliminary stage, to say nothing of the main practice, belongs to the unusual or special method of gaining direct contact with Reality. However, the first exercise, meditation on Vajrasattva and the muttering of his mantra, is sometimes considered to belong to the ordinary method, and then follow the ceremonial acts of taking refuge and adopting an enlightened attitude, to which may be added meditation on the four immeasurable feelings of benevolence, compassion, joyfulness, and equanimity. To whichever category one may reckon the meditation on Vajrasattva the practice is the same.[1]

First, one has to learn to visualize rDo-rje sems-dpa' (Vajrasattva) which involves three stages. rDo-rje sems-dpa' is white, has one face and two hands in which he holds a sceptre and a bell, symbolizing beneficial expediency and discriminative awareness. He sits cross-legged with the soles of his feet turned up in a posture known as Vajrāsana. On his lap is his spouse rDo-rje sñems-ma who is also white, has one face, and two hands in which she holds a knife and a skull filled with nectar. These are symbols of her function of tearing asunder ignorance and conferring bliss. With her legs she encircles rDo-rje sems-dpa' and with her arms clings to his neck. In their heads is the white letter *oṃ*, in their throats the red *āḥ* and in their hearts the blue *hūṃ*. From these focal points symbolized and indicated by the letters, a radiant

[1] See such works as Khsg 4*b* sq.; Dchzr 2*b* sqq.; Dchkh 2*b* sq.; Dchb 2b sq.

light bursts forth which shines in every direction and invites all the Buddhas and Bodhisattvas in their male–female forms. At this stage the following prayer is spoken: 'Exalted Ones, absolve and purify me and all sentient beings who are as limitless as the sky, from the impurities of evil such as failing to be true to authentic being in its basic and derivative forms, which we have committed in thought, word and deed since the beginningless cycle of births.' All this is the 'external rDo-rje sems-dpa'', the experience of a wider frame of reference in a certain emotionally moving form. It is also known as Kāyavajrayoga (*sku rdo-rje rnal-'byor*) or living up to authentic being-in-an-environment.

The next step concerns the disc of the moon in the heart region of the deities on which stands the letter *hūṃ* symbolizing the five types of transcending awareness.[1] This central letter is surrounded by 100 syllables forming the mantra of rDo-rje sems-dpa'. Though we speak of letters and syllables it is essential to be aware of them as powers vibrating with life. One mutters this mantra of 100 syllables the whole day for one month. This step is called the 'inner rDo-rje sems-dpa'', a still deeper experience than the one before, where the mantra is vibratory sensation rather than the spoken word or syllable. It is also called Vāgvajrayoga (*gsuṅ rdo-rje rnal-'byor*) or living up to authentic communication.

One should then feel how from the places where the letters and syllables join and from the points of contact between the male and female deities, a stream of higher awareness permeates one's whole body and brings about a sense of clarity and purity which is a sort of pure sensation and awareness. At this stage there is no idea of either a 'without' or a 'within'. Figuratively speaking all evil is expelled in the form of malignant demons and every place has been filled with the bliss of awareness. This is known as the 'mystic rDo-rje sems-dpa'', a total experience which appears as having been given all at once. Technically it is called Cittavajrayoga (*thugs rdo-rje rnal-'byor*) or living up to one's capacity to deal with situations authentically. In all three instances the term authentic is meant to refer to the fullness of one's being of which one is usually unaware in one's ordinary actions.

[1] See note 1, p. 73.

Of course, the various experiences are not separate in an absolute sense; they fuse into each other. This becomes evident from the last stage in the practice. After one has muttered the mantra of rDo-rje sems-dpa' and when the feeling of purity sets in, one prays: 'Lord, as my Guru and master protect me who have through ignorance and emotional unbalance, fallen from and violated all that to which I had committed myself. I take refuge in you, my Lord holding the sceptre, the embodiment of Great Compassion. I confess and atone for all my shortcomings in not having kept the major and minor commitments. Remove all evil and purify me from it.' When properly practised it is as if both deities, rDo-rje sems-dpa' and rDo-rje sñems-ma, were saying; 'All your evil has been purified.' At this moment the deities and oneself dissolve in an experience of ineffable light, and one may remain in this state of utter composure as long as one likes. This is called the 'ultimate rDo-rje sems-dpa', the experience of the Real as such. It is also named Jñānavajrayoga (*ye-śes rdo-rje rnal-'byor*), living up to transcending awareness as the ground of our whole being.[1]

This meditation is only a step in preparing us for further tasks with a similar aim. It opens our eyes to something more than our limitedness which for the most part is taken for granted and unalterable. It is never concentration on a static ideal of frozen absolute, but is itself a living symbol indicative of the intentional structure of all human experience. I cannot act without doing something and I cannot be aware without being aware of something. The subjective is given the same value as the objective. The act of being aware is present as an indeterminate relational form, grounded in the knowing agent. The object, however, is determinate and has apparently its own ground. This duality is overcome when the indeterminate, and hence empty, relational form, is terminated by the object. There is thus a peculiar relational union which in philosophical language is called noetic identity. Although the experience of rDo-rje sems-dpa' is cognitive, this does not mean that it is wholly unemotional. It is emotionally toned in an eminent sense. It is bliss in its very act of integrative awareness,

[1] A more detailed account is given in my *The Philosophical Background of Buddhist Tantrism.*

Its ecstasy is commensurate with its cognition. All these points are brought out in Padma dkar-po's definition of rDo-rje sems-dpa': 'The bliss of the indivisibility of the relational structures that make up man is rDo-rje (*vajra*) or noetic capacity, while sems-dpa' (*sattva*) or the three worlds together are the terminal object. The unalterableness of the union of the two is the intuitive grasp of meaningfulness'.[1] In the diction of modern philosophy the last sentence would mean that inasmuch as the differences of a continuous process are transcended by its essential unity, we can refer to its oneness and identity from beginning to end.

The perfection of the prerequisites for uniting with the spirituality of ultimate reality, which becomes accessible through the line of Gurus, has two sides. The first is called the perfection of merits, and the second that of transcending awareness. Ordinarily these perfection practices refer to the Mahāyānic perfections of liberality, ethics and manners, and others. But here we are concerned with meditational practices and move in a world of symbols. And so the first is practised by conceiving one's Guru as the incarnate reality of rDo-rje-'chaṅ (Vajradhara), Lord over the five Buddha-families, who in turn is the symbol of the basic oneness of all the constituents of reality. One has to imagine him sitting on a throne supported by eight lions symbolizing fearlessness and the conquest of all obnoxious powers, on a seat formed by lotus, moon, and sun, symbolizing respectively undefilement by evil, the dispersal of the darkness of spiritual ignorance, and the spread of light of transcending awareness. Further, one has to conceive of one's Guru as being deep blue in colour as a symbol of the unchanging reality (this colour being selected because of the ever blue sky in the tropics), holding in his crossed hands a sceptre and a bell, symbolizing the indivisibility of nothingness and compassion. Nothingness does not mean absolute negation but the indeterminate relational form of the act of being aware that may become terminated by any object. In order to be able to unite with any content it must be as nothing and must work freely without being warped and twisted by any bias. In symbolic form this is rDo-rje-'chaṅ's spouse, rDo-rje rnal-'byor-ma (Vajrayo-

[1] Sphyd 21*a*.

ginī), whose body is red; she embraces him in utter abandonment, symbolic of the highest intensity of feeling, joy, and ecstasy. She holds in her hands a knife and a skull, symbolizing the cutting off of our separateness in the subject-object division and the lavish endowment with bliss. The various ornaments worn by both rDor-je-'chaṅ and rDo-rje rnal-'byor-ma, represent the six perfections, and the major and minor bodily marks indicate that all qualities are present in them. Their garlands represent the sounds out of which are formed the words and sentences that refer to the profound and the common teaching of Buddhism. As possessing the five types of transcending awareness they are bathed in the light of five colours, which spread into all the regions of the world. But this is not enough. In front of them on a seat of lotus and sun on a throne supported by elephants there is 'Khor-lo sdom-pa (Cakrasaṃvara), the tutelary deity of the bKa'-brgyud-pa order, surrounded by a host of other deities; to the south of them on a seat of lotus and moon on a throne carried by horses is the historical Buddha Śākya thub-pa (Śākyamuni) surrounded by Buddhas of the past, present, and future; to the west on a similar seat on a throne supported by peacocks is the Great Mother (*yum chen-ma*), the embodiment of the perfection of discriminative-appreciative awareness, surrounded by the Buddhist scriptures; and to the north on a throne supported by śaṅ-śaṅ (fabulous winged creatures with bird's heads) is sPyan-ras-gzigs (Avalokiteśvara) surrounded by the followers of the three ways of life in Buddhism (Śrāvakas, Pratyekabuddhas, Bodhisattvas). And wherever there is free space one has to imagine the presence of the Protectors of the Religion and other helpful powers. The main object is thus to create a deeply moving atmosphere. When this has been achieved one pays homage to them with folded hands; offers them the whole world (this is done by folding the fingers in a certain form); confesses the evil one has done; evokes a feeling of joy over the good that others have done; requests the Buddhas to spread the Dharma; and begs them not to pass into Nirvāṇa as long as sentient beings still need their guidance. Finally, one renounces any claim on the good one may have gained by performing this ceremony and wishes it to become part of enlightenment. Thus again the perfection of merits is a step onward to the goal, not a means of self-aggrandizement.

After making this vow as often as one likes, one allows this vision to dissolve in one's Guru whose image fuses with oneself in another feeling of composure.

The acquisition of transcending awareness is indicated by two formulas which begin this phase of practice. They are: *oṃ svabhāvaśuddāḥ sarvadharmāḥ svabhāvaśuddho 'ham* and *oṃ śūnyatājñānavajrasvabhāvātmako 'haṃ*, which mean 'all entities are pure by nature and so am I' and 'I am by nature nothingness, transcending awareness and indestructibility'.[1]

From a purely philosophical point of view the first formula points out that all the entities which make up our world are 'pure' and stainless, because they are merely appearances and not independent entities as such. Yet they are not unreal. As a matter of fact, 'appearances' are the realities which we perceive and it is only by becoming an 'appearance' that anything can notify its existence to us. The important thing to note is the dynamic aspect of becoming an appearance which implies the incessant activity of mind which, in a certain sense, I am myself. Or, put otherwise, I as a mind create the world of objects which I knowingly grasp. However, creating the world is not so much creation *ex nihilo* as an arranging and revealing. There is a certain similarity to that which in Western terminology is called mentalistic solipsism, though not a complete one. The decisive point is that in this activity of mind that which appears before the mind is believed to be veridical or, as the texts declare, 'the sensa are existing in truth'. Most mentalistic (idealistic) systems both in the East and West stop short at this point, but while Western idealistic systems tend to define the sensa as being mental, most Buddhist systems reject this conclusion and merely content themselves with stating that sensa are experienceable and, while an experience is a mental phenomenon, it does not follow that that which is experienced is mental.

However, the analysis has to be carried further. This is done by the second formula which means that on closer inspection the subjective aspect, which has only meaning in relation to its ob-

[1] The significance of these two formulas is given in Dchkh 4*a* and Dc 13*b* sq.

jective reference, is meaningless because in postulating mentalism the subject has been turned into an object. By transcending the subjective and the objective instead of reducing the one to the other, we arrive at an act of becoming aware which is neither subjective nor objective, but an act of being aware in itself and brilliantly perspicuous in itself. This is the meaning of 'nothingness (*śūnyatā*) transcending awareness (*jñāna*) and indestructibility (*vajra*)' and the conviction that sensa are delusive.[1]

This whole procedure, however, is not merely an intellectual method; on the contrary, the intellectual formulation is the outcome of an immediate experience. Therefore, the moment the experience is referred to, another set of symbols is used. The experience beyond subject and object is pointed out by the word *nāda* which, because of its symbolic character, is not translated into Tibetan. Although the literal meaning is 'sound', to experience it is as if our whole being were vibrating in what can only be expressed, though inadequately, as a condition in which there is nothing but this nothingness, transcending awareness and indestructibility.[2] It is the experience of nothingness that becomes the foundation for union with the Guru, who is the embodiment of unique Buddhahood. Thus when all the external reference has subsided and one has reached a state of pure awareness one must become aware of oneself as rDo-rje rnal-'byor-ma, who in form resembles the spouse of rDo-rje-'chaṅ, but has a few other attributes and takes a different posture. Directly over the crown of her head one has to imagine one's own Guru in the shape of rDo-rje-'chaṅ, sitting on a richly adorned throne, and above him, one above the other, the line of Gurus who represent the tradition of the particular school; in the case of the bKa'-brgyud-pa there are now quite a number of them. Thus the purpose is through an identity with the discriminating, and at the same time inspiring, function to reach beyond oneself to the ultimately real which has been present in each Guru in a different way, so as to fulfil the different needs of every aspirant. Here again the conclusion is an experience of light in which all the manifested forms fuse.

This whole practice is a process of spiritual transformation. It

[1] See note D, p. 267 and note 2, p. 41. [2] Kylg 2*b*.

frees man from his limitations and awakens in him the awareness of his kinship with God, as the mystics would say, or to put it more prosaically, he learns to see himself in a different context, from higher dimensions which are not like those of current physics. He becomes aware of himself in terms of patterns or norms which cannot be defined quantitatively. Such patterns are those of *sku*, *gsuṅ*, *thugs* and *ye-śes*, words which are currently translated by Body, Speech, Mind (Spirit), and Knowledge, but have nothing to do with what we ordinarily understand by these terms. The fact is that our everyday language is not suited for translating experiences on higher levels, because it is geared to the three-dimensional level. As Noel Jaquin remarks: 'In many cases repeated attempts to explain certain symbols in three-dimensional terms have merely succeeded in creating an entirely false concept, and one that often has no relation to the actual meaning of the symbolic representation.'[1]

The transformation process, which is at the same time an ascent to higher levels and into greater spheres, needs confirmation by a competent Guru, who ultimately is reality itself. Although there are four confirmations this process is not to be understood numerically.

All that has been said so far is merely the preliminary to becoming able to practise the various stages in the total pattern of transformation, and thus is termed the way to maturity. The Developing Stage, the Fulfilment Stage, and the ultimate coincidence of the two, is the actual way of liberation. Liberation is a way of existing rather than a goal to be achieved.

The Developing Stage is essentially a means to experience oneself as a god, not in the sense of a superhuman being to be worshipped as having power over nature and human fortunes, but rather in that of an apparition having a luminosity of its own. sGam-po-pa explains the term 'Developing Stage' to signify configuration, transfiguration, and symbolization.[2] By the first term he understands that the shape of the god is a manifestation of an all-encompassing spirituality and as such as intangible as an apparition or a rainbow. By the second term he stresses the lumi-

[1] Noel Jaquin, *The Theory of Metaphysical Influence*, p. 29.
[2] sGam-po-pa, viii. 8*a* sq.

nous character of the divine shape after the preoccupation with oneself, as consisting of flesh and blood, has disappeared. And by the last term he refers to the awareness that although the divine figure is as real as any other apparition it does not stand for a thing but is merely a name, a symbol, a cipher or convention, and nothing in itself.[1] Padma dkar-po, on the other hand, defines 'Developing Stage' as a process-product word: ' "Developing" means the creation of a god in the same way as other sentient beings are born; "Stage" means to practise the creation of a god by gradually purifying and perfecting this procedure. Or, that which has been created is a god, and the stage is his entourage. Or, "Developing" is the actuality of the resident and his residence (i.e. the god and his palace) and "Stage" is the means to perceive it intuitively in one's own being-this-or-that. Therefore one speaks of a Developing Stage or a *maṇḍala*, because *maṇḍa* means essence and *la* to accept it.'[2]

This practice which comprises the three phases of any experience or process, its origination, its presence, and its fading away, commonly called birth, intermediate stage, and death, where intermediate stage admits of different interpretations according to the point from which it is viewed, is essentially a means for liberating man from his limitations and attuning him to something on a cosmic scale. Therefore it is said that 'there must be attunement of body-mind to the birth of a god in order to overcome the impurity of holding it in low esteem; for birth is the manifestation of a certain pattern or existential norm; there must be attunement of appearance (one's being-this-or-that) to the dream images in order to remove the impurity of believing it to be something solid; being-this-or-that is the manifestation of a mode of communication; and there must be attunement of sleep (i.e. the passing away from conscious wakefulness) to the primordial radiant light (as the source and nature of all life) in order to remove fear due to wrong ideas about death which is the manifestation of ultimateness (i.e. existing as an end fulfilled).'[3]

According to ancient belief there are four forms of birth: from a womb, an egg, the combination of heat and moisture, and a

[1] sGam-po-pa, viii. 8*a* sq.
[2] Sphžg 75*b*.
[3] Dchb 8*a*; Tsk 9*a*.

spontaneous one. Each form represents a specific method.[1] The most elaborate one is that of womb-birth; a medium one is the egg-birth which has been developed in particular by Nāropa and Maitripa. It has two types. In that of the bird the god himself is first produced and later his palace, similar to a bird which develops its feathers at a later stage, living, so to speak, within them. The other is the tortoise type, because here the god and his palace are created simultaneously, similar to a tortoise which has its shell the moment it leaves the egg.[2] A concise form, which is applied in other contexts also, is called the 'three-phase procedure'. This indicates the three stages of the ground, the seed resting on it, and its transformation into the final shape of the deity. The ground is an eight-petalled lotus on which is a certain letter standing on the disk of the moon. This is the seed which then becomes the deity one wishes to meditate upon and fuse with.

In the heat-moisture form of birth the lotus flower which has opened by the rays of the sun symbolizes heat, while the seed, a symbol for the noetic capacity in its intermediate state on the disk of the moon, symbolizes moisture.[3]

The most concise practice is a spontaneous visualization and experience without the use of mantric syllables which play an important part in the previously mentioned practices.

Although these syllables occur over and over again in the Developing Stage they are not the main feature, and any preoccupation with them defeats its own purpose. The decisive point is the awareness that has to be brought to utmost clarity. As a possibility it is already present in the process of the Developing Stage and its dawning is the assurance that this procedure has been successfully performed. The awareness itself is the Fulfilment Stage. The transition from the one stage to the other is as if the emphasis has been shifted from the objective to the subjective pole. But in this shifting another level and sphere are revealed. While the Developing Stage may be said to be oriented in ordinary space and time with the percipient as a fixed point of reference, the Fulfilment Stage with its cognitive and emotional components belongs to a four-dimensional field of space-time, to which as a fifth dimension the relation

[1] Dchkh 3*a*. [2] Dchžr 3*b*; Sphžg 78*b*. [3] Sphžg 75*b*.

of identity is added. This relation means that it is possible to know an *object* as it really is in itself, and not a mere semblance or an idea of it, and simply to *know*, not merely to respond to, the object or to undergo its influence. Thus the formal identity between the knower and the known, as referred to by logicians, is an experiential fact.

This attunement to some wider aspect of reality and this widening of the perceptive range entails certain modes of behaviour. The text lists seven of them. As is to be expected, food and drink are mentioned first, but it is important to note that no dietary restrictions are implied. To interpret the co-existent behaviour in such a way is to fall a victim to a three-dimensional distortion of a higher-dimensional experience, a 'misplaced concreteness'. The astute adept will enjoy food and drink out of a reality sphere which is not limited by an external reference, and without preconceived ideas, while the mediocre one will enjoy it as in a dream, and the lowest type as if making an offering to his tutelary deity.[1] The same experiential character attaches to the other modes of behaviour. In every case the contact with the divine has to be preserved.

2. ONE-VALUENESS

The instruction in one-valueness sums up the nature and purpose of all that has been practised before. It will be recalled that the practices referred to by the terms 'Developing Stage' and 'Fulfilment Stage' do not imply a preoccupation with the contents or objects of consciousness, although at the beginning consciousness appears to be connected with them. Nor is there any intention to build them into a conceptual system. To conceive of oneself as a god or a goddess is not to perceive oneself in space and time as something to which the term god as an object is appropriate, but to become aware of a wider context and of greater spheres which easily disregard the limitations of space and time. Contrary to our habitual way of objectifying thought which necessitates an ever increasing expansion of thought forms, the purpose of these practices is to arrive at a state of pure lucidity, luminosity, and radiancy in which the continuing phenomena may be present only

[1] Dchb 29*b* sq.

as empty forms, undistorted by any concepts. The emphasis thus seems to lie on the subject. However, this term is not primarily identical with the psycho-physical subject which is only the starting point and field of action reaching beyond itself. It refers to a reality which is there before there is any subject which later may face an object and thereby become that which we usually understand by 'subject'. In other words, the above practices aim at a complete de-objectification, including the subject which in Western thought 'tries to arrive at self-comprehension through objectifying conceptual thought'[1] and at immediately experiencing structured processes which at every moment in life reveal the potential source of new development which is equal to becoming aware of 'a unity of process seen in all particular forms and reconciling their differences.[2] This de-objectification is marked by an ever increasing lucidity and transparency which is both a progress of knowledge and an intensification of realization, in so far as realization means that the Real stands out more and more clearly and that one becomes more and more one with the Real, which, it is important to note, is never an objective Absolute. This process of realizing is summed up in the term 'attunement' which also includes the goal, a state of being tuned-in. It is thus, as are so many other terms in Buddhist philosophical thought, a process-product word. This is evident from its definition: 'Attunement is (i) to experience through the instruction in one-valueness that the many has but one value and (ii) to fortify this experience in a state of humility.'[3]

The reader must be warned against a possible misunderstanding. Attunement to that which precedes any subject and object might be thought of as a sort of submission, particularly as we are dealing not merely with abstract philosophical thought, but rather with that which affects the whole human life. Where this happens in the West we usually borrow from religion: 'Thy will be done'. This sort of submission is certainly not implied here, because such submission retains the separation of the individual subject from that which for want of a better term we may call the Subject (with a capital

[1] William S. Haas, op. cit., p. 181.
[2] Lancelot Law Whyte, *Accent on Form*, p. 191.
[3] Dchb 33*b*.

letter). Separation is the embarrassing character of the *unio mystica* in Western mysticism. As William S. Haas points out: 'When the Western structure seems to approach the state of pure consciousness there will always arise an irresistible temptation to experience this state as a possession. The subject would want to emerge from behind the state to assure itself of its attainment. This constellation is bound to return even in ecstatic states of the great Christian mystics. For whatever be their experience of God, in the act of supreme knowledge either they possess God or God possesses them.'[1] Possession is assuredly not attunement.

While attunement is of tremendous importance it is only one side of the picture. So one can even say that it is of no value unless something is done with it. Attunement must find its expression in conduct which, as the text clearly shows, is the second aspect of this instruction. One-valueness becomes thus a general term which does not imply anything static. One-valueness is a goal-ward process and a goal-inspired action. The reference to sense activities also shows that the information we receive through them functions not merely for the sake of pure awareness or barren contemplation, though that may often be its by-product, but in order that we may act.

Attunement may be described from various points of view. It may refer (i) to the process of experiencing, (ii) to the feeling-tone therein, and (iii) to structural patterns or existential norms.

(i) The first aspect is related to the four 'confirmations', each of which serves a different purpose, although all of them are interrelated. The purpose of the first confirmation is realization of the lucidity and transparency[2] that are inherent in one's awareness of oneself as a god or goddess during the Developing Stage. This is known as the 'jar-confirmation' whereby the purification of the 'body'-pattern is symbolized. It has to be remembered that in Tantric Buddhism 'body' does not mean the body as an object, as seen by the biologist, but the body as lived in by the subject; it is a shorthand expression for body-mind, a live structure. Just as the physical body may be cleansed by water so the psycho-organism—to use a Coghillian term—becomes 'pure' and transparent in the

[1] Op. cit., p. 188. [2] Dchb 33*b*.

god-experience. In this lucidity, objectness which is a *con*-struct of mind has been *de*-structed and, paradoxically speaking, in this destruction a more live and vivid pattern or structure is revealed,[1] which, as Lancelot Law Whyte remarks: 'has inherent developmental and explosive tendencies, attraction, and repulsion, and unpredictable possibilities.'[2]

The moment this lucidity has burst forth, the colour and the various characterizing marks of the god or goddess are seen and felt to be empty of any tangible content,[3] as a mere actuality. Again it seems paradoxical that to come to grips with that which is nothing by all ordinary standards is the nature of the 'mystery-confirmation'. This process is one of *de*-verbalization, a word always being tied up with a concrete content or object. When, however, another level and pattern is revealed, its freedom from restricting concepts and deadening words guarantees a wider field of action, expressiveness, and communication.

The process initiated by de-objectification passes through deverbalization into a feeling of appreciation in which lucidity and nothingness are experienced as indivisible. Since this feeling is not limited and differentiated, because there is nothing that can excite traces which cause specific modifications in the "mass" of feeling,[4] this appreciation and feeling is one of 'eternal delight', as the mystic Blake would say. It is associated with the level of mentation, which is not conscious thought but the matrix of all conscious emotive experience. What we call a conscious emotive experience is, according to Buddhist Tantrism, the loss of lucidity, nothingness, and 'eternal delight'; it is something frozen into opaqueness, concreteness, and a transient feeling of pleasure or pain. To come to the primordial point or state of eternal delight is the purpose of the third confirmation which is called 'transcending awareness through discrimination-appreciation'. Here discrimination has a particularly strong flavour of appreciative understanding; it is related to the Karmamudrā, the female partner, standing for the motor act as exemplified in sexual intercourse, and transcending awareness

[1] Sphžg 70*a*.
[2] Op. cit., p. 27.
[3] Dchb 34*a*.
[4] C. D. Broad, *The Mind and Its Place in Nature*, p. 216.

relates to the increasing feeling of delight or the emotive component of the motor act.[1]

The various phases in this process of experience are partial patterns of local activity, although the nature of localization is radically different from that of what biologists call the 'analytic apparatus'.[2] It is therefore a futile endeavour to identify the 'loci' of the experience phases with sections of the nervous system. To do so is, moreover, to relapse into objectifying thought which is to be overcome by the above practices. It is, however, most important to note that over and against these partial patterns there is integration, or the total pattern. These two kinds are primordial and essential components of every action system, be this an amoeba or a human being. Notwithstanding the differences between these two types, they are never dissociated in working. Integration becomes of primary importance because every partial pattern has the tendency to develop into a sort of independence, which produces a disturbance in the balanced relation of the parts to the whole and may be manifested as abnormal behaviour. Integration is the purpose of the fourth confirmation which consolidates the state of balance consisting of lucidity, nothingness, and eternal delight. This state is not produced by causal necessity, because here we are not concerned with a theoretical world conception in which causal necessity is the main principle of order, nor can it be terminated by any relations holding between different terms, because there is no 'term' which could modify this lucid nothingness and even feeling. Nor is this state a creator, an invention serving as the connecting link between the changeless and the ever changing.

In this way the Developing Stage, viewed as a whole, is an integrative, not an additive, process in which the various levels and patterns preserve their individuality and at the same time are related in such a way that they cohere in a unified whole. This is evident from the statement that 'by the practice of the Developing Stage the four confirmations are experienced as a unity: the lower limit is the "jar-confirmation", the upper one the fourth confirmation, and the "mystery" and "third" ones are the relating links'.[3] This

[1] Sphžg 69*a*.

[2] C. Judson Herrick, op. cit., p. 87.

[3] Dchb 34*a*.

unitary experience is referred to in the various Tantric texts[1] by the words 'knowing the one, becoming conversant with everything', which means that there is continuity from one step to the other, however abrupt the transition may appear.

While the 'confirmations' refer to the process of experience seen from without as it were, attunement to the freedom paths indicates the inner life of the process, so that one is tempted to speak of an experience in the act of being experienced. In European philosophy the problem of freedom, usually called freedom of the will, is a formidable one, so much more so since Kant convincingly demonstrated the theoretical impossibility of freedom in a world order governed by causal necessity, although he later smuggled freedom in as a postulate of practical reason. The problem of freedom is still obscure and unresolved. This is mainly because no one realized that the opposite of necessity is not freedom but contingency. William S. Haas rightly remarks: '. . . the opposite of causal necessity is not simply the absence of necessity which has been erroneously identified with an ill-defined idea of freedom, but contingency. And contingency is both a positive and tangible datum in thought no less than in experience. Freedom is the true opposite of compulsion by instinct. If there be anything which survives the elimination of instinct it must be freedom. But it is not the empty idea of freedom which Western philosophy opposes to necessity, a pseudo-freedom which must be saved by such formal terms as self-determination and the like.'[2] If freedom is to have any meaning it must prove its independent significance. This is done in Buddhist Tantrism where freedom is genuine, immediate, and lived, and is by no means a category of reason. In this respect there is a marked similarity with existentialist thought. As John Wild shows: 'Freedom is not to be approached as a kind of thing, or a kind of change, or even as a kind of possibility. It is a way of existing, . . .'[3] Just as we may speak of the existence of Mind before any content, so freedom exists before any concept about it and is identical with Mind. This has important consequences for the interpretation of the term 'freedom path' (*grol-lam*). It does not

[1] Dchb 34*a*; Tbkh 2*b*, &c.
[2] Op. cit., pp. 255 sq.
[3] Op. cit., pp. 116 sq.

mean a path to freedom, but freedom as the path of our actions. As such, freedom is basic to and interconnecting with the various 'freeing' phases. This is clear from the following explanation: 'The lucidity present in experiencing oneself as a god is the path of the Developing Stage. At and on this Stage attention should only be given to the radiant form. The emptiness of content (of this radiant form) is the path of the Fulfilment Stage. Here, too, there is nothing else to be attended to but the nothingness of anything tangible. The experience of eternal delight, of the non-duality of lucidity and nothingness, is the path of Coincidence (noetic identity). In this coincidence there is also nothing but the delight of non-duality. The fact that lucidity, nothingness, and eternal delight are indivisible, do not come and go, and are beyond determinate origination, annihilation, and an intermediate presence, is the path of Mahāmudrā. Here, too, there is nothing else but radiant light which neither comes nor goes, nor is present (like ordinary light). These four paths manifest themselves simultaneously through the practice of the Developing Stage in which they are traversed, the lower level being the Developing Stage, the upper being Mahāmudrā, while the Fulfilment and Coincidence Stages are the relating links. Thus by knowing the one one knows everything else.'[1]

Usually we tend to deal with an experience as an objective phenomenon, and in analysing it we can detect various phases which then, through the projection of language, appear to follow each other in a linear way. In so doing, however, we only too easily lose sight of the experiencing subject. The moment we include it we discover that it always finds itself in a situation. In ordinary life we, as experiencing subjects, solve a situation by interpreting it conceptually, only to find ourselves in another situation which equally demands a solution. While thus a solution turns out to be a construction, in this practice it is a de-struction, an unfreezing in which freedom asserts itself and takes the lead. And while we become fixed and committed to that which leads away from freedom in our attempt to solve a situation conceptually, here we have to commit ourselves to that which guarantees the continuity of freedom and is so to speak a situation that is solved by itself. In

[1] Dchb 34*a*.

this sense each confirmation is a partial commitment which converges in the final and unitary experience of lucidity, nothingness, and eternal delight, and thus becomes a long-range commitment which will have its repercussions in ordinary life.

Our usual preoccupation with the contents of consciousness rather than with consciousness itself, leads to the assumption that without contents consciousness must fade and fail and that we are left with nothing in the strictest sense of the word. Hence the assertion that de-objectification leads to the shining forth of a basic pattern or structure comes rather as a surprise. In addition we are confronted with another unsolved difficulty due to our dualistic mode of thinking which, since man himself is concerned, has created the body-mind problem in classical philosophy and psychology. Although modern psychology and medicine more and more abrogate the distinction between body and mind as two separate entities and realize that the establishment of an 'ideological reality' and a 'physical reality' 'explains nothing and closes the door to further scientific inquiry',[1] they are still a long way from the Tantric assertion that the body is neither the body nor the mind but body-mind as a surface phenomenon. Here it will be useful to introduce the idea of 'structure' which, according to Lancelot Law Whyte, 'is a name for the effective pattern of relationships in any situation'.[2] As human beings we observe ourselves moving, speaking, and thinking, and this triad of action, speech, and thought is a most effective pattern of relationships. Because of the overt character of act in this triadic pattern we speak of a 'body'-pattern. However, it cannot be repeated too often that 'body' (*lus*) always means the body as lived in by the subject and not the object studied by surgeons, so that the body-pattern becomes something like a life-pattern which we primarily view on the physical and material plane. But when 'physical' is not opposed to 'mental', and 'material' to 'formative', the usefulness of such terms as physical and material is exhausted and we had better avoid them. Similarly 'mental' is of little use and may become dangerous in so far as it might give rise to a theory of panpsychism and a subsequent inane idealism. Neither the one nor the other is guaranteed by any evidence. We have to do with formative processes

[1] Whyte, op. cit., p. 457. [2] Ibid., p. 27.

which become inadequately objectified into physical-material and mental-psychical part-conceptions. Another advantage of speaking merely of formative processes is that the problem of matter and form becomes meaningless, and thereby another philosophical stumbling-block of Aristotelian provenience has been removed.

The usefulness of the concept of 'structure' is demonstrated in still another way. Whyte observes that 'stable structures are end-states of processes and serve as records of them',[1] and 'stable structures dominate the picture, since the unstable disappear'.[1] The latter statement is borne out by the history of Western thought, which is littered with the corpses of abandoned conceptions, all of them at one time or another pretending to be objective and to cover reality as a whole. The fact that they had to be abandoned shows that they were unstable structures. The same holds good for life. Its ever-changing patterns reveal the presence of unstable structures. In the language of existentialist thinkers these unstable structures are man's unauthentic being-in-the-world, which is a constant threat to his real (authentic) existence. The aim of the various practices outlined in the instructions given to Nāropa is to arrive at stable structures or authentic being. Stability is achieved by shedding whatever there is of *con*-structions, by dismantling the maze of dead and deadening concepts, and by penetrating to a spaciousness that is pulsating with life. The first step is to experience one's being-in-the-world as a god or goddess in a mansion which has the character of a magic spell. It is the magic that is important, not the spell itself or its content.

All these features of a stable structure as the end-state of a process and the disappearance of unstable structures are recognizable in the statement that 'the attainment of stability where there is neither increase nor decrease in the lucidity of the empty form, through attending to the Developing Stage as a magic spell, is the result of the 'jar'-confirmation—Nirmāṇakāya'.[2]

When Whyte further states that 'the presence of a particular structure facilitates the formation of similar, complementary, or identical structures',[3] and that 'the properties of complex structures

[1] Whyte, p. 101.
[2] Dchb 35*a*. [3] Op. cit., p. 102.

often depend on the character of the structural pattern rather than on the individuality of the units that make up the pattern',[1] this again gives us a clue to an understanding of the following statements: 'Similarly the attainment of stability as to nothingness of tangible content is the result of the "mystery"-confirmation—Sambhogakāya (unlimited communication), and stability of eternal delight is the result of the "transcending awareness through discrimination-appreciation"-confirmation—Dharmakāya (the matrix of all conscious emotive experience). The radiant light which neither comes nor goes is the result of the fourth confirmation—Svābhāvikakāya (the integration of all structural patterns). And the fact that there is nothing but the stability of lucidity, nothingness, and eternal delight in experience and the transcendence of the Real beyond the passing phenomena of origination, annihilation, and intermediate presence gives rise to the total picture in which Svābhāvikakāya is the upper limit and Nirmāṇakāya the lower, while Sambhogakāya and Dharmakāya are the relating links.'[2]

(ii) The inherent emotive quality is referred to by 'four joys' or 'delights'. Whether they 'descend' or 'ascend' is primarily an index of their degrees of intensity. Each phase of the process of experience has a certain feeling-tone which more and more loses its distinct character of a particular feeling until it culminates in the feeling of eternal delight. More precisely, the term 'descending' means that with the *de*-struction of objectifying thought, with the dissolving of fixations, the basic feeling and sensitivity of life lived can assert itself and gradually spread through the whole organism, thereby gaining in intensity until it reaches its peak value. Although there are practices in which sex is not involved, the attribute 'descending' ultimately goes back to the experience of the orgasm which is gradually built up by a concentration of all sensitivity and feeling in the male organ, the lowest (not the vilest) focal point of experience in the human body. Various texts[3] have made a detailed

[1] Whyte, p. 102.
[2] Dchb 35*a*.
[3] Thus for instance *Caturmudrā-upadeśa*, 211*b* sqq. This text is not identical with the one in *Advayavajrasamgraha*, pp. 32 sq. The correct title of the latter is *Caturmudrā-niścaya*, and its author is Nāgārjuna, not Advayavajra.

study of the orgasm and distinguish between orgasm as the peak of sexual activity and the spasms and convulsions as the after-effect. Mr. Kinsey's[1] and his collaborators' findings confirm their statements. This distinction is important for understanding the meaning of 'ascending'. If one succeeds in preserving the peak value it will gradually 'ascend', that is, it will spread through the whole organism. The effect will be that one sees and feels oneself and one's environment transfigured. It is banal to talk of lovers seeing everything in a rosy light. But there is a certain truth in this saying.

The four delights of the goal attainment are an index of the transcendent delight of Buddhahood, every partial pattern preserving its own value and all of them fusing in a unitary experience.

(iii) The three structural patterns or existential norms are Dharmakāya, Sambhogakāya, and Nirmāṇakāya. Attunement to them at death means that we must try to realize a way of existing as an end fulfilled, which is Dharmakāya rising in all its splendour and light at the moment of death. Here death is not merely the physical stoppage we can observe from outside. It is an inner experience that may happen at any moment here and now. If this is not possible because of the presence of experientially initiated possibilities of experience, which prevent the complete attunement, then at least the attempt should be made to realize a more authentic way of communication, Sambhogakāya, and if this also is not possible, to remain with the Nirmāṇakāya or significant being-in-the-world. Any lapse into objectifying thought would result in our becoming fettered to various forms of life, some of which would stand in the way of attunement and the realization of the Real.[2]

Similarly sleep is to be linked up with these three norms. Usually we contrast sleep and dreams with the waking state and it needed psycho-analysis to make us aware of the close resemblance between the dream state and wakefulness. Sleep becomes a possible transition to the Dharmakāya and the other patterns, particularly through its special form of dream. The dream state is a particular topic of instruction and has been practically developed by Nāropa.[3]

[1] A. C. Kinsey and others, *Sexual Behaviour in the Human Female*, p. 627.

[2] A more detailed account is given in the discussion of the Intermediate State. See below 12, pp. 235 sqq.

[3] See below 6, pp. 183 sqq.

Attunement of the waking state to the three norms is linked up with the practice of the Developing Stage as discussed before.

Attunement of death to a way of existing as an end achieved, of the intermediate state to that of authentic communication, and of birth to authentic being-in-the-world, imply the same procedure but so to speak on a more cosmic level.

The fivefold attunement mentioned in the text needs special attention. It recurs under different names in other texts.[1] At first glance it seems that emotive factors have to be transformed. This is true, but this does not mean that we have here something similar to what is termed sublimation in psycho-analytic literature. Sublimation is a term for 'an unconscious process by which a sexual impulse, or its energy, is deflected, so as to express itself in some non-sexual, and socially acceptable, activity'.[2] This term suffers from a simultaneous overestimation and depreciation of sex—everything is sex and sex is sin—and in practical therapeutical use it is mostly an evasion. Moreover, there is no standard by which to gauge that which is 'socially acceptable', for what is 'acceptable' on one level is 'unacceptable' on another. But above all that which is 'socially acceptable' ignores the disposition and the requirements of the individual. Hence sublimation does not guarantee a 'form of relatively conflict-free behaviour',[3] because there is still far too much repression. The actual situation has been clearly estimated by Noel Jaquin: 'From my observation involving the examination and periodic check-up of hundreds of cases, I have no doubt at all that sexual repression has a disruptive effect at the physical level. And repression, in the sexual sense, may involve a deliberately supplied sublimation process, or it may be hidden by a process of evasion or disassociation: the individual is consciously aware of a sexual requirement, but will neither accept it nor bring it into its rightful perspective. He either refuses to think of it and it is pushed back into the darkness of the subconscious, or he tries to distract his attention from its existence by creating camouflage interests and requirements.'[4]

[1] For example Lzzl 24*b* sqq.

[2] James Drever, *A Dictionary of Psychology*, s.v.; in a slightly looser sense, J. C. Flügel, *Man, Morals and Society*, p. 289.

[3] J. C. Flügel, op. cit., p. 303.

[4] Op. cit., p. 167.

In all the practices that have been developed in Tantrism there is nothing which has the slightest resemblance to the creation of subterfuges. Over and over again it has been pointed out that the aim is a *de*-objectification and a release from bondage through genuine freedom. Man is continually creating systems that do not suit him and leave him disintegrated. He also has emotions which, if unharnessed, have the same effect. But life is a unity, and thought and emotion are not two separate things, however different they may appear in their final state. Therefore the practices of attunement begin with the emotional disposition rather than with the final frozen state. The fivefold division, therefore, implies the following.

(i) The disposition which is termed 'passion' can develop in different ways which yet seem to remain in the framework of what we call 'warmer' feelings. Because of this it can also be used in different ways. Generally speaking it develops into 'lust' for this or that and thus turns into a disturbing 'affect' in the sense that we are constantly affected by something else. Lust becomes a process of alienating us from ourselves and of plunging us into a greedy concern for others, all of which fails to give stability. It is different if 'passion' develops into love. Unfortunately the term love has been misused so often that it has become almost synonymous with lust. However, lust and love should be kept apart because the former is the very incapacity to love, even if for the moment it may make a show of 'warmth'. Love is a positive and enriching action lifting man above his pettiness and self-imposed restrictions. Following a valuable distinction made by Spinoza, Erich Fromm observes that 'love is an action, the practice of a human power, which can be practised only in freedom and never as the result of a compulsion. Love is an activity, not a passive effect; it is a "standing in", not a "falling for".'[1] Freedom, as we have seen, is basic to man but only when he has divested himself of his conceptual thought which is particularly harmful where the givenness of the instinctive forces of life are concerned. Love therefore coincides with pure awareness. This is not some abstract idea, but life throbbing in the warmth of a radiant light. Thus the attunement of 'passion' to the experience termed 'inner mystic heat' means a

[1] Erich Fromm, *The Art of Loving*, p. 22.

development of the capacity for love, which in the true sense of the word is felt to radiate warmth in every direction.

(ii) Just as 'passion' stands for attraction, amalgamation, and union, 'aversion' implies separation, loneliness, and anxiety. In most cases this disposition develops into a definite hostility towards and hatred of the object, thus deepening the gulf between subject and object. It is often said that hatred can only be overcome by love, but this statement becomes meaningless if we do not know what love really is and confuse it with some passing sentiment or with lust. Moreover, the essential requirement is not to overcome 'aversion' by something else, but to use it and turn it into a means of integration. The gulf between subject and object is bridged in the experience of what I have called the magic of a spell or a situation, distinguishing thus between the experience itself and its more or less irrelevant content. In the magic of the situation, subject and object (the god or goddess and his or her mansion in the Developing Stage) are not given as antagonistic to, but as together with, each other. There is thus no attempt to obliterate the one or the other, which produces only a sense of despair which in turn one tries to overcome by an intensified hostility, but the separateness of subject and object has turned into a juxtaposition which takes the sting out of 'aversion' and leaves it as the capacity to separate.

(iii) 'Bewilderment-errancy' is the maze of our thought which, precisely because it has come out of 'nothing' (though not in a *creatio ex nihilo*), can return into this nothing of which it partakes, by a process of de-objectification leading to the primordial radiant light. The attunement of bewilderment-errancy to this light is therefore different from what Greek philosophy calls the *noesis noeseos*, 'the thinking of thought', where thought has become its own object, an ideal which is of course never achieved. Attunement, however, can be achieved.

(iv) 'Haughtiness' is another way in which we express ourselves. Usually it becomes manifest in self-assertiveness which is a compensation for the inner feeling of insecurity. This insecurity is our unauthentic being-in-the-world, our belief that we are either this or that. However, when we return to ourselves by breaking through the façade we realize the exalted position we hold in our being identical with the Real. It is the Developing Stage with its god-experience as the formed expression of ultimate Buddhahood that dismantles our sham constructions and allows the primordial light to shine forth.

(v) Lastly, 'envy' has to be attuned to pure appearance. Envy in ordinary life stresses a coveting of that which belongs to another, be it possessions or attainments, or of that which has come to him, such as success or any other good fortune. Here again envy is tied up with a certain content. Pure appearance is without any concrete contents and envy attuned to it must necessarily lose its link with the object of its coveting. Since pure appearance cannot be said to belong either to me or to you exclusively, there is nothing to be coveted. All that is possible is that envy becomes the chagrin that others do not partake in what can never be an object of coveting.

If a person has succeeded in attuning the various emotive dispositions to that which is named pure awareness, primordial light, or which is referred to by any other index, this does not mean that he can no longer love, hate, and think as other ordinary beings or that he is 'self-less' and empty of any feeling. If he were all this he would be a monstrosity, not a sage. A man who is tuned-in is just as capable of love as of hate,[1] but these emotions are fed from a different dimension than those of ordinary life. We must never forget that attunement is only one phase and must find expression in conduct.

The teaching in attunement and conduct as the two aspects of one-valueness can be summed up in the words of William Ernest Hocking: '*Be what you are.* That is, be in action what you are in reality.'[2]

3. COMMITMENT

It has been shown previously that all practices aim at the realization of pure awareness in a process of de-objectification. Moreover it has been realized that the momentary contents of consciousness are impermanent and transitory and hence cannot provide a solid basis for action. To elevate something transitory into an immortal principle shows lack of wisdom. The consequence is that any line

[1] Phgdz 28*a*.

[2] Op. cit., p. 271.

of conduct based on the determinate and transitory character of things and principles built out of them must be erratic and doomed. It may be argued that commitment to selfish interests will be self-destructive in the end but that it is different with ideals. What is overlooked in such an argument is that all ideals, because of their determinate character, are impossible and hence must collapse. But is there no type of behaviour to which one must be true under all circumstances? There is, and as F. S. C. Northrop has shown, 'this constantly valid moral type of conduct has its basis in the indeterminate, all-embracing, undifferentiated aesthetic *continuum*, and the common bond of emotionally felt sympathy for all persons and all things which it provides, rather than laying down of one's life for a specific, determinately differentiated line of conduct. It is this which has given to Oriental religion a charity, an open-mindedness, a disinclination to force itself upon other people's attention, and a fellow-feeling not merely for all men but for all aesthetic natural objects of any kind whatever, which Western religion either in theory or in practice cannot claim for itself.'[1]

The text itself makes it quite clear that commitment must be to that which is left after the process of *de*-objectification has been completed. This implies that commitment is not an imposed duty but an outflow of the Real. In other words, commitment means to be true to what one is in reality oneself.

Several terms are introduced here. Some of them will be elucidated in the instructions to follow. Those which need special explanation are the terms 'Wish-Fulfilling Gem', 'Extent', 'Upper Gate', and 'Lower Gate', all of them characteristic of Buddhist Tantric philosophy.

'Wish-Fulfilling Gem' is not some objective entity but the name for an immediate situation and relation to reality. One distinguishes between an Ordinary Wish-Fulfilling Gem which is related to the Developing Stage in the experience of the 'jar-confirmation', and an Experientially Present Wish-Fulfilling Gem which refers to the subsequent experiences of the following confirmations and is related to the Fulfilment Stage or the union with the Real, and lastly a Wish-Fulfilling Gem of Commitment which applies to all

[1] Op. cit., p. 345.

confirmations and serves to keep the experiences alive and not to allow them to glide into objectifying thought about them.[1]

'Extent' is linked to the being-in-the-world and is a name for the peculiar experience of developing the divine in the Developing Stage which, starting from a small point, spreads to cosmic dimensions. Yet it would be a serious mistake to see in this something resembling the idea of man being a microcosm to be assimilated to or identified with a macrocosm. The fact of man's being-in-the-world and his transfiguration into a god or goddess in a mansion is not an objectively limited entity, but a formative developmental process that in its lucidity and nothingness cannot be determined in terms of ordinary size or by means of an equation.

'The Upper Gate' which is related to communication and hence to symbolic transformation (*mantra*) is the name for a purely meditational process in which the female element enters only as an idea. Communication is only possible between subjects, and the most intimate communication is the one between a man and a woman, which then serves as a symbol for inner experiences. Another name for it is 'instrumentality of one's own body-mind'.[2] The Six Liberation Practices here are detachment of the senses from their objects, musing, breath control, fixation of the meditation content, its inspection, and deep absorption.

'The Lower Gate' is an index of the experience of eternal delight by using sex as a means towards transcending awareness. It is related to the Karmamudrā which, as has been pointed out above,[3] is apart from being a real woman a symbol of the motor act and its inherent feeling-tone. Another name for this practice is 'the experience of discrimination-appreciation through the other's (the female's) body-mind'.[4] What is called in the text the 'mystic association with the Ḍāka' is termed in other works 'the messenger's path'. This is explained by Padma dkar-po in connexion with the Karmamudrā: 'Mudrā is *mu* "joy" and *ra* "receiving". That is to say, because one receives (experiences) the four joys in the acts of kissing and the other amorous acts, one speaks of Karmamudrā

[1] Tshk 3*b*.
[2] Sphžg 148*ab*; Sphyd 98*b*, 121*b*; Lzzl 37*a*.
[3] See note 1, p. 145.
[4] Sphžg 145*b*–161*b*; Sphyd 41*b*, 98*a*, 122*b*.

("Seal by Acts"). Because through her one reaches one's desired goal quickly, just as a messenger hurries to the castle, one speaks of her as "the messenger's path" or "the direct means"; and because this is concerned with psycho-somatic processes that are localized below (i.e. in the sex region) one also speaks of the path as "The Lower Gate".'[1]

It is refreshing to learn that in commitment as defined here there is no sense of guilt. Man is given his due dignity. He is not the chattel of some dark power which he will never understand, nor is he burdened with sin for which he after all cannot be held responsible. And so this instruction on commitment as being the natural expression of man's freedom comes as a valuable corrective of modern existentialist thought where guilt looms unresolvable.

4. THE MYSTIC HEAT

This instruction leads us into the middle of Buddhist Tantric practices and their underlying philosophy.

Since in the whole of Tantrism man is of immediate concern, it starts with giving us a sort of 'anatomy' of our being in a graded hierarchy. The difficulties we have in understanding this diagram of our existence are mainly due to our objectifying thought which tries to find correspondences between that which is essentially imaginable and that which is given by the various sciences about man. We further are accustomed to the body-mind duality and have developed certain hypotheses about their relation, such as interaction, parallelism, and others, all of which create almost insuperable difficulties. But Tantrism is not concerned with evolving hypotheses, it aims at realizations and therefore has to give man a tool which will serve this purpose. This means that we should aim at mental and bodily de-objectification. This, however, has nothing to do with a depreciation of the body. Our body as lived in by us is the most precious possession we have, as sGam-po-pa and others have been at pains to point out.[2] We must use it, not fight against it in some ill-conceived ascetism. Thus to point out the presence of our body-mind does not say anything about its reality

[1] Sphžg 91*a*.

[2] See my *Jewel Ornament of Liberation*, pp. 14 sq.

or unreality or whatever else it may be. This being-there of ours is a simple fact. Any attempt to read into it 'objective' findings repeatable at will in a laboratory, transcends this simple fact. What is presented here, however fantastic it may seem, is in the words of William S. Haas 'one of the most daring and ingenious conceptions of the human mind. This great adventure in consciousness is distinguished from all others in that consciousness deals with itself alone and with the sole aim of arriving at its own essence—pure consciousness. All other adventures, particularly those of the West, deal with qualified consciousness, be it religious, artistic, philosophical or scientific, and they achieve something concrete and determinable. Nevertheless, the fundamental assumption which underlies Yoga can certainly claim a higher degree of evidence than can the presuppositions of religion, philosophy, art or science of any denomination.'[1]

It will be easier for us to understand this when we bear in mind that the Buddhist Tantric conception of man's being starts from its thoroughly functional character. We act, speak, and think, and this is done mostly in an orderly way. And whether we like it or not, the most obvious content in consciousness is our body-mind. At the same time we see it change in growth and decay and as such it cannot serve as the starting-point for the development of what is most human in human beings—self-transcendence. To this purpose the stable pattern as outlined by the three structural pathways, a central one and two to the right and left of it, lends itself admirably. This pattern is both within man and beyond him, it guarantees his individuality and yet places him in a larger context: 'The three pathways point to the actuality of being-in-the-world, communication and situationality.'[2] It would be a serious mistake to assume that this means that man as a microcosm is the replica of the macrocosm. No such considerations enter into the picture, on the one hand because the relation is more intimate and on the other because such a determination would be an attempt at objectification.

A fuller account of the nature of this triadic pattern is given by Padma dkar-po who declares: 'The upper end of the central pathway goes up to the cranium and then turns forward into the space

[1] Op. cit., p. 228. [2] Ržd 151*a*.

between the eye-brows. Here nothingness enters and descends, which is of the nature of Akṣobhya. Other names for this end are Rāhu, Time and Pure Consciousness. Below the navel the central pathway proceeds straight to the perineum and at the sex region turns to the right. Here fertility ("semen") and awareness act, which are of the nature of Vajrasattva. Because at the time when the semen is emitted this lower end is in spasmodic movement it is also called "the all-jerky one", or as others say, since in a male it is filled with fluid which is whitish like the flower of jasmine or like the colour of a conch-shell, it is called "the one similar to a conch-shell". In women this lower end of the central pathway (i) looks like the tip of an elephant's trunk; (ii) is twisted like the turning of a triton shell, (iii) is closed by some soft mucus and (iv) opens and closes like a lotus flower. Hence it is called "of four types". Because at the time of the menstrual flow it must not be touched by a man it is similar to an untouchable woman and hence is called "untouchable woman" or "Ḍāka-face". It is filled with a red fluid.'[1]

This description plainly shows the contribution of the tactile sense to the formation of the image of our being. This is not by accident. Although this pattern will have to be visualized and incorporated mentally into the ordinary picture of our body, it is not meant to serve as a concept separating the subject from the object and giving rise to further objectifying concepts, as is the case with concepts evolved on the basis of the visual sense. It is the tactile sense that reaches deeply into the sphere of the instincts and their activities and creates the sense of togetherness rather than separateness. Sex drives in particular are associated with tactile sensations. It would be an easy task under these circumstances to identify certain characteristics of the pathways with physiological phenomena. But there are a number of other definitions which make us pause. First of all, what we consider the emission of semen or the secretion of mucus is termed *byaṅ-sems* (*bodhicitta*) which literally translated means 'enlightenment-mind'. The fact that a term can be used both in a mental-spiritual ('enlightenment') and physiological ('semen', 'mucus') sense shows that we move in a world which probably is neither physical nor mental, but may partake of

[1] Sphžg 28*b* sqq.

both (or be something completely different). Therefore we may render this ambiguous (if not obscure) term *byaṅ-sems* (*bodhicitta*) by the neutral word 'creativity', signifying in the physical sense what we understand by procreation and otherwise what we understand by 'a creative mind', which in its very creativity has transcended itself and thus is more of a translatory capacity, creating out of transcending awareness, which is beyond the ego and yet works through it into the three-dimensional realm of ordinary life. The unique moment of highest creativity and yet utter 'nothingness' is similar to the moment of orgasm where on the physical plane man becomes 'self-oblivious', which seems to be a sort of self-transcendence. However, I emphasize the word 'similar' in the previous sentence, because there is a subtle, if not a tremendous, difference. At the peak of orgasm (often inseparable from the emission of the semen and under favourable circumstances from fertilization), man succumbs to the objects of his own making. He does not free himself from them as is the case in the attainment of transcending awareness which coincides with what looks like orgasm on the physical plane.[1] This phase is symbolized by Vajrasattva.[2]

Transcending awareness is, as has been pointed out frequently, 'nothingness' and is present in our life as the nothingness of the noetic act, symbolized by the Buddha Akṣobhya, who thus is the mediating link between our consciousness with its tendency to objectify and pure transcendence which is lost in the procreative act as the end phase of objectification. Again this does not imply an evaluation of the sexual act. All that has been said so far goes to show that the central pathway cannot and must not be identified with the spinal cord or any other nerve trunk. This is once more emphasized by the reference to the four properties of this pathway. It is 'red like sealing-wax, lustrous like an oil lamp, straight like a plantain, and hollow like reed'.[3] Here the attribute 'hollow' must not mislead us into assuming that the central pathway is something like a tube.[4] 'Hollow like reed' is a metaphor for utter nothingness, because if we try to concretize it it will break in our hands. Lastly, sGam-po-pa

[1] Phgdz 57*a*; Sphyd 45*b*.
[2] See p. 134 for the symbolic meaning of this term.
[3] Sphkh 12*a*.
[4] Zmnd 38*b*.

is very clear on this point, that no identification with any part of the body is aimed at. He says: 'Within the body, which is hollow like an inflated bag, there is a central structural path with its upper end entering the mantra *Haṃ* in the cranium; but although its lower end is to be found in the sex region one has to imagine it four inches away from and not touching it. For it has been said that if one were to imagine it as touching the sex region lust would increase.'[1]

While the lower end of the central pathway relates man to his biological field of action which, as the texts make clear, is never 'nothing-but-sex' but permeated with awareness, the upper end connects him with cosmic spheres. Not only is Akṣobhya a symbol of consciousness through which man can reach beyond himself into the nothingness of pure transcendence, but the other names of the upper end equally point to the same. Thus Rāhu connects him with the stellar world, for Rāhu is a term of astrology and according to the Indian conception of it this factor has no existence of its own, is in other words 'nothing', yet is capable of bestowing its own effect and will deputize for other planets whose houses he occupies. Finally, as 'Time', it links man to time not in the sense of being a content in time but of being time. To understand what is meant by this it will help to refer to Martin Heidegger's penetrating analysis of time which John Wild sums up in the words: 'Time is an existential structure which pervades man's being-in-the-world. The human person is not a thing or a set of events *in* time. His being is stretched out into a future, past, and present which Heidegger calls the *ecstasies* of time. He is not something first confined to a given moment, and *then* stretched out into a past and future. From the very beginning, his being is stretched out into possibilities ahead of himself, and a past which he must take over if he is to be with things at a factual present. Thus in existing, he temporalizes himself in ways that are authentic or unauthentic. But in either case, the three *ecstasies* of time are integrated in the unity of his being. He is not *in* time, but he rather *is* it, and exists it.'[2]

From this central pathway two others branch off. Their salient features are: 'From the central pathway, under the dominance of temperature or the female creative power, there is a branch called

[1] sGam-po-pa, xiii. 6*a*; Ržd 151*a*. [2] Op. cit., pp. 206 sq.

"sun" or "the pale one" or *ro-ma* (*rasanā*). Along it passes warmth-temperature. It represents the object-polarity and is of the nature of Ratnasambhava. It divides into two, the one above the sex-region, the other below it. The one becomes the urinary tract and the pathway for motility (and the motor act), the other is related to the flow of blood. Both are of the nature of Amoghasiddhi. Under the dominance of the male stabilizing force, there is to the left of the central pathway one which is called "moon" or "aries" or *rkyaṅ-ma* (*lalanā*). On it operates cohesion. It represents the subject-polarity and is of the nature of Amitābha. Below, it also divides into two. The one is the conduct of faeces and solidification, the other that of the fertilizing power ("the white *bodhicitta*", *byaṅ-sems dkar-po*). Both are of the nature of Vairocana.'[1]

This description continues the picture of man's relatedness to the cosmos. Sun and moon are astrological terms; the sun as the richness of life and the gifts and objects it has to offer; the moon as the expression of the personality which as a subject co-ordinates the objects of his experience.

Just as the central pathway was a dynamic picture rather than a static model, so also these two branches are not static patterns, as the connexion with the materiality-producing forces and their end-forms might suggest. They, too, are intimately bound up with the second aspect of the total picture: motility. Thus it is said[2] that along the central pathway there passes awareness-motility, while along the *ro-ma* (*rasanā*) passes that which ends in the establishment of the object polarity, also called 'sun motility', and while along the *rkyaṅ-ma* (*lalanā*) there passes that which will end in the subject polarity or 'moon motility'. The object polarity consists of the five forces: solidification, cohesion, temperature, movement, and spaciality; the subject polarity of consciousness, motivation, feeling, sensation, and formative phases. While the two branches are also connected with vital functions on the biological level, it would be just as futile as in the case of the central pathway to hunt for correspondences in the picture which medical science has created.

[1] Sphžg 29*ab*. Essentially the same, though less detailed, is the account in sGam-po-pa, xvii. 2*b* and xxxi. 3*b*.

[2] Sphžg 39*a*.

There can be no doubt that this picture of our 'body' or rather of our psycho-organism is an admirable help to a mind which is concerned with realizations. It links man with the most sublime but at the same time does not fight shy of the natural functions of defecation, urination, and procreation. It does not shroud him in an ugly garb of sin, but reveals through the symbols of the various Buddhas man's affinity and ultimate identity with Buddhahood which he first comes to experience in the practice of the Developing Stage.

Alfred North Whitehead has remarked that 'human experience is an act of self-origination including the whole of nature, limited to the perspective of a focal region, located within the body . . .'.[1] These words are particularly applicable to the idea of focal points, among which the 'heart focal point' is of singular importance.[2] Here again it will be necessary to remember that the 'heart' is not to be equated with the physical organ; in fact the 'heart focal point' need not be localized in the heart but may be anywhere in the breast. However, the experience of increased palpitation in the events of anger, fear, pain, and above all of sex response, contributed to selecting the heart as one of the more, if not the most, important focal points of experience. In Tantrism the 'heart' becomes the combined symbol of man's triadic composition as manifest in overt behaviour, an acting, speaking, and thinking organism, and of the forces that contribute to the formation of the organism, but also of his orientation in a world of phenomena. The 'heart focal point' is conceived in the form of an eight-petalled lotus: 'To the East a petal called *Sum-skor-ma* (*traivṛttā*) and representing solidification (earth); to the South *'Dod-ma* (*Kāminī*), cohesion (water); to the West *Khyim-ma* (*gehā*), temperature (fire); and to the North *gTum-mo* (*caṇḍāli*), movement (wind). To the south-east, starting from *Sum-skor-ma*, form and shape; to the south-west, counting from *'Dod-ma*, fragrance; to the north-west, beginning from *Khyim-ma*, flavour; and to the north-east, starting from *gTum-mo*,

[1] A. N. Whitehead, *Modes of Thought*, p. 290.

[2] According to Ržd 152*b* the 'head' focal point represents bewilderment, the 'throat' focal point passion-lust, the 'heart' focal point aversion, the 'navel' focal point haughtiness, and the 'sex' focal point envy. Each of these focal points is characterized by a certain mantric syllable having a certain colour.

the tactile',[1] and 'in each of the eight petals there is present the triple set of situationality, communication, and being-in-the-world, the former derived from motility, the two others from the 'white' and 'red' materiality-producing forces respectively'.[2] Thus the heart focal point serves as an integrative pattern over and against the analytic patterns in a sort of interlocking directorate. In this way also the whole body forms a unity in spite of its division into twenty-four parts (8 × 3) which again may be divided into an almost infinite number, all of which indicate the sensitive nature of the whole organism and the importance of the tactile element.

In the course of this analysis of the pathways we have had occasion to refer to another important feature in the picture of man's being, that is, motility (*rluṅ*, *vāyu*), which is defined as 'that which makes everything move'.[3] It serves as the vehicle of the creative potentiality along the pathways. The basic meaning of the word *rluṅ* (*vāyu*) is 'wind', and as breath, perceptible only at low temperatures, this easily suggests its use as a symbol of that which mediates between the invisible and the visible. However, breathing is only one form of motility which we can observe or sense throughout the working of our body. Here, too, it would not be difficult to identify the various forms of motility described in the texts with what we call the circulatory, respiratory, digestive, eliminative, reproductive, endocrine, nervous, and muscular systems. The texts themselves assert that between this picture of man's being and that of medicine there is a certain similarity. But this is not so much a problem of anatomy as of function, and in this connexion it is interesting to note that the conative aspect of mind is stressed. Tantrism thus anticipates a trend in modern psychology.[4]

In the same way as the pathways pointed to motility, the latter refers beyond itself to creative potentiality to which reference has already been made by one of the names of the upper end of the central pathway, 'Pure Consciousness'. It is essential to note that *yid* (*manas*) always denotes mind before it has crystallized into consciousness in the sense in which we understand this latter term.

[1] Ssrdz 35*b* sq. [2] See Note I, pp. 277 sq. [3] Sphžg 38*a*.
[4] Ibid. 34*b* sq. G. F. Stout, *A Manual of Psychology*, pp. 212 sqq. W. H. Sheldon, *On the Nature of Mind*, pp. 197–207.

In relation to creative potentiality, motility is seen from two angles, awareness-motility which serves as the vehicle of the three reaction potentialities, and action-motility which is the carrier of the eighty reaction patterns. The distinction between the pathways motility and creative potentiality is, of course, not so strict as language seems to suggest. Actually all the three terms refer to one and the same process viewed from various angles. So also, what the text calls the 'common feature of psycho-organism and spirituality', and defines as the subtle identity and the reaction potentialities,[1] out of which in course of evolution conscious experience develops, is the unique character of sentient life which in its awareness moves along certain ways. The Tantric texts again seem to have anticipated what Judson C. Herrick says on the basis of psycho-biology: 'Overt behaviour is movement of some sort. Movement is primordial and mentation arises within it not to cause behaviour but to regulate it, direct it, and improve its efficiency. Conscious emotive experience reinforces the action system with additional driving power, and in proportion as intelligence guides the direction taken in its expression, the efficiency of the behaviour is improved. In both embryological and phylogenetic development, intrinsically activated motility precedes reaction to external stimulation. The body acts before it reacts. In embryo-genesis myogenic movement precedes neurogenic action. Muscles can act and react before they have any nervous connections.'[2] In the light of these findings the Tantric conception of an embryo's development, as intrinsically connected with motility in its various forms and movement along certain pathways, is less fantastic than the wording makes it appear.[3]

Judson C. Herrick makes another significant statement which may perhaps help to explain Tantric ideas. He says: 'Mind emerges from the non-mental, and it may in turn control not only the behaviour of the body but also its structural organization. It is recognized by everybody that disorder of bodily structure may disturb the mind. The converse is equally evident, as painfully illustrated by the prevalence of gastric ulcer associated with chronic anxiety or

[1] Sphžg 12*a* sq.; Ssrdz 34*b*.
[2] Op. cit., p. 312.
[3] See the description in Ssrdz 38*b*.

worry. Equally striking changes in the physical structure of bodily tissue and its chemical processes have been induced by hypnotic suggestion. The ulcers or hypnotically induced blisters are not caused by a non-physical entity called a mind but by a psycho-neural bodily process that is organically related with the other vital functions.'[1] In the Tantric texts that which is called 'creative potentiality' (*thig-le*) is certainly not a mind in our sense, which is the end-phase of a long evolutionary process. Neither is it physical, although it becomes observable only in the physical organization commonly called a body. It is a unitary principle that may be viewed either as structure or as motility or as the controlling and structuring process.[2] Conversely it is group-patterned by the carry-over of experience traces or as C. D. Broad more exactly calls them 'experientially initiated potentialities of experience.'[3] The same author cautiously advances a theory which is a corner-stone in Tantrism. He says: 'We must therefore consider seriously the possibility that each person's experiences initiate more or less permanent modifications of structure or process in something which is neither his mind nor his brain. There is no reason to suppose that this Substratum would be anything to which possessive adjectives, such as "mine" and "yours" and "his" could properly be applied, as they can be to minds and to animated bodies',[4] and 'as we know nothing about the intrinsic nature of the experientially initiated potentialities of experience, we cannot say anything definite about the intrinsic nature of the common Substratum of which we have assumed them to be modifications. As there is no reason whatever to think that such potentialities of experience are, or could be, themselves experiences, there is no reason whatever to suppose that the Substratum is a mind. On the other hand, it could hardly be any particular body. It does not seem impossible that it should be some kind of extended pervasive medium, capable of receiving and retaining modifications of local structure or internal motion.'[4] All this puts a new interpretation on the word 'creative'. In this context its meaning is not that of an

[1] Op. cit., p. 282.

[2] Sphkh 5*a*; Sphyd 51*a*, 56*a*.

[3] C. D. Broad, *Religion, Philosophy and Psychical Research*, p. 66.

[4] Ibid., p. 67.

act of construction, since it is neither wholly active nor wholly passive. It is rather best described as 'responsiveness'.

Just as the pathways linked man with something greater than himself, so also motility is not restricted to his limited existence but shares in a wider context. This is indicated by the reference to the vibratory rate in relation to the houses or signs of the zodiac, which operates in connexion with the motor activity of the body when the cusps are reached. In other words our conscious life, which has a strongly conative character, is constantly, though mostly imperceptibly, fed by what defies determination and only figuratively is expressed in terms of astrology, or hinted at by the highly technical term 'awareness-motility'.

The creative potentiality can be viewed from various angles, either with relation to the pathways and motility as the structuring and controlling process, or as the presence of something spiritual in man. The use of the words 'spiritual' and 'spirituality' does not imply any sort of so-called 'spiritualism'. I understand these words merely as working concepts, indexes. There is thus a close resemblance to the use of this word by Noel Jaquin who declares: 'I do not wish to use the word "spiritual" in this connexion in any religious or mystic sense, but rather as implying that part of man's being which is a directive counterpart of his physical being in terms of a higher-dimensional existence. This means that our approach to the continued examination of the physical structure and its activities must be made with a full awareness of these unexplored possibilities.'[1]

With reference to the physical side of man as detailed by the Tantric texts as pathways and motility, potential creativity is a principle that, genetically speaking, is the coalescence of the affinities of the male and female creative forces which have been symbolized by the colours white and red respectively.[2] This coalescence is the most subtle aspect, as the present text says, and crystallizes into its subtle or indestructible and indissolvable creative (responsive) principle, out of which in the course of evolutionary development the crude form of the ego results.[3] The coalescence

[1] Op. cit., p. 18.

[2] Ssrdz 39*a*. See also note 302.

[3] Sphžg 28*a*; Sphkh 5*a et passim*. According to Dnz 48*ab*: 'The most subtle

of the male and female energies is both an end and a beginning. It is an end in the sense that it is the possibility of the beginning of a new evolutionary process in the form of the growth of a child. It is a beginning in so far as the thus group-patterned principle, which the text defines as 'the primordial light modified by experientially initiated possibilities of experience',[1] proceeds as and by motility along the pathways that are evolved in the course of this unitary process, to the fully developed human being. Creative potentiality is thus a term for a process-product and product-process. What the Tantric texts describe in a highly technical language, Noel Jaquin analyses as follows: 'The point of conception makes the first major attunement of the individual with this particular episode in his evolutionary progression, and there occurs an automatic carry-over of the previously acquired affinities. This major attunement is quite an automatic process, the sexual approach of two people to each other sets in motion, or brings into being, a focal point. This we may regard as the crystallization of the two wave bands; they become fused in harmony or disharmony to a degree of exactitude that is beyond normal human comprehension. The exactitude of the composition of the focal point of fusion at that moment is perfection; that is, it holds the exact degrees of balance and variation contributed by the two people involved, in degrees of relative strengths that are complete and perfect within the period of its existence.'[2] The same author then continues: 'In its composition are focal points, which we can term "basic affinities", that are particular to itself alone, and which constitute the attraction or "call sign", for the inception of a third being. Thus the physical processes of fusion that occur on the cellular and chemical planes are the parallel physical processes that enable the "called in" entity to "take hold"— to gain control.

influences in the psycho-organism are the four types of nothingness and in particular motility which has become the vehicle of the primordial radiant light which is complete nothingness' and 'the most subtle in spirituality-mentality is spirituality which has become the actuality of the primordial radiant light which is complete nothingness. Although the most subtle, motility and spirituality, are different and yet forming one and the same actuality; they have never been apart, whether Buddhahood has been realized or not, and hence they are also known as "co-emergence" (*lhan-skyes*), "genuineness" (*gñug-ma*), or 'indestructible possibility" (*mi-śigs-pa'i thig-le*).'

[1] Sphžg 10*b*.

[2] Op. cit., pp. 37 sq.

Truly this is a matter of "like attracts like". It means that the "called in" entity is attracted by the similarity of affinities—it becomes an automatic attunement. The parents *A* and *B*, by their indulgence in sexual intercourse, create physical conditions that make it possible for the reproduction of the third being *C*, their child.'[1] However, since we have to do with truly metaphysical processes which reach into the physical, any numerical reference can only be taken figuratively. Similarly, 'parallel' must not be understood in the orthodox sense of psycho-physical parallelism. Otherwise the account tallies completely with the Buddhist Tantric conception of the inception of a new being, which in rudimentary form is already present in the canonical literature.[2]

While creative potentiality becomes observable in the physical as directive control, it has its mental-spiritual counterpart in the 'three reaction potentialities', which 'entering into conscious emotive and behaviour experiences produce Saṃsāra. This production, however, is not like that of a jar by a potter, which may persist even if there is no longer a potter, but like clay turning into a jar.'[3] This triad is the precursor of conscious emotive behaviour and derives its name from overt behaviour. Hence they are named by the misleading terms 'passion-lust', 'aversion-hatred', and 'bewilderment-errancy'—misleading because we associate with them concrete contents. These three potentialities are always together, although the one or the other may be in the ascendant over the others.[4] This makes for the variety of types which we in fact actually meet with in ordinary life, and we may boldly state that each man is predestined metaphysically, though not by an arbitrary outside force but by his own attunement. Since this is a matter of practical concern, through an attunement to and regrouping of the reaction potentialities it should become possible to alter the trend in one's destiny.[5] However, whether or not this can be achieved is unpredictable and can be demonstrated only by experience.

This triad has the character of light shining in every direction.[6] Yet there are degrees in it. The lowest is a mere soft light com-

[1] Sphžg 37 sq.
[2] *Majjhimanikāya*, i. 265 sq.
[3] Sphžg 10*b*.
[4] Ibid. 15*b*.
[5] See also Noel Jaquin, op. cit., p. 115.
[6] Sphžg 10*b*, 11*b* sq.; 38*b*, 200*a*.

pared with that of the moon in a clear autumn sky, and is associated with the prototype of aversion-hatred; the next is an intense light like that of the sun in a brilliant sky, and is associated with the prototype of passion-lust; and the third is a hidden glow which to all outward appearance is mere darkness, related to bewilderment-errancy.[1] This description is of course only an attempt to convey something of the experience of emptying consciousness of every content in a language intelligible to others who may attempt to arrive at the same goal. The process and experience of consciousness becoming empty and ever more translucent and radiant is further indicated by the various degrees of 'nothingness'. Thus the mere light which is sensed and felt, after the subject-object polarity has given way, is called 'nothingness', while the subsequent phases are called an 'intense nothingness', and 'great nothingness'. However, since every account we can give is bound to the subject-object polarity, so also consciousness, even as pure awareness, is referred to as somehow sharing this polarity, although the polarity does not exist in the ordinary form. Thus the symbols of sun and moon and of utter darkness do not mean that their light is the content of consciousness, but that consciousness is of such brilliancy as can best be illustrated by the light of sun and moon which shines everywhere. Similarly this external reference has its internal counterpart which is symbolized by smoke, a glow-worm, and a lamp in a container.[2] This last stage of what outwardly appears as utter darkness and inwardly as an intense self-reflecting light is a critical moment. From here it becomes possible to enter the primordial and ineffable light which is the complete emptying of every content or 'complete nothingness' and which outwardly is compared with the strange glow just before sun-rise where everything stands out clearly in its own light, as it were, and inwardly with a cloudless sky. If it should not be possible to enter into this experience yet the projective power of the experientially initiated potentialities of experience will begin to work and through various experiences will bring us back into the world of common events.[3]

[1] Barb 4*ab*; Bargd 11*b*; Sphžg 15*a* sq.; Sphkh 58*ab*; Spgyd 100*ab*.
[2] Sphžg 187*a* sq.
[3] Ibid. 187*b*.

The temptation is great to see in the reference to utter darkness just before the dawn of the primordial brilliant light something like that which Saint John of the Cross describes as 'the dark night of the soul'. There is in this experience in Tantrism nothing of the anxiety and agonies associated with the dark night. If some comparison with feeling may be allowed, there is here a feeling of contentment and self-sufficiency which is almost indistinguishable from a serenity and peace of mind that cannot be shaken and is referred to in the texts as eternal delight. After all, there is here no longer a subject or an object and thus there is nothing to communicate with. The difference between the two viewpoints (Tantric-Buddhist and Christian) is therefore tremendous. William S. Haas has admirably assessed this difference when he declares that the process of emptying consciousness 'does not involve the same devastating psychological effect as the destruction of everything objective would necessarily produce in the Western mind. For there, the radical elimination of the object would dry up the very life-stream of the subject. The philosophical idea of an Absolute or the scientific construction of an objective world are congenial to the Western mind. So likewise is any kind of relationship of the subject with these conceptions such as subordination, union, identification, or absorption, because any form of participation in the Absolute means objectivation which is to say reality. In the East on the contrary the subject discovers reality in theoretical and active withdrawal from every object, which in turn is to say, in the dismantling of all other data and in the corresponding discovery of an ever more real existence of itself as consciousness.'[1] Buddhist Tantrism even goes one step further in refusing to commit itself to any ontology. It does not accept the statement 'consciousness exists' as ultimate. In this respect Buddhist Tantrism endorses the words of Karl Jaspers: 'Ontology purports to be a doctrine of being itself as such and as a whole. In practice, however, it inevitably becomes a particular knowledge of something within being, not a knowledge of being itself.'[2]

The triad of the reaction potentialities cannot be called an

[1] Op. cit., pp. 232 sq.

[2] Karl Jaspers, *The Perennial Scope of Philosophy*, p. 143.

entity in the proper sense of the word. Being thoroughly dynamic and in a constant flux it is ultimately connected with motility and through it becomes split up into the eighty self-contained reaction patterns, of which thirty-three are related to the prototype of aversion-hatred, forty to passion-lust, and the remaining seven to bewilderment-errancy. 'Although the triad of pure consciousness is not an entity having a foundation somewhere it is endowed with light, and although motility has no definite shape it yet produces movement; these two (consciousness and motility) are fused like oil with oil and in the twinkling of an eye become a light that shines everywhere, out of which in a fraction of a moment the (eighty) reaction patterns evolve, the one or the other in ephemeral ascendence.'[1] This evolution involves a division into the subject-object polarity and inasmuch as the organism acts before it reacts these patterns determine the overt behaviour, which moves exclusively in the realm of the I and It, rather than in that of the I and Thou, and in this lifeless 'objectivity'—object as that which is opposed to the subject—becomes either good or evil.[2]

As so often, here too, a word of caution becomes necessary. The reaction patterns are pre-conscious and therefore seem to have a close resemblance to Carl Gustav Jung's archetypes. Jung's contribution to psychology is tremendous and he has done much in clarifying the working of the human psyche. But in his own words he recognizes the psyche as an 'object' of the natural sciences.[3] And it is only in this respect that the term *arche* can have any meaning. It denotes something like principle and above all beginning. That is, it names that from which something proceeds, and in Greek philosophy, with which C. G. Jung is well acquainted, this beginning is astonishment. As a matter of fact, the whole of Greek philosophy is supported and pervaded by astonishment,[4] but astonishment clearly separates man in his act of wondering from the object of his wonder.[5] Certainly the reaction patterns in Buddhist Tantrism have no direct connexion with astonishment or wonder. They are signs of a total situation in which the object

[1] Sphžg 11*a*. [2] Ibid. 11*b*.
[3] See the critique in Medard Boss, *The Analysis of Dreams*, pp. 52 sqq.
[4] Martin Heidegger, *What is Philosophy?*, p. 81.
[5] William S. Haas, op. cit., p. 123.

pole is not necessarily opposed to the subject, rather there is a togetherness; and so the reaction patterns are not objects of objectifying thought but the living medium of possible experiences.

This diagram of man's being is, in spite of its many schematizations, a living picture and thus fulfils its purpose in keeping man in the realm of experiences. And to the extent that it is efficient it is real. How to implement this picture in connexion with the breathing technique can be learned only through instruction by a competent Guru. Much of what has been said above in the text gives an idea of what happens within this practice. However, the experience of the various degrees of light are not the object of one's attention but the concomitant aspects of the properly performed practice.

5. APPARITION

This instruction is intimately connected with the experiences during the Developing and Fulfilment Stages which are a special setting in a larger programme.[1] It deals with experiential facts that in the Western world have hardly been touched upon or are scorned by the matter-of-fact disciplines. It is based on a particular technique which begins with the contemplation of a mirror image.[2] In the first instance this is the reflection of one's own person and the purpose is to transcend the belief in physical objects as the sole reality and to arrive at pure sensation. A mirror image is particularly suited for this because it presents a peculiar situation. C. D. Broad points out that 'in visual perception we have to consider an emitting region, a region of projection, a pervaded region, and a pervading shade of colour. The pervaded region is immediately determined by events in and near the region of projection. These events also determine immediately the pervading shade and colour. And they are themselves determined by microscopic events in the emitting region. In the cases that arise most often in everyday practical life the pervaded region and the emitting region roughly coincide. But, in the case of mirror-images and the visual situations which arise when we are surrounded by non-homogeneous media,

[1] sGam-po-pa, viii. 12*a*. Sphžg 164*a*. A further distinction between a 'pure' and 'impure' apparitional existence will be discussed in the Bar-do chapter.

[2] sGam-po-pa, xiii. 9*b*; xviii. 7*b*.

the pervaded region and the emitting region cease to coincide and may be very distant from each other. The pervaded region may then contain no physical events at all; and, if it does, they will be quite irrelevant',[1] and he continues: 'If I look at the reflection of a luminous point in a plane mirror the region which is pervaded from where I am standing is somewhere behind the mirror; it is the place where a luminous point would have to be put in order to present the actual appearance, if viewed directly and without a mirror, from where I am standing. And of course nothing physically relevant is happening at this place behind the mirror.'[2] Thus a mirror-image greatly undermines our belief in physical objects. The moment the reflection of oneself appears in the mirror it is critically appraised by exalting and blaming it until it neither attracts nor repulses one. After this, the image is contemplated as standing 'in between the mirror and oneself' which is a further marked loss in the external reference causing the belief in physical objects. And lastly the difference between oneself and the image is abolished in an act of pure sensation. In the same way the six remaining topics with which we are concerned in everyday life are dealt with and lose their hold over us. They are: gain and loss, fame and disgrace, and pleasure and pain.[3]

That which is indicated by the technical term *sgyu-lus* (*māyā-kāya*) and translated by 'apparition' is a special aspect in a wider context termed *sgyu-ma* (*māyā*).[4] The basic meaning of this word covers what we call 'illusion' and 'hallucination'. As this is one of the key-terms in Tantric philosophy—the practice outlined here is even called 'the axle-tree of the Path'[5]—and as it is likely to give rise to unwarranted conclusions, it is necessary to give a somewhat detailed analysis.

We have to distinguish clearly between an illusion and a hallucination, even if sometimes the two overlap. An illusion consists in jumping to wrong conclusions from given sense-data. For instance, if in the mountains I look at the ground and, sensing something, take it for a piece of silver, when it is but a brilliant

[1] C. D. Broad, *The Mind and Its Place in Nature*, pp. 168 sq.

[2] Ibid., p. 166.

[3] Sphžg 45*b*.

[4] sGam-po-pa, vi. 14*a*; xxix. 3*a*; xxxi. 22*b*.

[5] Sphžg 163*b*; Sphkh 45*a*.

piece of mica, that is a case of illusion. A peculiar feature of illusions is that the expectation that there might be some silver, because silver is usually found in mountains, caused the wrong perceptual act to be built upon a concrete foundation. This is clearly indicated by the observed fact that people do see pebbles and pieces of wood as persons and houses, or whatever they may have expected. In the same way ordinary people are said to see the world in the light of their expectations.

This word 'illusion' has had a most unfortunate influence on the presentation of Eastern thought, for it has generally been understood that the texts categorically asserted that the world is an illusion. In this way a perfectly sensible contention was twisted into a meaningless proposition and an alleged idealism was supposed to have grown up from this shaky basis. There is nothing illusory about the world as such. It becomes an illusion when I expect from it more than it can give. And since all my expectations are bound to come to naught if I fail to grasp the given, as it is given, I shall have to suffer in consequence. The expectation in such cases is indeed pure illusion. But the frustration of my expectations can hardly be said to entail the flat statement that the world itself is an illusion. The purpose of Buddhism, and of Tantrism in particular, is to teach man not to expect more than is possible, and to avoid creating the illusion of the illusion of the world. In one of his Vajragītis Nāropa puts it as follows:

> These drunkards who are caught
> By the demon of their habit-making thoughts
> See gold in stones and trees—
> But they are neither gold nor gems.
> Following this demon of their thoughts
> They are fettered.
> Try then to conquer it
> By compassion and awareness that discriminates.[1]

A hallucination, on the other hand, does not imply a perceptual error. The sense-data are actually there, although the physical sense-organs had nothing to do with their production. Such, for instance, are the pink elephants the drunkard is alleged to see;

[1] *bsTan-'gyur* (Derge ed.), *rgyud*, vol. ži, fol. 152*b*.

while they may be attributed to the presence of poisonous materials in his blood, such as alcohol, the fact that there are genuine hallucinations, as for instance in cases of apparitions, makes this explanation rather inadequate. G. N. M. Tyrrell offers a much better interpretation. He says: 'An apparition lacks physical, causal properties and cannot affect the physical organs of perception. Yet sense-data, exactly similar to those which occur in normal perception, arise; and not bare sense-data only—complete acts of visual, auditory, and tactual *perceptions* are built on the basis of these sense-data. Perception, then, clearly need not be dependent on the operation of the physical sense-organs or any physical processes whatever in the external world. "Hallucinations", which reach the standard of normal percepts in principle, even if they are to some extent imperfect on any given occasion, can be originated by *psychological* factors in the personality. This is an important discovery.'[1] The consequence is that the whole process of sense-perception has to be revised; it can, as Tyrrell further points out, be 'thrown into operation in two distinct ways, (*a*) from "below" (by normal, physical means), and (*b*) from "above" (in response to a controlling idea)'.[2] In this case the physical processes, assumed to play a decisive role, would be reduced to guiding and conditioning rather than to causative forces. In view of the Tantric conception of the structure of the human being this theory becomes very tempting. It will be remembered that the structural pathways, which superficially have a physical correspondence, are in no way causative.

The hallucinatory character of that which is termed *sgyu-ma* (*māyā*) is easily recognized in the case of Śrāvakas, Pratyekabuddhas, and Bodhisattvas, who see the world where there is actually nothing, but who unlike ordinary people avoid jumping at wrong conclusions. In the example of the magician and his onlookers there is more of a partial hallucination. The audience is expecting to see something, and the magician is suggesting the idea of men and houses and other desirable things. There seems thus to be a joint working of illusion and telepathic hallucination.

The idea that the whole world is some extraordinary large-scale

[1] G. N. M. Tyrrell, *Apparitions*, p. 92. [2] Ibid., p. 93.

hallucination, turning hallucinatory even the physical which we consider the unique criterion for distinguishing between veridical and delusive perceptual situations, seems to be fantastic. But may this apparent fantastry not be due to our bias towards taking the physical for granted, and to our inability to perceive that in assigning reality solely to the physical we not only elevate a mere belief into an infallible principle, but also fail to appreciate a very important and significant aspect of reality as a whole? The problem may be approached from yet another angle. Might it not be possible to look at the hallucinatory character of the world and the apparitional one of its inhabitants as equally exceptional to something which cannot be characterized, as it is to our customary physical setting? The text is clearly in favour of this viewpoint, as is evident from its reference to the Buddha-level on which there are neither hallucinations nor illusions. In this context a hallucination is no longer something abnormal or paranormal but a unique means of approach to Reality (not as an Absolute, of course) from which we have allowed ourselves to become isolated into some partial reality, and thereby have fallen into the error against which Bernard Bosanquet warned us—namely, that of taking something for more than it is.

Another point to note is that the hallucinatory character of the world is not necessarily to be thought of as the work of some demiurge. It need not be 'thoughts in the mind of God', to use a Berkeleian expression. Rather is this hallucination due to a reciprocity; it is a drama constructed by all beings in collaboration.[1]

The idea that the human personality in this drama is a graded hierarchy is also met with in this context and is of great importance. At the lowest level we have the physical aspect of body-mind, being the end-phase of a structuring process which, however, does not exhaust itself in its product. Rather it remains as an ever-present potentiality which from the low-level viewpoint looks like motility and mentality. They are one, not two, but even the one is not to be taken numerically. To a certain extent this potential

[1] *Abhidharmakośa*, iv. 1, declares that the world is the product of the Karma of all sentient being. Collectiveness is also recognized by G. N. M. Tyrrell, op. cit., p. 109, and elsewhere.

factor corresponds to what in philosophical language is called the existential self. This, however, is not an immutable entity but is something group-patterned by the traces of former experiences and out of this 'dress' controls and makes possible new experiences. In this respect it is different from the pure mentality-motility potentiality inasmuch as it is already an activated potentiality, cast into the familiar patterns of emotively toned bodily act, speech, and thought, which are filled with a definite content on the lowest physical level. Thus are three strata:

(*a*) pure potentiality, mere motility-mentality, or the real personality;

(*b*) a post-potential but pre-physical ens, which is 'the three reaction potentialities having taken on the character of the patterns of possible bodily act, speech, and thought; being a psychological ens or the very subtle personality;'[1] and

(*c*) the lowest or physical self which is the ego, the outcome of a primary, though ephemeral, structuring process.

It is the pure potentiality of motility-mentality that is the foundation of the apparitional personality. Although it has certain features which are characteristic of apparitions, being luminous and intangible in a physical sense,[2] it cannot be exactly equated with them. Apparitions as they are known to us are, so to speak, too personal; the apparitional being is non-personal because it is the expression of formulation of the total subject. Subject here, of course, has nothing to do with what we normally label 'merely subjective'.

The technique of producing an apparition and the apparitional character of the environment is related to breath-control, which proceeds from a more marked form to a more and more subtle; one symbolized by three mantric syllables: *oṃ* for what on a coarse level would be inhaling, *hūṃ* for retaining and *āḥ* for exhaling.[3] These symbols are not contents of breathing. They imply that the external reference and its association with words subsides more and more. The respiratory changes indicated here are very similar to those which Trigant Burrow describes on the basis of

[1] Sphžg 15*ab*.
[2] See also G. N. M. Tyrrell, op. cit., pp. 77 sq.
[3] Sphžg 96*b*.

his and his associates' experiments in 'cotention' and 'ditention'. According to Burrow, 'ditention' is a 'term used to indicate the intrusion of affect-elements or bias in ordinary attention'.[1] In particular it involves what he calls the '"I"-persona' or 'the artificial system of prefabricated affects and prejudices that underlies man's present level of "normal" feeling and thinking.'[2] 'Cotention', on the other hand, is 'the neurodynamic relation of organism to environment as it exists natively and undifferentiated within the cerebro-sympathetic system. Cotention represents the balance of internal tension and stress that primarily relates the organism kinesthetically to the outer world. It is the phylo-organism's basic tensional constellation or its total matrix of sensation in its relation to the environment. This tensional mode represents the non-differentiated pattern of motivation that mediates primarily between man's organisms and the external world.'[3] This total pattern is marked by the exclusion of mental images and is itself not a verbal process.[4] This is precisely what the Tantric texts declare.

The experiments by Trigant Burrow are of particular interest as regards the respiratory phenomena. Thus there is 'a marked and consistent slowing of the respiratory rate in cotention as compared with ditention, the decrease in rate in cotention being accompanied by an increase in the thoracic and abdominal amplitude of the respiratory movements.'[5] This is easily recognizable in the texts which insist that breathing becomes more even and that movement ceases in the abdominal region.

Another interesting feature of T. Burrow's experiments is that there is 'a reduction in number of eye-movements in cotention. This reduction during cotention occurs not only when the eyes are closed, or when they are directed straight ahead and no specific task or stimulation is imposed, but also under a wide variety of stimulus conditions.'[5] This suggests the fixed glance of Tilopa and other yogis, a characteristic that is mentioned in all Tantric texts. Steadying the eyes is one of the foremost prerequisites.[6] It

[1] Op. cit., p. 527. [2] Ibid., p. 291. [3] Ibid., p. 347.
[4] Ibid., pp. 93 sq. [5] Ibid., p. 395.
[6] Ibid., p. 372.

is a well-known fact that respiratory difficulties and restless eye-movements are closely associated with the emotively toned thinking and feeling of men, be they 'normal' or neurotic—such a classification being only statistical, not intrinsic. Hence it is no wonder that primary attention should be directed to breathing and eye-movements. Other phenomena in cotention which are of tremendous importance, but of no immediate concern in this context, are listed by Burrow.[1]

Breathing and eye-movements are physiological, but tell us nothing about the psychology and experience cotention. In the text these are indicated by the two types of meditation. The one, 'dissolution', is described as the visionary experience of a pure Buddha-pattern that has arisen from motility-mentality. It is the realization of a value which demands expression and so transforms itself into the white form of the spiritual Buddha Akṣobhya, in whose heart the letter *hūṃ* radiates in a pure white light that gradually dissolves every formed aspect in its own brilliancy and finally disappears itself. This process is likened to the gradual melting of a snow-flake until only a drop of water remains. The second meditative experience, 'evaporation', is the emanation of light from the same letter *hūṃ*, dissolving the whole world and the beings therein in its brilliancy, a process that is likened to the fading of breath on a mirror.[2]

While this description refers to the content of consciousness, though there is hardly any content worth this name, the accompanying feeling-tone is indicated by the reference to experience-feeling-patterns, of which some are unmistakably related to sex. This is due to the fact that in Tantrism sex is a recognized means and it is therefore possible to refer to the spiritual in terms of the sexual and vice versa. Tantric practices involve the whole man, not some partial aspect of him that on the basis of one prejudice or another is deemed to be of a 'nobler' kind.

The purpose of this practice is to achieve a change in one's attitude towards oneself and towards one's environment at large. It is the attainment of the awareness of the unitary character of all our experiences. Coincidence is not mere juxtaposition of what

[1] Ibid., pp. 487–523.
[2] See notes 2 and 3 pp. 64 sqq.

is usually termed an ultimate truth and a relative one, but their essential identity. Unfortunately, identity is an ambiguous and misleading word. Here it does not mean the sort of identity that the idealist logicians speak of when they declare that any relation between two distinct entities necessarily involves a higher unity or identity in difference. Coincidence as the cognitive relation of identity here means that, if it be possible for a person to know something as it is, he must both be able to know *it* (i.e. the object) and must be able to *know* it. To know *it* means to know the object itself, not a mere semblance or copy of idea of it; and to *know* it means simply to know, not merely to respond or to react to the object or being acted upon by it. Yet coincidence is more than this. It is a step into a world of values that reflects back on the world of facts. For the world in which a man can live depends upon the values with which he can fill the physical outline of bare facts and is thus a world which remains superior to and more satisfactory than the physical limitations. This is indicated by the seven features of the Sambhogakāya, which is not an entity but a symbol for unlimited communication and its awareness of the deeper significance of life and more satisfactory feeling-tone. These seven features are (i) the richness of value, through the unification of the ultimate truth which is ultimate in the sense that it cannot be resolved into anything else, and the relative truth as supported by the ultimate one before it becomes a partitive and partial truth; (ii) the enjoyment of the bliss of this unitary character; (iii) the unsurpassableness of this bliss because it is not a conditioned pleasure; (iv) the absence of anything that might claim existence exclusively within itself because it is not affected by the delusiveness of the postulates of subject and object; (v) its transcending compassionateness because it manifests itself in a being-for-and-with-others, although the constructs of subject (self) and object (other) do not obtain (i.e. infinite compassion is not a sentimentality vented upon men, but something that comprises all that lives and thus reaches into the very vanity and hallucinatoriness of the world); (vi) its continuity, the endless unfolding of a world of facts and values; and lastly (vii) its imperishableness, because it remains above all change.[1]

[1] Sphžg 132*ab*; Sphyd 6*b*.

6. DREAM

It will come rather as a surprise that dreaming is said to be an active means in the attainment of one's goal, enlightenment. This is due to the current theories which fail to take a dream as such and always prejudge it from the waking state. The instruction, given here, makes it abundantly clear that a dream is not a passive surrender to a stream of images of which the dreamer is the unwitting plaything and that it also cannot be judged as complementary to and compensatory for the waking state. This at once disposes of the dream theories of Freud and Jung.[1] There is no sharp division between waking and dreaming. On the basis of a strictly phenomenological investigation Medard Boss can say: 'Yet, so far, we have been unable to determine a criterion whereby the essence of our dream life as a whole could be distinguished from waking life.'[2] Further on he declares: 'Neither waking nor dreaming can be adequately described as independent interconnections of experiences or conceptions. Whether man is awake or dreaming he always fulfils one and the same existence.'[3] A dream is as much an immediate reality as is the waking state and the relations we have to our environment, to things and men and to what we call the divine, are no less absorbing than those in our waking life. It is even possible to see the world more clearly in our dreams than in the waking state. The life-possibilities of the dream are potentially present in the waking state as are those of the latter in the former. Therefore the practices of 'apparitions' and of 'dreams' are on the same level, because both of them function to 'purify' the low-level attitudes and conceptions of a rigid sense of ego.[4]

The 'place' where dreams originate is the total man, the existential self or, as the texts unanimously assert, 'the stirring of motility in the primordial radiant light'. This is particularly significant. It shows that dreams are not psycho-genetic, the psyche being

[1] Nevertheless the fact remains that it was psycho-analysis that revealed the closeness of the dream state to waking consciousness. See also William S. Haas, op.cit., p. 169. The way in which sGam-po-pa, x. 13*b*, analyses his dreams can be called 'psycho-analytic' in the best sense of the word.

[2] Op. cit., p. 208.

[3] Ibid, p. 209.

[4] Sphyd 20*b*; sGam-po-pa, xxxi. 6*b*, 8b; xv. 9*a*.

conceived as another entity in interaction with a physical continuum; similarly, sensory stimuli and sense impressions, which a materialistic conception of dreams considers of primary importance, are not causal at all, but rather the mould through which the mental-spiritual[1] is processed and turned into a deeply frozen product. Ever and again we find references to our waking life being a state of frozenness and that it is necessary to 'unfreeze' this state, 'to loosen the rigid interconnexions of the pathways'. Thus, for instance, sKye-med bde-chen says:

'When the sphere of non-memory has been stirred up by the ever-changing memory, it is solidified into the interpretative constructions of the mind. Just as water that has been stirred up by the cold storm of winter is turned into ice, so also, when the interpretative constructions of the mind have entered into that which is not these constructions, it is going to grow into Saṃsāra. Therefore Saraha says: "When the water has been stirred up, because the wind has dived into it."

'However, when the wind does not dive into the water, the latter remains gentle and does not suffer; but when the cold wind, the condition for the disturbance, does so, the water becomes rock-like ice. So also, when the interpretative constructions of the mind due to memory do not invade non-memory, there is not the painfulness of emotional reactivity and, since there is no construction of different characteristics, its gentleness is preserved. But when out of non-memory memory rises, and when this is conceived of as some permanently existing entity, emotional reactions become more and more intensified and the interpretative constructions of the mind are not likely to pass away. Hence Saraha continues: "Even the gentle water assumes the shape and texture of a rock."

'Further, when one knows that in its initial phase memory starts from non-memory, that in its middle phase it is rooted in non-memory, and that in its end-phase it dissolves into non-memory, everything that has arisen as memory is like the snow which has fallen into a lake. But when those who do not understand it in this way take memory as a permanent, and eternal, and independent, entity, it is like the snow that has fallen on the surface of a

[1] This term is meant only as an index, not as a characterization.

glacier. Inasmuch as in this way the interpretative constructions of the mind become more and more pronounced and, since the individual who does not recognize reality stirs up non-memory by memory, he only causes Saṃsāra. And therefore Saraha exclaims: "Oh you fools, stirred up by interpretative constructions of the mind the Unpatterned . . ."

'Further, when one understands as ultimate reality the pathways, the mystic sound, the creative potentiality, the inner mystic heat, the quietistic state of (wishful) nothingness, and other such topics, although they are mere products of imagination, by becoming more and more involved in such constructs, this activity is not likely to subside. Therefore Saraha concludes: "Becomes extremely hard and solid." '[1]

About the approach to great bliss as a process of unfreezing, Saraha says:

> 'First appearance is felt as nothing:
> This is like recognizing ice as water.
> Then, without appearance disappearing,
> Nothingness is indistinguishable from bliss:
> 'Tis like ice turning into water.
> When memory dissolves in non-memory and this in that which has no origin,
> When everything is indistinguishably one in bliss supreme:
> This is like ice dissolved in water.'[2]

Although in many cases in dream one merely re-lives one's wishes of the day, dreaming cannot be confined to such experiences. At best they emphasize the fact that there is no strict borderline between dream and the waking state. In a wider context the dream state, as in between the events of falling asleep and awakening, is significantly compared with the intermediate state between death and rebirth. Falling asleep is a kind of dying, and only when the old form breaks up can the individual be re-formed into newer and more mature structures whose possibilities are, as it were, envisaged in dream and factually shaped in waking.

[1] *Dohākośa-nāma-caryāgīti-arthapradipa-nāma-ṭikā*, 43*b*.
[2] *Kāyakośāmṛtavajragīti*, 112*a*.

How dream is born after the old patterns have been broken up, the text itself has pointed out. But it has been described more elaborately by Padma dkar-po: 'When the vibrations of the psycho-somatic constituents, the materializing forces and their interactional fields, become subliminal and gather in the "heart", the various phenomena of falling asleep, which resemble the meditative progress from a soft glow to a spread of light and beyond, dissolve in what is called the spread of light, which in turn dissolves in the darkness of the inner glow, the foundation of sleep, because mind overcome by darkness resembles this darkness of the inner glow. Out of this darkness then breaks forth the primordial radiant light, a momentary awareness which is absolutely free from all obscurations and all mental constructs. It is from this light that the various phenomena of dreaming proceed. Although the dream has no independent existence of its own it appears as something being-itself, and according to its nature, is capable of performing various functions. And so it is with the whole of entitative reality. Therefore by means of dreams one can individually experience and apprehend the whole of entitative reality as a divine pattern which is a semblance (of the radiant light).'[1]

In this passage the term 'momentary awareness' deserves particular attention, because it is of the highest philosophical significance. It does not mean a momentary event which is always an event *in* time, but that we can only in such a moment enjoy the elevation above the limits of ordinary body-mind, which is independent of temporal duration. In other words, that which is named 'momentary awareness' is in its temporal aspect time at the root of sentient life. It is out of this that we temporalize our experiences into events succeeding each other. In its noetic aspect it is nothingness that can be filled with any content. And so its definition runs as follows: 'Not proceeding from one instant to another but remaining unaltered as to its former and later presence',[2] and '"momentary" here is not to be understood as a particular perishable entity.'[3] In this conception Tantric philosophy has anticipated what in modern existentialist thought is called the

[1] Sphžg 171*a*. [2] Nbdztsh 9*a*. [3] Ibid.

'existential moment' and which has been most clearly discussed by Søren Kierkegaard and Karl Jaspers.[1]

It is important to note that it is not the radiant light which is the cause of dreams, but motility stirring in it. This motility then develops through the experientially initiated possibilities of experience into both dreams and the waking life. This again shows that the waking state and the dream state belong to the same nature within the all-encompassing light.

The reference to the 'throat' focal point relates dreaming to meditative processes. The 'throat' is not only the place of speech through which we establish relations with others more easily than by bodily act, it also points beyond to the value inherent in the widening of relationships and to authentic communication. Similarly the 'heart' focal point points to man's being-oneself which must find its reflection in communication and authentic Being in-the-world. The dream as a means to realize one's potentialities is therefore also induced by imaging oneself as Samayasattva (commitment-being) in whose 'throat' resides Jñānasattva (awareness-being), in whose 'heart' is found Samādhisattva (absorption-being).[2] This triple hierarchy again emphasizes the necessity of man's ascent from a spiritless Being-in-the-world to spirituality-permeated being-oneself.

Another point of this instruction is to learn to recognize the fact that one is dreaming while one dreams. This is not in order to come to the reassuring conviction, 'Thank goodness, it is only a dream', but to arrive at an understanding transcending our everyday experience of 'objects'. Among the techniques to achieve this end we find the development of the dream content into a number of contents of the same nature or the change of a certain content into its opposite. However, here we must be careful not to read something into the dreaming experience which in waking life we would have to consider as a sort of escapism or shallow optimism based on repression. Nothing could be more fatal than to have recourse to repression, because any attempt to do so would

[1] Karl Jaspers, *Philosophie*, i, p. 18; Otto Friedrich Bollnow, *Existenzphilosophie*, p. 111.

[2] Sphkh 51*a*.

only strengthen the ties from which one wants to become free. Padma dkar-po is quite explicit in declaring that in dreaming of fire and its extinction by water, or of the evaporation of the latter by the former, the purpose is not to counteract the one by the other and then rest content with what has been done, but 'by becoming aware of the infinite modes to counter one thing by another, as in the case of diseases by medicines, not to become confused as to the proper means and in recognizing the mystery of the inseparableness of the opposites to clarify the state of bewilderment-errancy and to attain a state of non-bewilderment'.[1] Bewilderment is essentially the attempt to 'explain', to reduce a living reality to a dead formula; it is the endless construction of ideas about the mysterious background of all that is, while non-bewilderment is to grant each appearance its full reality, a direct appearance of the Real revealed in the light of the individual's understanding.[2]

7. THE RADIANT LIGHT

The instruction on the radiant light reaches back to the conception of the radiant mind which is already found in the Pāli Canon. This idea has been interpreted variously. While certain schools believed in the radiant mind as an entity remaining unchanged behind the accidental veilings of its light, the general trend, however, has been to consider it merely as an instrumental concept.[3] Similarly all other terms referring to the radiant light, such as a shining jewel or a burning lamp, are not qualifications but indexes, suggestions which we must be grateful to receive, but cautious to substantiate.

Another point to note is that in Tantrism the ordinary world of

[1] Sphžg 173*a*.

[2] There are thus four stages in the dream practice. The first is to to take hold of a dream, the next is to develop the dream by recognizing it to be a dream. Then follows the attempt to overcome any fear one might have in the dream situation. Lastly, one has to come to the realization that the apparitional character of the dream is basically one's own mentality which is not an entity, and hence cannot be said to have come into existence at any time. The dream, and man's whole life, partakes of this nature, because his dreams are but the formulations of something that precedes any formulation. See sGam-po-pa, xiii. 8*b* sq.; xvii. 2*b* sqq.; xxxv. 2*b* sq.

[3] See *Vijñaptimātratāsiddhi*, pp. 109–13.

appearance is not unreal but the ultimate in a limited and restricted way, and thus a challenge to man to perfect and enhance it with beauty and value which is more than earthly. Buddhist Tantrism is on the whole (there are of course exceptions) what William Pepperell Montague calls 'positive mysticism' and describes as: 'The positive mystic is one whose revelation of the invisible and transcendent serves not to blind him to the concrete details and duties of visible existence, but rather to illuminate and strengthen his earthly life. His outlook on the world is devoid of illusionism, pessimism, asceticism, and occultism. To mystics of this higher type nature seems more real rather than less real, and beautiful rather than ugly. And instead of devoting their lives to the negation of the will to live and to a repudiation of earthly existence and its duties, they use their inner light to supplement the outer light of common sense and of science, and strive to incarnate the kingdom of heaven in this world.'[1]

The idea of the unity of reality is expressed in the relation between the ground, the goal, and the path to it, or in terms relating to the luminous character of all our experiences, the ground or the light of common sensibility, ultimacy, or the primordial radiancy, and the semblant light which in the narrower sense of the word is our actual experience of daily life. Both ultimacy and semblance must coincide in a unitary experience or the goal lived in everyday life. Technically this is known as the coincidence of ultimate truth and relative truth.[2] The goal is in no way different from the foundation or starting-point, and the path, therefore, also is not some separate entity leading from one extreme to another. The idea behind this, at first sight extraordinary, conception which often is expressed in the words that

> 'The effect is to be sealed by the cause,
> But also the latter by the former',[3]

is the principle of circular causation. It can best be illustrated by the device by which a guided missile is directed towards a moving target by sound-waves, light rays or other emanations from the

[1] William Pepperell Montague, *The Ways of Knowing*, p. 63.
[2] Sphžg 175*a*, 197*a*.
[3] Phgdz 27*a*. See also *Sekoddeśaṭikā*, p. 70.

target. There is a sort of 'feed-back' from the goal and the end does control the means. The action, however, is here and now, although the goal to be reached is in a future as yet undetermined. Hence Padma dkar-po can say: 'As to the foundation or starting point, the ultimate is pure and that which partakes of the ultimate is pure and inseparable from the former. Therefore the relation between the two is like that between the water and its ripples.'[1] The path is essentially the attempt to 'unfreeze' the common state of hardened prejudices and opinions and to endow the smallest thing with pulsating life in a transcendent glow of ineffable beauty and value. This comes about by a process of de-objectification, which was most obvious in the practice of apparitional existence. So also Padma dkar-po continues: 'As to the path, it is the experience of attuning one's apparitional existence to the radiant light.'[1] The goal is the realization of reality as unitary and as life out of this sphere which in normal behaviour becomes one with a living transcending awareness as a positive contribution to human life, not a flight from it, or as Padma dkar-po puts it: 'As to the goal, it is the realization of spontaneous (unlearnable) coincidence, the indivisibility of authentic Being-in-the-world and noetic being as such.'[1]

For ordinary man the depth of vision is shallow and clarity is obscured by pre-judgements, while in the mystic depth and clarity are the most characteristic features, and he uses them to illumine his earthly life which he clothes in a garb of value.[2] Depth and clarity[3] are the recurrent attributes of the unitary experience of the mystic. 'Since depth and clarity cannot be separated as water and ice, they coincide, or are non-dual transcending awareness.'[4] It is the depth of the mystic's vision that lifts him above the shallow-

[1] Sphžg 174*b*.

[2] According to sGam-po-pa, xi. 2*a*, this term (*zab*) is used differently. Atīśa understood by it the attention to the impermanent character of our world including ourselves; others denote by it meditation on one's tutelary deity (and in this sense it is widely used today), while Mi-la-ras-pa understood by it the practice of the mystic heat (*gtum-mo*) and the Mahāmudrā or anything which might bring about this experience.

[3] According to sGam-po-pa, iv. 8*a*, this term (*gsal*) describes the intuitive nature of the relevant experience. In Sphžg 129*b*, Padma dkar-po speaks of the 'co-emergence of depth and clarity'.

[4] Sphžg 59*a*.

ness of ordinary consciousness, and thereby generates the idea of an 'ultimate truth'. It must, however, be noted that it would go against the spirit of Buddhist Tantrism to assert that ultimate truth is this or that. 'Ultimate truth' is not an entity, but merely an index. Neither is 'conventional truth' a well-defined entity; it is the light that may shine everywhere and be terminated by any content without itself being limited in any way. The idea of a double truth is thus essentially different from the one which in the Western world found its specific formulation as that of reason and revelation at about A.D. 1270 by Siger of Brabant. Although condemned by the Church in 1276–7 by Bishop Stephen Tempier, it lived on and was accepted by Francis Bacon (1561–1626) and, as the double truth of science and faith, it was re-stated by Kant who was the first also to see its implications. His attempt at reconciliation is now generally held to have failed. Neither have his successors, Hegel, Bradley, Bosanquet, Royce, and Stace succeeded. The conflict still continues and most people live in 'a kind of schizoid dissociation'[1] which often assumes pathological dimensions.

The demand of Tantrism that ultimate truth and relative truth must coincide and, in a certain sense, were in a state of coincidence before they were split up by a mind, is not so much a novelty as a new sphere which has as much an affective as a cognitive range. It is experienceable as the experience process itself, not as the content of the experience. The coincidence and hence identity between ultimate truth and conventional truth or between depth and clarity is indicated as follows by Padma dkar-po: 'The actuality of the radiant light is said to be depth or ultimate truth, because as the ultimacy of spirituality in all sentient beings it is pure in its being itself; and the spontaneous shining forth (of this light) everywhere and unimpeded is called clarity or conventional truth. The inability to differentiate between the two (as separate entities) because its absolutely specific character can be experienced only individually, is coincidence and declared as Being-as-such (*gśis*) incomprehensible by any other means than by itself.'[2] It is

[1] Kimball Young, *Personality and Problems of Adjustment*, p. 469.
[2] Sphžg 175*b*.

important to note that only the unity and, ultimately, identity of ultimate truth and conventional truth is termed Being-as-such. This term again is only an instrumental concept, no predication of an absolute truth. We deal with and out of something which cannot be determined as truth in opposition to something false; since we have to do with reality we cannot arbitrarily denounce our reality dealing as falsehood. This reality conception is summed up in the statement that Being-as-such (*gśis*) is ultimately devoid of truth, but as its lucid manifestation (*gdaṅs*) it is conventionally devoid of falsehood, and this peculiarity of the unity of the unfathomable and fathomable is the very fact of co-emergence.[1] The Real is thus beginning and end, and though it needs constant striving to arrive at its total experience it is present to us as semblance or index wherever we move. To call the world we live in a semblance of the Real is in line with positive mysticism which enriches the given by its transcending vision. For the positive mystic the problem of evil and falsehood arises with the failure to enhance the given and to perfect it.

The striving itself is inseparable from the radiant light as our Being-oneself in the being-this-or-that. Becoming directly aware of this light so as to live out of its sphere, is termed 'intuition'. In Western thought this word has been badly mauled by indiscriminate usage. In Tantric Buddhism it is not so much a 'looking at' or 'viewing', and certainly not 'instinct' in the sense in which the word is used by Henri Bergson. It denotes rather the successful attainment of a state of peace and composure in which a complete harmony between the within and the without has been achieved and whereby the range of vision has not only been widened but has also been cleared. It always refers to an 'experience more intimate and immediate than that of thought, and more clearly analogous to a pure feeling or emotion in which the distinction between the self and its objects is no longer present'.[2] The certainty that goes with intuition is not itself a criterion of objective truth; truth is for the Tantrics (as for certain existentialist thinkers) subjectivity. Certainty is merely the expression of success in having stepped

[1] Phgdz 35*b*.
[2] William Pepperell Montague, op. cit., p. 54.

beyond the disquieting part-reality of ordinary life, mostly sensory and external, and having gained access to a realm of immediate values which cannot be derived from perception. As Montague points out: 'The mystic is one to whom these inner experiences appeal as vital and real. He pictures the world in terms of them, and the picture is precious in that it embodies and makes visible in objective form the hidden depth of the human spirit. Even ordinary perception and reasoning is largely based upon subconscious stores of memory and instinct. They furnish the meaning with which our sensations are clothed, and the motives by which our reasonings are driven. The intuitions of creative imagination as expressed in the cosmic revelations of the philosophic and religious mystics, and even in the less generic visions of the great poets, owe their grandeur und uniqueness to the fact that in them the subconscious functions move spontaneously, more nearly as a unified whole. In normal experience intuition is the servant of the specific, external situation, and there is evoked only that part of the subconscious which is relevant to that situation, while in the real mystic intuition the inner self in its entirety is the controlling factor.'[1] In this last sense the Tantric texts also speak of a 'great intuition' which takes in the whole of Reality.[2]

'Effulgence' and 'non-effulgence' are names for experiences during the process of the realization of the inner light. The former is the completion of the process and the beatific vision turned into a healthy and beneficent purpose, while the latter is the critical moment when the mystic may rise to the beatific vision or relapse into a world of ordinary sensory experiences. Tilopa expresses this in the following words:

> Just as a light within a pitcher
> Does not shine outside,
> But when the latter is smashed
> The light will spread,
> So is it with our lives, a pitcher,
> And the radiant light, the lamp (therein).

[1] Ibid., p. 57. [2] Sphyd 90*b*; Sphžg 62*b*.

When by the Guru's teaching that pitcher has been broken
The Buddha's transcending awareness forth radiates.[1]

The progress towards light is intimately related to the stages in the concentration process. There are four such stages which are subdivided into three according to the nature of the stability of the respective experience. This subdivision is attributed to Phag-mo gru-pa, a disciple of sGam-po-pa, and considered authoritative for the bKa'-rgyud-pas. The text mentions these subdivisions with their respective names of a low-, medium-, and high-grade quality, the former indicating a meditative and concentrative stage that has not yet become stable, the second a slight stability, and the last one complete stability.[2] Another equally authoritative subdivision is into sixteen aspects, each having four sub-stages due to the fact that the various stages interpenetrate. The first stage is called 'unitary experience', the second 'non-diffusion', the third 'one-valueness' and the fourth, not mentioned in the text because as the culmination it is beyond words, 'unmeditatable'. The two former are of a more common nature and correspond to the older ideas of 'tranquillity' and 'insight', while the latter two go beyond these.[3] Each of these concentrative stages has, as it were, an inner and outer reference which in our language it is difficult to describe, because to do so we must 'objectify' while the meditative process itself is a 'de-objectifying' one. What I have called the inner reference is with respect to that which is termed 'unitary experience', a feeling of bliss which in itself is nothing because it is not determined by specific modifications in the general mass of feeling due to the arousal of experience traces. The 'unitary experience' approximates to what we call 'pure sensation', i.e. a situation in which a certain sensum is intuitively apprehended, but in which there is no external reference. It is therefore also called an 'absorption in which bliss and nothingness prevail'. Outwardly this experience is expressed in the doctrine of pure mentalism which, because it transcends the subject-object division, cannot forthwith be equated with the Western system of Subjectivism and

[1] Tilopa, op cit., 5*b*.
[2] Phntm 5*b*; Rzd 63*b* sq.
[3] Phzb 2*a*; 6*a*.

its postulation of an absolute self. The experience is described as follows: 'There is no dividedness; the noetic capacity is awareness and clarity; and its feeling-tone is one of bliss. Bliss, clarity, and non-dividedness form a unit.'[1]

Similarly, 'non-diffusion' is marked by an increased clarity which in itself also is nothing. While in the preceding stage the state of being torn between a subjective and an objective pole has been removed and a deep peace has been realized, this peace in turn provides the solid foundation for a wider view which is not based on the prejudgements of opposites such as being and non-being, eternity and annihilation, singularity and plurality; technically known as the 'Middle View'. The wider view which has been made possible by a state of peace and restfulness is one of the utmost clarity and luminosity and termed 'non-diffusion', because 'diffusion' is the opposite of concentration, is 'negativity, emptiness, giving way to unchecked flows of thought which prevent a restful attitude'.[2]

'One-valueness' is the experience of everything that appears as nothing though not in the sense that appearance is mere illusion and that, since all we meet in life is illusory, there is no need for serious action. On the contrary, one-valueness is the spontaneous interest in the several situations of life which man encounters. This interest has been purified of all vested interests through the preceding phases of the concentrative process, and hence is more suited for beneficial activity. However, as this stage is not yet the final realization, although no other path has to be taken up, one still has to learn the meaning and application of the logical relation of coincidence. 'At the stage of one-valueness the intuitive understanding of coincidence that has still to be learned in order to be practised, has been perfected. Value remains the same in the singular intuitive understanding that, as regards everything apprehendable, subsumed under the headings of Saṃsāra and Nirvāṇa, there is nothing to be eliminated or postulated, rejected or accepted, and lessened or augmented.'[3]

[1] Phntm 6*b*; 11*b*.

[2] Thérèse Bross, *Altruism and Creativity as Biological Factors of Human Evolution*, pp. 131 sq.

[3] Phntm 11*b*.

It is out of this state that the final realization of the unity of 'the world of facts and the world of values'—to use A. N. Whitehead's words—may be born, which liberates him who has this experience from the fear of this world and the hope for another one, and itself is nothing that can be attended to as an entity. In poetical language Saraha says:

> Since all joys and sorrows in our dreams
> Do not exist when we awaken,
> What thought of negating or affirming either can be held
> When they have arisen from thoughts of hope and fear?
>
> Since all the things in Saṃsāra and Nirvāṇa
> Are nothing when we have seen the Ultimate,
> What efforts should we make to accept or reject them,
> When the particularizing mind with its hopes and fears has ceased to move?[1]

The actual practice of the light as the path is the emptying of consciousness from every content. Outwardly this is a process of dying, while inwardly it is an increase and gathering of light, passing through the non-effulgent state of unknowing into the radiant light which cannot be predicated in any way and hence is referred to as 'complete nothingness', provided one is fully aware of the various phases in this process. These are the same as have been described previously.[2] The differentiation between a path of the night and one of the day is, on the one hand, an indication that every experience of ordinary life, whether with our senses wide awake or in states of sleep and dream, can be used as a springboard for arriving at fulness of being, which as goal achievement, the light as the result of our striving, brings about a transfiguration of the man indicated by the symbol of the rainbow. On the other hand, the path of the day and that of the night are also names for the direction of the process.[3] Accordingly, the path of the day is the passing from the radiant light through the outer darkness of the inner glow and the intense light of expansion into the soft glow from which the

1 Phntm 11*b*.
2 *Dohākośa-nāma-mahāmudrā-upadeśa*, 123*a*.
3 See p. 197.

conscious world springs forth; and the path of the night is the same procedure in an inverse order. However, since man cannot live without values, the approach to the world of values, the path of the night, is considered the procedure following the natural order, while the entanglement in a world of facts with its increasing loss in value is procedure of an unnatural order. This distinction does not imply an evaluation as to good or bad, necessitating a rejection of the one or the other. Man lives in and out of a sphere of light, but his life is more like a rhythm symbolized by the phenomena of day and night, birth and death. Moreover, since reality can only be one, the relation of the poles between which man's life is swinging is one of circular causality. As Tilopa and Padma dkar-po explain, in one instance the triad of the soft glow, the intense light and the inner glow are cause of the radiant light, while in the other the latter is the cause of the three former.[1]

The attainment of the goal is an access to a sphere of life larger and more powerful and divinely inspired than the normal conscious life. Not only does it make us happy, it also sheds its light through us on others who, awakened by it, may also follow its path.

8. TRANSFERENCE

This is a technique with which every initiate is familiar. It is practised for a limited period and then remembered at the moment of death. Hence it is also called a technique to arrive at Buddhahood or enlightenment without meditation.[2] Since death means to exist as fulfilment, the purpose of this technique is to be ready for death, and through this readiness to avoid unfavourable situations of rebirth.

The last part of the instruction in the body of the text is found verbatim in the 'Oral Transmission' texts and is explained as follows:[3]

'The explanation of transference in detail consists of two sections: (i) the time of transference (which is when the signs of death appear) and (ii) the method of transference. The latter has three stages: (*a*) a preliminary one, preparing oneself as does an expert archer; (*b*) the actual procedure, shooting the powerful

[1] Tshk 6*a*. [2] sGam-po-pa, xxxii. 10*b*. [3] Tshk 6*a*.

arrow of noetic capacity at the desired target; and (*c*) a summing up: hitting the mark.

'(*a*) The preliminary stage is twofold: (1) ordinary and (2) extraordinary.

'(1) The former is twofold: (i *a*) conceiving of qualities of the future realm of existence and developing a yearning for it; (i *b*) becoming aware of the shortcomings of the pleasures of this life and discarding the hankering after them.

'(2) The extraordinary stage is threefold: (i *a*) closing the gate to the path of the world by the mystic view of the nature of body-mind;[1] (i *b*) opening the gate to the path of tranquillity by a powerful lever;[2] (i *c*) sending up the messenger of one's prayer as the designing agency.

'The actual procedure is fourfold: (*a*) filling the charge;[3] (*b*) overcoming the hindrances of unfavourable conditions;[4] (*c*) outlining the path of favourable conditions;[5] and (*d*) shooting the noetic capacity off like an arrow.

'The summing up is threefold: (*a*) The superior type realizes authentic being as such; (*b*) the mediocre one, that of authentic communication;[6] and (*c*) the inferior one, that of authentic being-in-the-world.'

In substance the same process is described by sGam-po-pa and others. sGam-po-pa distinguishes three degrees in transference. The highest one is to transfer oneself to the realm of the radiant light, a mediocre one is transference into an apparitional existence, and the lowest one is the practice of the Developing Stage.[7] In this

[1] This means according to Padma dkar-po, who refers to Nāropa's teaching, to allow the noetic capacity to pass only through the fontanel opening and not through any other opening of the body. Sphžg 191*b*. According to sGam-po-pa, xv. 16*b*, the navel, the space between the eyebrows, and the crown of the head, are the best gates through which transference is able to take place; nose, ears, and eyes are of medium quality, while mouth, anus, and the urinary passage are the worst possible gates.

[2] i.e. the creative potentiality (*thig-le*).

[3] i.e. the syllable *hūṃ* is made to dissolve into pure motility.

[4] i.e. muttering the mantra *kṣa*.

[5] i.e. preparing the exit of the noetic capacity through the fontanel opening by closing all other possible exits with certain mantric syllables.

[6] Here the meaning of Sambhogakāya as an existential norm is most evident. One is in communication with the Ultimate in the shape of the Guru.

[7] sGam-po-pa, xiii. 10*a*; xviii. 4*a*.

respect transference is closely linked to the general trend in Buddhist meditation to arrive at a trans-objective and trans-subjective reality. In this context it is particularly important to note the difference between the mantric syllables. The *hūṃ* is connected with experiences of an apparitional nature during the processes of the Developing and Fulfilment Stages. The *hik* is reserved for a technique preparatory to physical death, which is known as the 'forceful means'. This technique, much practised today, is as follows:[1]

After one has created a suitable mental climate by uttering and pondering over the Mahāyānic formula of Taking Refuge and by making the firm resolution to develop and to practise an Enlightened Attitude for the sake of everything alive, one conceives of oneself as the female deity rDo-rje phag-mo (Vajravārāhī) or rDo-rje-rnal-'byor-ma (Vajrayoginī) with all her emblems. Above her is rDo-rje-'chaṅ (Vajradhara), also richly adorned, but having the distinct features of one's Guru. The purpose of this practice is clear. It is a preparation for transcending the subjective level and for establishing an immediate contact with the Ultimate which for the time being is still pictured in individual shapes (one's Guru) pointing beyond themselves. This is still more emphasized by the Gurus who succeed one another in a long line, each of whom represents the sum total of the philosophical quest of his period. The idea behind this is what Karl Jaspers calls 'philosophical faith' and which he describes in the words: 'Nowhere is the truth ready made; it is an inexhaustible stream that flows from the history of philosophy as a whole from China to the West, yet flows only when the primal source is captured for new realizations in the present.'[2] Thus the stream of the Ultimate flows through the great philosophers in tradition, Tilopa, Nāropa, Mar-pa, Mi-la-ras-pa, Śakyaśrī, and lastly one's Guru. Then after the invocation of these philosophers in tradition, which is repeated *ad libitum*, the next step is to arrive at a stage of pure sensation where all objective reference, be it to an 'objective' or 'subjective' pole, is obliterated. At this moment a new vista is opened which I shall call 'the dimension of structure'. It is here that the meaning of the pathways, motility, and creative potentiality

[1] The account is based on Lzph.

[2] Karl Jaspers, *The Perennial Scope of Philosophy*, p. 26.

is revealed as forming a unitary experience in the sense that, as modern psycho-biology has shown, motility is the cradle of mind and mentation, or as Judson C. Herrick puts it: 'Movement is primordial and mentation arises within it not to cause behaviour but to regulate it, direct it, and improve its efficiency.'[1] The inseparability of motility and mentality is a recurrent theme of Buddhist Tantrism and discussed at (rather complicated) length in the Pañcakrama and most lucidly by sGam-po-pa who, in answer to Phag-mo gru-pa's question whether motility and mentality are two entities or one phenomenon, replies that 'motility and mentality are one. When motility stirs mentality becomes the various contents of mind. The two cannot be spoken of as being different from each other. When mentality-spirituality is understood motility becomes pure in itself and this is the co-emergence of non-dual noeticness and nothingness.'[2]

The indivisibility of motility and mentality as a creative power, as yet in a state of non-creativity—hence one speaks of its potential state—is supposed to be found in the heart focal region, which it has to be noted is not to be considered spatially. We are here faced with a difficulty of language which creates the impression of independently existing entities in time and space, while actually we deal with a realm which *is* time-space but not *in* time-space. In other words, we move in between two worlds, an individual one and an ultimate one which is not in opposition to but encompasses the worlds of individuality and generality. The task is now to achieve the shift from the individual level to the encompassing ultimate one. The driving force in this shift is the mantric syllable *hik* which in actual practice is uttered twenty-one times. Since the practice is preparatory to death, the aim is essentially to facilitate death when it comes, and hence, for the time being, one returns to the individual level by means of the mantric syllable *ka* which is also uttered twenty-one times. sGam-po-pa illustrates the practice by the training of race-horses. They are galloped up and down the race-course so as to become acquainted with it.[3]

[1] C. Judson Herrick, op. cit., p. 312.

[2] sGam-po-pa, xi. 10*b*.

[3] Ibid. xv. 17*a*.

After the mantras *hik* and *ka* have been uttered twenty-one times the practice is discontinued for the day and resumed on each following day until lymph or blood appears at the fontanel opening. Then the practice is discontinued completely and only repeated once at the exact moment of physical death. The oozing of blood or lymph at the fontanel opening is a phenomenon as yet unexplained by the medical sciences, though well attested by all who have performed this practice. Another peculiar phenomenon is that, when a competent Guru imparts this instruction to his disciple, the region of the fontanel opening becomes highly sensitive to touch and remains so for some time. Moreover, when after the instruction he touches this region with Kusa-grass, symbolically representing the opening of the passage to the ultimate, the distinct sensation of being pierced from top to bottom is created. Needless to say, this practice is not without its dangers and under no circumstances can it be performed when there is any deformation in the bones of the skull or in the spinal cord.

9. RESURRECTION

Resurrection means, properly speaking, to endow a corpse with life. In this sense resurrection is said to have been in vogue up to the time of Mar-pa, whose son mDo-sde-pa is said to have been the last to perform this rite. Such at least is the official version. Unofficially it is admitted that this rite is till practised sometimes, and sGam-po-pa gives a detailed account of it which is nothing short of black magic.[1] This may be why later, though beginning with sGam-po-pa, any association with black magic was rejected and resurrection equated with transference as a perfectly legitimate meditational practice. Nāropa himself still seems to have considered resurrection as a separate technique, because it is one of his Six Topics. But otherwise it is expressly stated that 'the bKa'-brgyud-pa Gurus reckon transference and resurrection as one topic and in order to make up for the Six Topics of Nāropa add the intermediate state'.[2] This statement, which we have no reason to doubt, would suggest that Nāropa

[1] sGam-po-pa, xv. 5*b*; xviii. 8*a*. [2] Tshk 6*b*.

himself still dabbled with black magic, but that with the emphasis on the spiritual side of Buddhist Tantrism, as particularly stressed by sGam-po-pa, the historical organizer of the bKa'-brgyud-pa order, any reference to black magic was banned and thus Tantrism became a positive discipline again.

10. ETERNAL DELIGHT

The instructions on this topic are, in a sense, preliminary to the following one on Mahāmudrā. They may be regarded as an attempt to sublimate the physical sex impulse into something spiritual. Although 'sublimation' has become a household word under the influence of psycho-analysis, we should be cautious in accepting it at its face value. In this respect Havelock Ellis's words are relevant: 'In the field of sexual psychology, "sublimation" is understood to imply that the physical impulse, or libido in the narrow sense, can be so transformed into some impulse of higher psychic activity that it ceases to be urgent as a physical need. The conception is now widely current in popular psychology. Those who adopt it, however, do not always seem to realize that this process of "sublimation" is even in its original imagery a process involving much expenditure of force, and in its metaphorical and spiritual form far easier to talk about than to achieve. That it stands for a real psychic transformation of physical impulses, by which the grosser physical desires are lifted on to a plane where their keenness is lost in the gratification of desires which correspond to the physical but are more, as we say, "spiritual" in nature, may be accepted. But that transformation, though possible, is not easy nor of swift attainment, and perhaps only possible at all for those natures which are of finer than average nervous texture.'[1] It is the contention of the adherents of the mystic Mahāmudrā philosophy that they are truer to reality, because they do not repress sex but recognize it as an occasion of the greatest of human illuminations.[2]

Technically the sex relation is known as Karmamudrā, 'Seal by Acts'. This means that we start with acts and not with thoughts. Acts are overt, symbolic, and covert. Overt activity involves the body in

[1] Havelock Ellis, *Psychology of Sex*, p. 262.

[2] Phgdz 78*a*.

more or less direct contact with other persons or things. Symbolic activity relates to the field of communication, which is largely verbal and preparatory to overt activity. In relation to these two there is also activity within the organism or the covert world of thoughts, attitudes, and values. All three levels should operate in unison.

Now overt action takes place between individuals, who are male and female. Man moves in this world. He is both male and female in the sense that in the womb the rudimentary beginnings of both sets of sexual equipment were present, not in the sense that there is a sexless nucleus to which male and female attributes attach themselves but that there is an ambivalent possibility of an otherwise well-knit system. This dual nature, which is both within man and also makes up his environment, gains more and more importance and significance in the course of his growth and development. Further, on the level of communication where words set up expectations and incipient reactions, the action occurs between the members of the two sexes. Finally, on the level of covert act, thinking takes on the nature of an inner forum in which social acts in symbolic form are manipulated in the same way as our more overt actions. Thus, wherever there is activity in the human sphere, it occurs, broadly speaking, between members of the two sexes. Because of this bisexual nature of man and his environment it is only natural that sexuality as an inalienable part of man's nature should play an important, if not often decisive, role. As psycho-analysts have observed time and again, at various stages sexuality does not 'raise its ugly head', but is ready to help man onward on his difficult path of integration.

In this respect the age of the persons involved, ranging between twelve and twenty-five years (according to other sources between eleven and twenty-four),[1] is significant. Puberty, which marks the awakening of the emotion of love for one of the opposite sex, the prime of youth, and the full-blown state of the physically mature organism are the critical moments when man's path may be smoothed and be made happy or when he may be thrown off his balance. Sexuality even in the narrowest sense of the word is never an isolated, self-sufficient urge; it is an impulse and sustaining

[1] Tilopa, op. cit. 4*a*.

power or motive permeating the whole of man's emotional and intellectual life, together with its specific emotion of love, and it not only facilitates social interaction but also assists all sorts of learning processes in a most positive way. The puritan's distrust and professed horror of sex, in which he nevertheless merrily engages, is basically the expression of the fear of being compelled to outgrow the seemingly happy era of infantilism and to attain maturity.

Fear is the great inhibitor of action and is linked to avoidance and ultimately to hatred; having become obsessive, it even prevents necessary activities. And there is nothing more fatal than repression due to fear, because the energy charge of the repressed content adds itself to that of the repressing factor, whose operation is stimulated beyond limits, accounting, according to the nature of the repressed content, for the well-known types of the 'purity'-fanatic (mostly hypocritical) and the sex fanatic (mostly frustrated). However, when sexuality is recognized as an inalienable part of man, neither to be despised nor exaggerated, the meaning and purpose of the union between a man and a woman takes on a different character. It is to be found not only in the biological sphere of the continuation of the species but also in the development towards spiritual maturity and its accompanying feeling of happy contentedness, both of which, it will be readily admitted, are in most people conspicuous by their absence.

To regard sexual intercourse as a coarse and animal-like activity and to see in it the working of the devil and the origin of evil is utterly to misconstrue its nature; and the punishment is emotional distress and serious unbalance. In reality it can and often does lead to a formerly undreamed-of enrichment of man's nature, to completeness and fullness of life.

The basic error of the negative view of sex is that it singles out only one aspect of love (a highly ambiguous term), physical passion, and contrasts it with spiritual passion which it frantically tries to keep free from all associations with the concrete, the physical and, in the narrower sense of the word, the sexual. The result is a sort of schizoid mentality. But love is never such a monstrosity; it is neither the one nor the other exclusively; it is so vast, so encompassing, and so radiant that, frightened by its brilliancy, lesser people have closed their eyes before its splendour and have tried to run away from it into some padded cell of alleged dispassionateness which turned out to be a hatred of all, with all the dire consequences resulting therefrom. Or, failing to understand the essence of love, others conceived of it as a mere sensual enjoyment and in their ignorance misused the object of their 'love' for selfish ends.

Genuine love neither presupposes a judgement nor is it a sentimentality. Its unique feature is that it is always love for a person; it is directed towards the person as reality. But what is reality? Certainly it is the other's physical charms, but also the other's mental-spiritual qualities, and over and above these there always remains that which is unfathomable. This is the true object of love. In proceeding towards its object love makes everything of value achieve the highest possible value ideally destined for it; and in this way it brings out the highlights of another's worth. Love elevates, it never degrades; at its highest pitch it is not love for something alien, but participation in it as something inalienable. Strictly speaking, at this point love has gone beyond a referential situation. It is important to note that this triple division is Nāropa's doctrine. The first aspect or Karmamudrā proper is a concrete woman, the second is a mental-spiritual process, and the third is the culmination or Mahāmudrā.[1] In other words, since love proceeds from the concrete person to that which is unfathomable, co-existent, in or co-emergent with the concrete, the 'lure of the flesh' turns out to be 'transcending awareness in and through discrimination and appreciation' as a transcending function (Überleitungsfunktion). In this connexion Devacandra's answer to the argument of the haters of love is worth mentioning:

'(The opponent): "Passion and similar emotions are the reasons why we have to wander about in evil forms of life for a long time in Saṃsāra. Having long succumbed to desires and expectations, sentient beings are born bewildered as to their birth in agonizing misery. By performing unwholesome deeds that should better have been avoided, they are going to experience great distress in

[1] Phgdz 20*b*.

such evil forms of life as animals, spirits, and denizens of hell. Do you not see that to praise passion and other emotions is to spread poison, as when you make a poisoned person drink milk?"

'(Devacandra): "This is true, but only in so far as those who have no spiritual friends or advisers are concerned. By indulging in passion and other emotional outbreaks they will surely suffer. To this effect much has been said by the adherents of the Śrāvaka and Pratyekabuddha ways of life. But—he who is utterly loveless will suffer much more, because he hates love. It is for such people that passion-love has been taught. As is said:

> Admire not those who have no passion
> Because they have renounced it, but still
> Hesitate to renounce
> Lovelessness as well.

' "And the Exalted One has said:

> In the three worlds there is no greater sin
> Than to be without love.
> Therefore you must never
> Be without it.

' "To those who are not loveless, genuine love (Great Love) is taught. So it has been stated:

> Some enjoy things passionately,
> Others renounce them out of lovelessness;
> The yogi with an unsullied mind
> Does not renounce what he has not appropriated.

' "And Saraha declared:

> Some are fettered
> By renouncing things;
> Others by these same things
> Gain unsurpassable enlightenment.

' "Therefore, to induce passionate people to be dispassionate, to teach loveless people passion-love as a mediator, and to bring people who have passion-love as a mediator to genuine love, this unsurpassable and extremely profound teaching of 'transcending awareness in and through discrimination and appreciation' is given to highly developed beings." '[1]

The Karmamudrā or 'seal by acts' is, therefore, first of all, a concrete person with whom a relation can be established on any of the three levels of action. But since all the three levels are interrelated, the Karmamudrā is not merely a sexually attractive woman, she is just as much a spiritual factor.[2]

The description of the Karmamudrā according to the four types, Padminī, Śankhinī, Citriṇī, Mṛginī (Hastinī), defining her nature by similitudes with animals or plants on the basis of the texture of the skin, the size of the genital organs, the gait or movement, continues the long tradition of the science of erotics.[3] But so far it locates the 'object' with its properties and qualities perceived or conceived, merely in space and time. It is therefore largely denotative.

[1] *Prajñājñānaprakāśa,* 84*a* sqq. The Tibetan term *'dod-chags,* which is the translation of Sanskrit *rāga,* comprises all that we term 'sensuality', 'lust', 'passion', 'love'. While the haters of love will understand this word only as 'lust' and 'passion', always darkening their minds by associations with evil and sin, those who affirm life and are not afraid of love will insist on the positive meaning. Love reaches out to sentient beings by participating in them, this participation being compassion (as an active emotion, not as a passive sentimentality). Thus Anangavajra says in his *Prajñopāyaviniścayasiddhi,* i. 15:

'That which liberates all and everything from the ocean of suffering
And from its cause
Is Compassion; by reaching out to sentient beings
It is praised as Love.'

This verse is also quoted in Phgdz 4*b*, and the translation is based on the Tibetan version.

[2] This is plainly evident from the discussion in Dnz 49*a* sq.

[3] These names are well known from the Kāmaśāstra literature. Which four types are accepted seems to depend on the attitude and predilection of the author. bDe-ba'i rdo-rje's account, the dNos-po'i gnas-lugs bsgom-pa, 206*b*, for instance, tallies with the one given by Padma dkar-po, while Amoghavajra's classification in the Karmamudrā-parīkṣā-upadeśa 123*ab*, is like the one given in Ssrdz 40*ab*. Amoghavajra who classifies the women suitable for this practice according to their complexion and deportment linked to caste (*rigs*), the size and shape of their sex organs (*bhaga*), and the nature and chance of the consummatory experience (*rtsa*) says: 'Thus from the three types of superiorness, mediocrity, and inferiorness of the class, the sex organs, and their sex experience, the superior and mediocre types may be resorted to; but the inferior type has always to be avoided. By the inferior type one's health deteriorates, thereby pleasure diminishes, and sublime absorption vanishes. Therefore, the wise avoid the inferior type.'

However, the Karmamudrā has both an objective and an inner or subjective meaning. To grasp this dual meaning in all its ramifications is of primary importance. Failure to do so will result in a complete misunderstanding of the role the Karmamudrā plays in our life.

It is well known that the meaning of an object is our incipient reaction to it, together with our feeling-emotional tone. For instance, in following the contours of an object with our eyes and exploring its texture with our hands, we perceive the object in relation to our body and this in turn in relation to other objects in space, all of which is known as an awareness of the relation of externality; but we do this in a certain mood, which can only be separated from the sense perception for descriptive purposes. Similarly, sounds are originally part of the total complex of reactions to specific situations. So they also have a reference to the outside, the object and the situation, and to the inside, the feelings, emotions, motivations, and attitudes.[1] Finally, there is the world of meaning, the inner anticipatory process which functions in the rise of all organized life and in the pre-direction of overt and symbolic responses. And so it follows that our response to a person of the opposite sex is not the isolation of ourselves as a self-contained subject and of her as an equally self-contained object, but a relation in which 'I' and 'she' are merely terms. Of importance is the relation, which is that of co-emergence or co-existence. But this co-existence is only 'shadowy', as kLu-sgrub sñiṅ-po[2] points

[1] Words should not be restricted to meaning only discursive language. In our experiences there are many things which do not fit the grammatical scheme of expression, and yet become verbalized. It is unfortunate that that which requires to be conceived through some symbolist schema or other than discursive language and rules of grammar, often happens to coincide with language proper. This is all for the worse. To give an example, the first moment when a man says to his beloved 'my love', this verbalization is pregnant with meaning and feeling. It is certainly not the mere feeling which Rudolf Carnap, *Philosophy and Logical Syntax*, p. 28, Bertrand Russell and Ludwig Wittgenstein in their earlier writings, and others, would like to see this expression reduced to. But this same expression becomes a meaningless noise when the man continues addressing his wife by 'my love', even when his love has grown cold and he is on his way to a divorce court. For a critique of the narrow view of language see Susanne K. Langer, *Philosophy in a New Key*, chapter Discursive and Presentational Forms.

[2] *Caturmudrāniścaya*. The Sanskrit original of this text is found in *Advaya-*

out, because at the beginning it relates to the subject-object dichotomy and fails to realize that this duality is only a term in a wider relation of co-emergence encompassing that which we habitually divide into transcendence and appearance.

Although the emphasis is always placed on the relation and not on its terms we fail to grasp the relation because the terms stand out so conspicuously. Certainly, to make love is something delightful[1] and sex pleasure is a sort of magic spell. But essentially the relation between a man and a woman is an awareness in which appreciation of the 'objective' qualities and 'subjective' responses plays an enormous role. Each moment of the amorous play reveals new and varied experiences. The general feeling of delight, however, is not only the 'subjective' reference; as the 'objective' reference it is the delight in the various techniques brought into play. Since out of the complex situation we can single out one aspect or another, we can reserve the feeling tone for the subjective reference and describe the objective reference or situation apart from it. This accounts for the fact that every phase of the relation has a certain feeling-tone and a particular 'moment'. Moment here does not mean so much a time unit, rather it is the whole situation which may be momentary, for nowhere are moments so precious as in sex play. The variety of delightful experiences is so attractive that we usually attempt to prolong the play or to reinstate it at the next best moment. Therefore, it fails to mature into the uniqueness of the real man–woman relation. The Karmamudrā remains on the level of expectations and frustrations, anticipations and responses. On this level the union of men and women is bound to break up, and this separation is all the more distressing because it isolates each participant. Focused on the subject-object dichotomy it accepts only this dichotomy, thus mistaking what is 'appearance' for the ultimate.

vajrasamgraha, pp. 32 sq. In the preface, p. x, the editor, Haraprasad Shastri, says that 'it has a Tibetan translation where the work is attributed to Advayavajra'. This is incorrect. The work by Advayavajra, *Caturmudrā-upadeśa*, is completely different. It contains a reference to kLu-sgrub sñiṅ-po's dissertation on the Four Seals.

[1] Thus Advayavajra says in his *Caturmudrā-upadeśa*, 214*a*: 'Karmamudrā is delight', and 213*b*: 'Kisses, embraces, and other caresses are variety and delight.'

In the transition from, let us say, sensuality to spirituality, from a partial response to a total response, several points have to be noted. First of all, sexual response and sex relationship depend as much upon tactile as upon psychological stimulation. Tactile stimulation will as much influence the mood of the situation as the mood set up by psychological stimulation will affect sexual responses. Sexual in this sense has a wider connotation than a purely genital response, it relates to the whole of phenomena, mental and bodily, occurring in the course of male–female relations. However, the problem does not consist in setting up a point-for-point correspondence between psychological and tactile stimulations, nor does it consist in equating the four focal points of experience (the crown of the head, the throat, the heart and the abdominal region) in which certain experiences appear to have the highest intensity and functional importance, with the four sections of the nervous system as they are known to us in physiology (cervical, thoracic, lumbar, and sacral)—a chance numerical coincidence which is highly intriguing for those who misunderstand and misrepresent Tantric aims. The problem consists in recognizing the possibilities which a sex relationship offers and in making use of them for gaining a more balanced and more healthy outlook. It cannot be repeated too often that the relation a man has with a woman (Karmamudrā) is not merely biological, a release of tensions, the easing of a locally circumscribed urge; it is much more 'projective', outlining possible ways to a larger whole. That the release of tension often coincides with the attainment of a larger whole does not entitle us to the premature conclusion that after all it is 'nothing but' a biological safety valve.

Stimulation, from whatever source it may come, tears the individual out of his withdrawal from man and is the best means to shatter his naïve belief in man as a self-contained and self-sufficient monad and to make him find the road to truth. The more man comes out of his solitude the more he will observe that his sense of egoness dwindles in proportion to his growing intimacy in communication with others. Particularly when there is the reality of love as the fundamental actualization of the sublime in man and as a movement towards a sensual transcendent without which man will be lost in loveless worldliness, egoness quickly loses its hold over him, and in a corresponding way also the idea of the other as an isolated entity disappears. The movement of love is at first an approach to an equilibrium in which there is neither a subject nor an object and where excitement has given way to a feeling of reciprocity. But only when the man's impetuosity belongs to the woman just as her appreciative and inspiring discrimination belongs to him, only when the treasure of virility and femininity are reflected in each other within the fire of an all-consuming love, only then has there been established and realized a relation whose harmony is based on the moment's charm which is in truth all bliss and yet nothing. In the symbolic language of the Tantras, the gradual disappearance of the subject-object dichotomy and the realization of the non-dichotomic satisfaction which is as much knowledge as feeling, is spoken of as a descent or downward movement of 'enlightenment'. Enlightenment is pure creative potency, manifesting itself on many levels and modes, underlying all cognition and awareness, and having no determinate foundation to restrict the range of its possible terms.[1] This downward movement of 'enlightenment' which, of course, is no descent in the literal sense of the word, but a stretching out to the farthest limits of human existence, allows itself in its expanding to be filled with a definite structure, the structure of male–female relationship finding its tangible expression in the sexual act.[2] In lucid words Padma dkar-po describes this process as follows:[3]

'When enlightenment extends from the crown of the head to the

[1] This is expressly stated in Sphyd 57*b*: 'Being the basis for its abiding in itself and not rising as the bewilderment of the subject-object dichotomy of sentient beings it is the central pathway (*dbu-ma*); from the viewpoint of its rising without becoming diminished in something else, it is non-dichotomic motility (*rluṅ*); since it is found only as a point-instant of brilliancy it is potentiality (*thig-le*), and because of the indivisibility of the reaction potentialities it is indissolvable potency (*mi-śigs-pa'i thig-le*).'

[2] This is also reflected in the language used to describe this process. As long as pure potency which has no structure of its own, is the topic, the terms *thig-le* (*tilaka*) or *byaṅ-sems* (*bodhicitta*) are used, but in the manifest form of the sexual act where this potency is felt as the emission of semen the term *khu-ba* (*śukra*) is employed or, due to the primitive belief that it is the menstrual blood that contributes to the formation of an embryo, *rakta* is used for the female counterpart.

[3] Sphyd 44*b* sq.

throat, body-mind feels somewhat pleasant. The gradual disappearance of the coarse subject-object dichotomy is a joyous excitement known as "delight stable from above". Since this is operating in a variety of erotic activities, the situation is one of variety. After that, enlightenment extends to the heart. Body-mind on the whole feels pleasant. The disappearance of the coarse idea of self is "ecstatic delight". Since there is little endeavour to procure delight but intense pleasantness, the situation is one of maturation. Thereafter enlightenment extends to the navel. Pleasantness diffuses the whole of body-mind. The disappearance of the idea of the partner is "absence of excitement" or "a special delight". Since this pleasantness in which subject and object are as one is the fermentation of the relation (between the two partners), the situation is one of ferment. Enlightenment then extends to the extreme of the sex region. Here it meets the corresponding force of discrimination-appreciation.[1] All that exists of appearance takes on the character of pleasantness and the idea of the three types of joyous excitement disappears. Having the character of the equality of value as far as passion-love and passionlessness are concerned, having come about from the co-emergence of virility with pleasure, this is "co-emergence delight", the intuitive understanding of the non-duality of bliss and nothingness through an individual awareness which is the noetic act as such.' To retain this latter delight and make it spread throughout one's being is the aim of the practice of sex.

It is now abundantly clear that when 'enlightenment' as pure potency achieves determination in the Karmamudrā, the latter is filled to overflowing. The awareness that is now present is not the production of some new thing within a 'container'-mind, because awareness is never within a container, but is always relational—towards something with which formal identity is achieved. In this way the Karmamudrā is both 'appearance' and 'transcendence'. It is in its experience that transcendence may suddenly shine forth, only to vanish before it can be fixed. The *cognitive* mode of

[1] That in this process it is not merely the biological aspect that is of importance, is made clear by the use of the term *śes-rab* (*prajñā*) 'discrimination-appreciation-inspiration' instead of *bud-med* (*strī*) 'woman'. The language thus expresses the shift from the object to the relational operation of awareness.

what goes by the name of Karmamudrā or 'transcending awareness in and through discrimination-appreciation' also marks it off from the *thing*-Karmamudrā, the object of our desires and intentions, so predominant in our ordinary object thinking. And it is this object thinking that is the cause of the confusion about the meaning of Karmamudrā and thereby also our failure to attain enlightenment. The confusion that prevails has been systematically pointed out by Advayavajra (gÑis-med rdo-rje), a contemporary of Nāropa, who states that 'transcending awareness in and through discrimination-appreciation' can be interpreted in three different ways. Two interpretations fail to see the purpose of the initiation into the male–female relationship as an index to transcendence and instead concentrate upon the 'object'. Of these two interpretations one is given by a man who is dominated by his impulses and urges, who is completely enmeshed in sensuality and who, lacking the subtler emotion of love and reciprocity, seeks domination rather than fusion. The other is given by a man who has misunderstood his initiation, because he too fails to see that the relation is of importance and instead concentrates upon the terminal object. Although in both types the sexual act in the natural sense is of paramount interest, each type has a different conception about the course it takes, and hence the classification is rather instructive as to the individual's feeling-awareness and appreciation of the sex situation. Thus Advayavajra says: 'The sensualist declares that love-making beginning with kisses and embraces is joyous excitement and variety. The copulatory act is maturation and ecstatic delight. The experience of the orgasm is the absence of distinct characteristics and the recession of excitement. The emission of the semen is ferment and co-emergence delight.'[1]

Although most people are unable to observe how they behave at and immediately after orgasm and hence are not very informative, the general trend of the above description is clear. As the responding individual approaches the peak of sexual activity he becomes momentarily unconscious at the moment of orgasm and is unable to give any information as to the character of the situation and the feeling-tone which is at least different from the

[1] *Caturmudrā-upadeśa*, 213*a*.

gradual build-up from excitement to ecstatic delight. The state into which the individual is thrown as a result of the tension release provides the satisfaction that usually results from sexual experience.[1] The determination of this state as 'co-emergence' delight seems to be based on a deep-rooted sentiment of many males. Knowing that full sex enjoyment is intimately related to the responses of the woman, yet ignorant of her sexuality and sex enjoyment, they naïvely believe that the full enjoyment for her is a matter of timing. The fact is that this enjoyment depends on the total situation which must be such that the distinctness of herself and of her lover is abolished, so that it becomes a fusion of her and her lover into one. Advayavajra's charge that the sensualist does not know what sex means, is therefore fully justified.

As far as the course of sex activity is concerned the person who has misunderstood his initiation is superior to the sensualist, although he too fails in a very important aspect. This type of person is characterized as follows: 'Love-making with kisses and embraces is variety and joyous excitement. The copulatory act is maturation and ecstatic delight. The experience of orgasm is the absence of distinct characteristics and co-emergence delight. Emission of the semen is ferment and recession of excitement.'[2] Advayavajra then adds: 'However, there is no difference between this type of man and other ordinary people. The reason is that he considers the subjective experience of orgasm as the ultimate.'[3]

This last statement is of the utmost importance, because it again clearly shows what the Karmamudrā is not and what it is also not meant to be. Certainly, it is not the appeasement of a physiological disturbance measurable by quantitative methods, nor is it some sort of hedonism; and certainly it is not meant to be just these together. Hence the two types of interpretation as given by the sensualist, who concentrates on the Karmamudrā as a mere object in a sort of pan-objectivism, and the man who has misunderstood his initiation, because he attempts to reduce intercourse to a purely subjective state, overlook the fact that the Karmamudrā is

[1] The text distinguishes between orgasm as the peak of sexual activity and the spasms and convulsions as the after-effect. The same distinction is made by A. C. Kinsey and others, op. cit., p. 627.

[2] *Catumudrā-upadeśa*, 213*ab*.

[3] Ibid.

a complex referential structure in which both the subjective and objective poles are always found together, and hence does not allow itself to be oversimplified in this way.

There is absolutely no reason for giving preference to the one pole or the other or for denying either. It is only when the individual frees himself from all bias and removes himself to a point whence he can apprehend reality as it is without internal warping, that the Karmamudrā will be properly understood. This is done by and in meditation in the Buddhist sense of the word, as a hard discipline by which the subjective pole is made to approach the nothingness of pure indeterminacy, so that it can give itself more completely to the 'object' or appearance with which it becomes one by terminal identification. Here no attempt is made to achieve ownership or to determine the object by understanding it as a mere object and thereby actually to misunderstand it completely. What happens is rather a determination of pure potency of awareness by the object in an intentional structure comprising both subject and object. To realize this pure potency in all cognitive and feeling enterprises as basic to them, to realize that this potency has no limits and that everything may become its 'terminal object', is the real problem of the Karmamudrā. Therefore Advayavajra says of him who properly understands his initiation into male–female relationship that he will understand sex as follows:

'The outward activity (beginning with kisses and) ending with coital movements is variety and joyous excitement. The experience of orgasm is maturation and ecstatic delight. The moment when each partner's quadruple potency[1]— quadruple it has already been called by the Exalted One—resides in the male organ (*vajra*) and in the female organ (*padma*) respectively, there is absence of determinate characteristics and co-emergence delight. When the two mingle in the female organ there is ferment and recession of excitement.'[2] Advayavajra then sums up his discussion of the three ways in which the Karmamudrā and the initiation into male–female relationship can be understood, in the words: 'Thus the sensualist's relation with a woman is lacking in the Akṣobhya-seal; he who

[1] See Note J, pp. 727 sq. [2] *Catürmudrā-upadeśa*, 213*b*.

has misunderstood his initiation is lacking in the Vajrasattva-seal and in the Vajradhara-respiration. But he who understands it has Akṣobhya sealed by Vajrasattva. This is the Middle Path.'[1]

The seals mentioned here in connexion with the ways of understanding the Karmamudrā, reveal better than any other words the philosophical attitude of the three types of people who practise the Karmamudrā. 'Lacking in the Akṣobhya-seal' means that the sensualist both fails to see that the object is always related to the subject—no subject no object—and does not realize that the epistemological object of his perceptual and thought situation does not guarantee the existence of a physical object corresponding accurately to the epistemological object. The idea of a physical object is nothing primary, but, though not arrived at by inference, is made up of postulates. On the other hand, 'lacking in the Vajrasattva-seal' means that the person who has misunderstood his initiation does not make the mistake of believing in the existence of physical objects apart from the postulates that define that belief, but does make the mistake of conceiving his subjective perceptions as the ultimate answer to the problem of reality. All that he has done is but to subordinate the objective to the subjective pole; both of which are present in experience. But since there is also no subject without an object, his position is as untenable as is the sensualist's point of view. Stated in more philosophical terms, idealism (mentalism) is as mistaken a philosophy as is realism. It is only when we regain that noetic nothingness which is the basis for the attainment of knowledge, and when all our awareness and all our actions are sealed by this nothingness, that we follow the middle path which leads us out of the prison of our own constructions. This is the Vajrasattva-seal.[2]

Padma dkar-po points out that the various phases of the sexual act are related to the Paths of Preparation, Application, Seeing, and Concentrative Attention.[3] As a result the intermingling of the physical and the spiritual in the framework of the Karmamudrā is also evident from the reference to respiration. It is well recognized

[1] *Caturmudrā-upadeśa*, 213*b*.

[2] Ibid. Vajrasattva is very similar to the existentialist's 'intentional structure.' For the meaning of the latter see John Wild, op. cit., pp. 232 sqq.

[3] Sphyd 44*b* sq.

that breathing becomes shallow, rapid, and to some extent even arrested during sexual excitement. The same phenomena occur in intense concentration. On closer inspection, however, we find that the ordinary respiration has given way to another one which is distinguishable as to its depth and which with increasing depth gives a higher feeling of pleasantness and peace.[1] This again shows that to think of the Karmamudrā as a suitable object for relieving oneself of one's tensions is to misconceive and even to degrade it. Sex is doubtless involved, but only as a partial phase in something which includes much more besides.

Like all other human experiences the Karmamudrā cannot be understood without also taking into consideration its intentional structure, on which the outcome of our endeavours as mutual creation or destruction ultimately depends. As such an intentional object of anticipation the Karmamudrā is a presence rather than an object to be manipulated like a thing, and this presence is a reality even if there should be no physical object present. This is implied by the statement that in dealing with the Karmamudrā we may also start with our own being.[2]

While the Karmamudrā is an integral part of and, indeed, a unique opportunity for the noetic enterprise of man, who seeks to understand himself and everything with him, such understanding can ultimately come only from a point of view which is no point of view at all, because if definite it is biased. As long as this enterprise speaks through the Karmamudrā only from the human point of view, it necessarily remains unfulfilled. Although in the loving communion of a man and a woman 'intersubjectivity'—to use a term of Gabriel Marcel—is admirably fulfilled, it is a reduced fulfilment, because it lacks the dimension of the whole of which it is a misunderstood index. This lack is indicated by Saraha and his commentator gÑis-med avadhūti.[3] Saraha's words are:

> He who does not know his entire being believes
> That he will find Great Bliss in copulation.

[1] Respiratory changes in that which approximates to meditation have been investigated by Trigant Burrow, op. cit., pp. 487 sqq.

[2] *raṅ-lus thabs-ldan.* See Sphžg 148*ab*; Sphyd 98*b*.

[3] *Dohākośa-hṛdaya-arthagīti-ṭīkā*, 100*b*.

Like a thirsty man running after a mirage
Will he ever reach the water of celestial space before he dies?
The pleasure in the Padma and the Vajra—
Of what higher bliss is it the merriment ?
Since the former's ground is powerless
How will the aspirations of the three worlds be fulfilled?

gÑis-med avadhūti now says: 'Since most people do not know that that which has no origin and encompasses all sentient beings is Sambhogakāya, Saraha says: "he who does not know his entire being." This is because he is ignorant of the sustaining power of Mahāmudrā, and since at the time of his initiation into male–female relationship[1] the bliss that he feels is not Great Bliss, Saraha elaborates on his ignorance and continues: "believes that he will find Great Bliss in copulation". As the experience of the Karmamudrā which is on the level of mentation, is not the Mahāmudrā experience proper, Saraha refers to it with the words: "like a thirsty man running after a mirage". Such a man will not quench his thirst by fancying as water that which is not water. Similarly he who does not know that Mahāmudrā is beyond all ideas of diversity, infinite like celestial space, and inaccessible to discursive thought, he will run after that which discursive thought and habit-forming memory wants to be the ultimately real. Therefore Saraha asks: "will he ever reach the water of celestial space before he dies?" Both the male and female organs (Vajra and Padma) are ephemeral, and the appearance of "enlightenment" therein is but an ephemeral movement of this "Mind",[2] and since the moment of the situation is not different from this movement, time also is but ephemeral. When the fourfold creativity[3] descends (in the man and the woman)

[1] Lit.: 'at the time of transcending awareness through discrimination-appreciation confirmation'.

[2] *sems, citta.* The context makes it clear that it is not a mind in our sense, although in course of its development it may become this and, at the same time, the feeling of vitality. On the other hand, the physical is a surface phenomenon. Because of the inseparability of the physical and mental, the phenomenon described here is ephemeral. It belongs to the determinate field-character and thus in its determinateness points beyond itself.

[3] See also Note J, pp. 272 sq. The statement that 'two descend and vanish and two become balanced' does not refer to any of the four aspects of the quadruple

passion-desire subsides, when it becomes balanced (between them) there is no absence of passion-desire, it only means that the one stays at the end of the male, and the other in the female, organ. This situation is referred to by Saraha in his words: "the pleasure in the padma and the vajra." This pleasure is but a semblance of the real co-emergence delight. Since one strives for it in the belief that it is the ultimately true, Saraha asks: "of what higher bliss is it the merriment?" If someone were to ask why should this not be the real bliss, the answer would have to be that while the bliss of Mahāmudrā, which is as infinite as celestial space, does not need any prop and is the ground of all that is, the bliss referred to technically as "descent of two and balance of two" is ephemeral, because its basis (the sex region) is powerless,[1] and so Saraha says: "since the former's ground is powerless". While the bliss of Mahāmudrā, which is never on the level of thought, fulfils by its encompassing nature all the aspirations of the three worlds, the pleasure felt in the descent and balance of the two potencies is biased as far as the world of sensual desires is concerned. Therefore Saraha concludes: "how will the aspirations of the three worlds be fulfilled?" '

In the rapture of the Karmamudrā which is the fulfilment of intersubjectivity, the relation between subjects, and not between a subject and an object, the common differences between subject and object, between external and internal, have been transcended. Man is no longer in a world of things which at best have some utility value, but in a world which makes for mutual recognition and respect and hence is full of pulsating life. In the communion with the Karmamudrā there is no desire for domination, no intolerance as to the other's influence. As a matter of fact, this influence is sought for and appreciated. This is implied by the saying that one absorbs the other's being. In this newly won participation everything that has made us miserable, because it excluded us from

potentiality. It relates to the experience of both partners in each of whom the idea of the other as an object disappears. The complete disappearance of this idea is called the balance of the two. This again emphasizes the fact that the Karmamudrā is not a one-sided affair but an intersubjective communion. sGam-po-pa, xix. 15*a*; Sphžg 156*b*–158*b*; Sphyd 45*a* sq.

[1] The physical being but a surface phenomenon cannot serve as a solid basis.

participation on account of our inveterate belief that as a self-contained subject we are thrown into a world of hostile things, has disappeared. In the more poetical language of Saraha, in the communion with the Karmamudrā the glaring sun of brutal worldliness which does not know of mutuality and only lets the differences between us and others stand out more conspicuously, has set. There is, as it were, a twilight period, in which the limits and limitations of subject and object, which after all may have been a subject all the time without our knowing and recognizing it, become blurred and fuse in a refreshing shadowiness. But man cannot content himself with the enjoyment of a relation that goes merely from person to person in the world; he must relate his life in the world to transcendence. This, however, he has not yet done in the intersubjectivity of the Karmamudrā. Therefore Saraha says that the moon has not yet risen. When she does, and with her the stars, we begin to see and to become open to infinite potentialities. It is through these potentialities that man lives. Thus Saraha declares:[1]

> When the painfully scorching sun sets
> The Lord of the Stars and the planets rise together.
> Remaining in the ultimate wondrous manifestations, yet
>   appear;
> They are the ultimately real mystic circles.

And gÑis-med avadhūti explains:

'People who are afflicted by the heat cannot bear to look with their eyes into the orb of the sun. Similarly, certain people, by looking through their physical existence which is as sensitive as the eyes, at the sun of the world which is only dreadfulness, think about the time when this sun will set. With the setting of the sun there rises the cooling light of the Lord of the Stars, pervading with his light the whole sky, and together with their Lord rise the stars and planets. The yogi also only thinks about the time when habit-forming memory, the cause of the world, similar to the painfully scorching sun, will fade. Therefore Saraha sings: "when the painfully scorching sun sets." It is like this. When at the time

[1] *Dohākośa-hṛdaya-arthagīti-ṭīkā*, 101*b*–102*a*.

of the full moon the sun sets, the stars, the moon and the planets rise together. When in the yogi habit-forming memory subsides all-encompassing non-memory, then formless unoriginatedness and unswerving transcendence rise together, and this happens immediately after the Guru's instruction. And so Saraha continues: "the Lord of the Stars and the planets rise together". Yet remaining in the sphere of non-memory, unoriginatedness, and transcendence, it is out of this that the exuberance of wondrous manifestations appears. As Saraha says: "remaining in the ultimate wondrous manifestations yet appear". Non-memory as the mystic circle of Nirmāṇakāya, because out of it the variety of appearance comes forth; unoriginatedness as the mystic circle of Sambhogakāya, because it is understood and felt that the former remains in the sphere of the latter; and transcendence as the mystic circle of Dharmakāya, because being transcendent it cannot be produced (artificially) by meditative-imaginative processes—are the three ultimately real circles; and so Saraha sums up: "these are the ultimately real mystic circles".'

As a unique incitement to the quest for meaning and for the attainment of fullness of life, the Karmamudrā is of tremendous significance:

> Without Karmamudrā
> No Mahāmudrā.[1]

The subsequent instruction in the equality of value in all forms of perceptiveness is the exposition of the nature of mystic philosophy of which William Ernest Hocking concisely says: 'Realism separates object and knower; idealism holds that all objects belong to some knower; mysticism holds that all the objects and the knowers belong to each other,—they are the same reality, they are one.'[2] This oneness is thoroughly dynamic and transforms itself into the reality of subjects and objects as partial aspects of it. And not being an entity this oneness is beyond the idealist's one mind. The transformation described in the body of the text is the same as given by Padma dkar-po.[3]

[1] *Prajñājñānaprakāśa*, 89*a*.
[2] William Ernest Hocking, op. cit., p. 255.
[3] See my *Jewel Ornament of Liberation*, pp. 11 sq. (note 19).

II. MAHĀMUDRĀ

Mahāmudrā (*phyag-rgya-chen-po, phyag-rgya-chen-mo*) is at the heart of and the unifying principle in Buddhist Tantrism. It is the key to and the pre-requisite for everything. It may be said to be a value-system which is at the bottom of or is the ground from which all human endeavour starts and also the path along which this endeavour proceeds in order to be successful, while, as the solution of man's existential problem, it must be experienced in order to be known.

The shortest analysis of the meaning of the word Mahāmudrā is as follows:

> *phyag*: the acquisition of non-dual knowledge;
> *rgya*: bliss since Saṃsāra's tangled skein is disentangled;
> *chen-po*: authentic being (Dharmakāya), free in itself and being the shining lamp of coincidence.[1]

A fuller definition, introducing several points of philosophical interest, is given by Advayavajra:[2]

'Mahāmudrā is the fact that all entities coincide with unoriginatedness, that the interpretative categories of subject and object do not obtain *per se*, that the veils of emotional instability and of primitive beliefs about reality have been torn, and the absolutely specific characteristics (of everything) are known as they are.[3] Hence Mahāmudrā is said to be the immaculate effect. Its actuality is that (i) it has neither colour nor shape as have all other determinate entities which have a beginning, a middle, and an end, that (ii) it is all-encompassing, that (iii) it is unchanging, and that (iv) it

[1] *Karṇatantravajrapada*, 304*a*. This text is not the same as Tshk, which is an 'Oral Transmission' text and only exists in manuscript.

[2] *Caturmudrā-upadeśa*, 214*a*.

[3] *raṅ-gi mtshan-ñid, svalakṣaṇa*. This plays an important role in Buddhist philosophy and has been interpreted variously by the different schools of thought. Scholars who let philosophy come to an end with Kant, equate it with the latter's awkward Thing-in-itself, which is said to be unknowable, although it is the cause of our sensations. In Buddhism it is known directly in a self-revealing mode. The analysis of this problem by the Svātantrikas and Prāsaṅgikas is similar to Bertrand Russell's theory of description which says that '"this is a conch" is true for a suitable this', but we cannot say that 'this' 'exists'. See Bertrand Russell, *A History of Western Philosophy*, p. 895.

stretches across the whole of time. Therefore Mahāmudrā is instantaneous awakening to Buddhahood, which means that the four time-situations and the four delight-intensities are not disrupted.'[1]

From a historical point of view, this definition is taken almost *verbatim* from Saraha, who, though considered as of greatest authority, does not figure in the line of the spiritual teachers of the bKa'-brgyud-pa school whose leitmotif is Mahāmudrā. Saraha declared:

> Having no shape or colour, being all-encompassing,
> Unchanging, and stretching across the whole of time.
> Like celestial space without end or beginning,
> With no real meaning as when a rope is seen to be a snake,
> Being the indivisibility of Dharmakāya, Sambhogakāya, and Nirmāṇakāya,
> Its actuality transcends the regions of the intellect.
> Mahāmudrā which is instantaneous experience of Buddhahood
> Manifests itself in Sambhogakāya and Nirmāṇakāya for the benefit of sentient beings.[2]

The four properties, mentioned in the latter part of Advayavajra's and in the first of Saraha's definitions, are of special interest. All-encompassing, Mahāmudrā transcends the limits of the knowable in the subject-object dichotomy, and without itself being knowable or unknowable, is the source from which everything has sprung, which therefore also is the path to it. sKye-med bde-chen defines this term as follows: '"All-encompassing" means the foundation of all and everything: it encompasses Saṃsāra and Nirvāṇa, cause and effect, appearance and nothingness, and everything else.'[3] sGam-po-pa uses a simile to illustrate its meaning and says: 'all-encompassing is to be like celestial space; in its

[1] They are the same as mentioned previously. Graphically they are:

variedness	joyous excitement
maturation	ecstatic delight
absence of distinct characteristics	co-emergence delight
ferment	recession of excitement.

[2] *Kāyakośāmṛtavajragīti*, 110*b*.

[3] *Dohākośa-nāma-caryāgīti-arthapradīpa-nāma-ṭīkā*, 51*b*.

unoriginatedness it encompasses the world as outer vessel and the sentient beings as the essence contained in that vessel.'[1]

This foundation has neither colour nor shape; only the tangible content of ideas, their definite objects, and the sensible character of all that exists for us have a certain shape and, due to it, a certain peculiarity which distinguishes one thing from another, but in so far as all this takes its life from its foundation it participates in the latter which cannot be said to have an origin or an end unless it is not all-encompassing but merely an event in time. Thus sKye-med bde-chen declares: '"having no colour or shape" means that, although in relation to each other and under certain conditions there is an appearance of the psycho-somatic constituents, of other constituting elements, and of all determinate entities, there is nothing tangible in them, there is unoriginatedness as such.'[2]

Being all-encompassing and indeterminate Mahāmudrā is also unchanging. Only that which is determinate changes and this occurs in something unchanging as the background against which everything stands out in its changeability.

Of particular significance, however, is the definition of Mahāmudrā as stretching across the whole of time. Mahāmudrā is not an event *in* time, it rather *is* time, not restricted to a precious now, but including the past and the future which we usually think of as non-existent. This is a gross error which the Buddhist Tantrics must be credited with not having committed, while in the Western world it needed existentialism to make philosophers aware of their error of conceiving time as a succession of nows. Time is the basic structure of our being alive; it temporalizes itself as a future ahead of us in the form of a goal; as a past in which we have already been but still carry with us; and as a present with which we are concerned in following a certain path of activity, which is full of risks. Stated otherwise, it is from the future that we interpret the past and so direct our present action or, in terms of Tantrism, in view of the goal we lay the foundation for being on our way to that goal. Thus the three aspects of time—or as Heidegger would say, the three ecstasies of time—fit into an integrated union. The past is not

[1] sGam-po-pa, x. 24*b*.

[2] *Dohākośa-nāma-caryāgīti-arthapradīpa-nāma-ṭīkā*, 51*b*.

something that once was but is now cut off and gone, and the future is not merely a not-yet-now that until then is nothing. This existentialist conception of time is precisely the view of sKye-med bde-chen who asserts: '"stretching across the whole of time" means that Mahāmudrā is not something cut off or non-existent like the horns of a hare or a barren woman's child; Mahāmudrā remains the indivisibility of nothingness and compassion for the whole of time.'[1] The last part of this quotation in particular assists us in understanding the meaning and purport of Mahāmudrā as a guiding principle. Although past, present, and future do not exist apart from each other and although there is no cogent reason to give absolute priority to the present, it is the present which offers us an opportunity to choose either to grasp the possibilities that are ahead of us or to maintain and to repeat our past possibilities. If we choose to grasp the possibilities stretching ahead of us and to lead them to decisive action which expresses itself in and is sustained by a feeling of compassion, we live out of the sphere of possibilities which from the ordinary, though mistaken, point of view is nothing as such, but which precisely because of its nothingness prevents us from having our minds filled with dubious ideas and ideals. In this way, being completely open, we link the unfinished possibilities ahead of us in the future with the unfinished possibilities which we have taken over from the past, in meaningful integrity. If, on the other hand, we choose to maintain or to repeat our past possibilities, we fail to provide the link, and the whole structure breaks apart; instead of meaning there is bewilderment-errancy. It is true, we cannot see the past, the future, or the present—indeed, we cannot see time itself; we can only see events in time on the level of a spatial dimension, but we can know time subjectively and practically from within. It is the meaningful integrity that is stressed by sGam-po-pa when he says: 'Mahāmudrā has four characteristics: all-encompassing, without colour or shape, because it is the actuality of transcending awareness, stretching across the whole of time, and neither coming nor going. When it is present in a man he will not consider Saṃsāra to be something that has to be renounced and therefore he will not

[1] Ibid.

shun what is said not to be conducive to enlightenment. Neither will he hold Nirvāṇa to be something restful, and therefore he will not rely on what is said to counter worldliness and so has neither wishful dreams nor thoughts of despair as to the outcome.'[1]

Since Mahāmudrā is not in time, but rather time itself, we can know it either as authenticity in so far as the process holds integrity, or as unauthenticity in so far as there is bewilderment. This latter also is not in time, but is time with the difference that in it, due to our pan-objectivistic tendencies which go by the name of 'ignorance', 'unknowing' time is dissolved into a succession of events and things. Mahāmudrā as authenticity and unauthenticity is referred to by Padma dkar-po in the following words: 'being as such which is unchanging, is the cause of purity itself; its creativity and manifestations are termed the basis and fount of the pure and impure, because it is capable of turning into everything and anything. By virtue of this changeability, it becomes impure in the presence of the condition of ignorance. Therefore rGyal-ba Yaṅ-dgon-pa has made the distinction between authentic Mahāmudrā and bewilderment, (unauthentic) Mahāmudrā, the former being the ground without bewilderment and the latter temporality or bewilderment since time turned into temporality.'[2]

The same distinction is made by sGam-po-pa who terms authenticity 'immaculate Mahāmudrā' and unauthenticity 'maculate Mahāmudrā'. He says: 'Maculate means that one knows Mahāmudrā on the surface only, there is not immediate experience of it; it means that the fetter of wishful thinking and despair as to concrete things has not been loosened.—Immaculate means that it is like a sun-rise in a cloudless sky; that there is neither wishful thinking nor despair, that there is no premeditation, that it is beyond words, that it cannot be turned and twisted into something determinate. It is goal-completion.'[3]

It is with authenticity that sGam-po-pa and the other philosophers of Tantric Buddhism are mostly concerned. For Tantrism is not content with positing a certain ideology, but aims at educating man in such a way that he can do something with or about the

[1] sGam-po-pa, xxvii. 10*a*.

[2] Sphyd 66*a*.

[3] sGam-po-pa, xx. 5*b*.

values it reveals in a comprehensive vision, and thus also at conduct that yields the highest quality of satisfaction. And so it demands what mysticism, the perennial philosophy all over the world, asks man to do. As Hocking puts it: 'The principle of all mystic codes of ethics may be stated in this simple form: *Be what you are*. That is, be in action what you are in reality.'[1] Thus sGam-po-pa says about Mahāmudrā as man's guiding principle in life:

'Mahāmudrā is maculate and immaculate. Here I shall discuss the immaculate form. It is threefold: immaculate (*a*) foundation, (*b*) path, and (*c*) goal. The former (*a*) means that Reality is in itself absolutely pure; the second (*b*) means to take co-emergent spiritual awareness as the path; and the third (*c*) means not to become alienated from the integrity of the indivisibility of ultimateness and awareness.

'In order to make the path immaculate and straightforward I teach this "lotus"-instruction. Here the word "immaculate" means to be free from mind's impurity or the belief in independently existing subjects and objects. And the instruction, which purports to make the path straightforward, is like a lotus flower because, by having determined the immaculate as the ground by philosophical insight and by making it the path (along which to proceed), the immaculate goal is reached. Here a simile: although a lotus flower grows from a swamp, its stem, leaves, and blossoms are not soiled by the swamp. Similarly, first one determines the immaculate (as the) ground; then by attending to its significance when it becomes an intimate experience, one takes the immaculate (as the) path, the radiant light; and this, when the goal is in view, becomes the means of attaining the immaculate (as the) goal, Dharmakāya (authenticity). This "lotus"-instruction comprises four topics:

'(i) The determination of Mahāmudrā by philosophical insight into the immaculate and straightforward:

'The whole of reality is appearance of co-emergent awareness. This is triple:

'(*a*) outer, (*b*) inner, and (*c*) mystic co-emergence.

'(*a*) The former means that the whole of appearance, the outer

[1] William Ernest Hocking, op. cit., p. 271.

objects of the six types of perception, is co-emergent with ultimate reality or nothingness and that ultimate reality or nothingness is co-emergent with appearance. The two do not appear at different times nor are they differentiated into good or bad entities, they are just born together. So also Saraha said: "understand appearance as a teacher; understand the many to have but one value; understand the entities to be co-emergent." Thus, as long as co-emergence is not understood there is belief in an (independently existing) outer object. If co-emergence is understood it is called by virtue of its actuality "co-emergent awareness"; by virtue of its noetic capacity (acting in) an objective reference and owner of the objective reference, it is called "awareness which sees Reality as it becomes manifest".

'(*b*) The noetic capacity, which creates the belief in an ego, is co-emergent with the radiant light or nothingness, and spirituality, the radiant light or nothingness, is co-emergent with the noetic capacity creating the belief in an ego. The two do not rise at different times nor are they differentiated into good or bad entities, they are just born together. As long as this is not understood there is the belief in an ego; but if it is understood then by virtue of its actuality it is called "co-emergent awareness"; and by virtue of its acting in the capacity of an objective reference and of an owner of the objective reference, it is called "awareness which sees Reality as it becomes manifest". So also Saraha declares: "dichotomy is supreme awareness; the five poisons (of emotionality) are (their own) remedy; the objective and subjective poles are rDo-rje-'chaṅ (Vajradhara)."

'(*c*) The noetic capacity which destroys all imputations, positive and negative, is co-emergent with ultimateness. As long as it is not understood, there are imputations, but if it is understood then, sustained by the awareness which is the ultimate, the dichotomy of sensation becomes pure. This indivisibility of ultimateness and awareness is called "awareness which sees Reality as it is" or "non-dichotomic awareness". But in reality it is no awareness (i.e. nothing ontological). So also Saraha says: "(there is) no way, no awareness."

'However, it is not sufficient merely to determine co-emergence by philosophical insight. One has to attend to (what one has seen) and to take it to heart. Hence

'(ii) Attending to (what one has seen) or taking the radiant light as the way:

'The whole of reality has been from the very beginning radiant light, nothingness, unoriginatedness, Dharmakāya. From the very beginning it has been pure and beyond all the limits of words and thoughts. As is stated in a Sūtra: "deep, peaceful, beyond thought, radiant, uncreated." Thus, understanding the whole of reality as unoriginated and in its own sphere as being free of a dichotomizing mind which distinguishes between meditation and non-meditation, existence and non-existence, and other contraries, as postulates, it is to be placed in the sphere which is free of mind in such a way that there is no subject (behind the world of subject and object). So also the great Brahmin (Saraha) said: "let the noetic capacity which is beyond thought stay in the ultimate which is beyond thought", and "let genuine noetic capacity act like a child."

'(iii) Conduct: To take whatever appears, final and free in itself, as the way:

'Whatever one sees with one's eyes, be it great or small, beautiful or ugly, or whatever it may be—whatever one hears with one's ears or whatever belongs to the field of the six types of perception, one determines as before by philosophical insight and attends to it by co-emergent awareness. Then by the power of attention to what one has perceived, at the stage of the subsequent presentational knowledge, whatever one has met with as appearance is understood to be co-emergent awareness and the objects of the six types of perception are thus left free in themselves. It is like recognizing a man one has known before. So also the great Brahmin (Saraha) says:

> The intuition as Mahāmudrā
> Of what appears at the time of its appearance
> Is recognized as simultaneous.

'(iv) To come to the conviction that the goal is self-authenticated and beyond wishful thinking and despair:

'Here "goal" means Dharmakāya; "self-authenticated" to understand that the whole of reality never had an origin and is Dharmakāya, and to comprehend intuitively the non-duality of Saṃsāra and Nirvāṇa.

'(Note: if someone is to ask what goal has been reached by thus taking to heart what has been discerned by philosophical insight, attended to by meditative concentration, and practised in conduct, the following words are relevant): there is neither wishful thinking nor despair. By understanding that Saṃsāra is Nirvāṇa and there can be no wishful thinking as to the attainment of Nirvāṇa apart from Saṃsāra, and by understanding that Nirvāṇa is Saṃsāra, there can be no despair as to falling into Saṃsāra as something evil. So also the great Brahmin (Saraha) declared:

> The three worlds have ever been Buddhahood,
> And so Saṃsāra has been Nirvāṇa.

'To come to this conviction means that all imputations have been destroyed from within and that out of the depth of one's being the assurance about the real is born. Hence there cannot be any wishful thinking or despair as to Saṃsāra and Nirvāṇa, be it only as much as a sesame grain.'[1]

Although here too the achievement of a goal is spoken of, we must not assume that it is in time. Mahāmudrā is never an event in time, rather it is time itself which becomes disrupted if the attempt is made to objectify that which can never become an object of thought. Hence it follows that Mahāmudrā is not restricted to the one or the other phase of the process, but is all phases in an integrated union. This means that Mahāmudrā is inherent in the Karmamudrā which we have seen to be an index, a cipher in Pascal's and Jaspers's terminology. Similarly the feeling intensities which keep the process going and which were discussed in connexion with the Karmamudrā, are not a succession of punctuated quantities, but form a structural whole. This is also what Advayavajra means in his statement cited above that the four time-situations and the four delight-intensities are not disrupted and that the Buddhahood experience is an instantaneous experience in the sense that it stretches across the whole of the process which we

[1] sGam-po-pa, v. 26*b* sq.

erroneously believe to begin and end at certain times, thus converting that which is not in time into something in time. In passing it may be remarked that this error is due to the fact that for descriptive purposes the process can be split up into separate phases, and in this procedure of splintering a well-knit whole into parts, we are apt to overlook the unitary character of the process and to be led into and confirmed in bewilderment-errancy.

As an integrated process Mahāmudrā remains a task rather than being an achievement. Only in so far as the performance of the task has the character of authenticity, can it be said to be an achievement, which again becomes an ever-lasting task, because otherwise it would be an event in time and, as we have seen, Mahāmudrā is not in time. That Mahāmudrā is a task becomes evident not only from the fact that it has to be attended to by meditation and practised in conduct, but also from its name 'Great Seal'. This name has been analysed by Padma dkar-po as follows.[1]

'The term *mudrā* has the double meaning of "to seal" and of "not to go beyond". The first is given by Maitripa who says:

' "The five psycho-somatic constituents are the Five Tathāgatas.[2] In order that four of them may also be understood as mere consciousness they are sealed by Akṣobhya. Inasmuch as in this way it is established that there is no external object (i.e. an ontological object corresponding to the epistemological object of the particular perceptual situation), because the objective constituent of the perceptual situation having a certain external reference is only mind, then also the apprehending subject is nothing (i.e. there is no Pure Ego which would correspond to or be the objective constituent of an introspective situation); however, recognizing some stuff which is neither subject nor object (but the common basis of both), leaves us with pure sensation (or pure experience in William James's terminology). The adherents of that branch of mentalism

[1] Phgdz 26*a*.

[2] The five psycho-somatic constituents and the five Tathāgatas are:

corporeality	Vairocana
feeling	Ratnasambhava
sensation	Amitābha
motivation	Amoghasiddhi
consciousness	Akṣobhya

which speaks of this stuff as being undifferentiated like the cloudless pure expanse of an autumn sky, call it the basic consciousness.'[1]

'Further it has been stated:

> Knowledge devoid of the habit-forming thoughts which
> cause belief in things,
> Is the Akṣobhya-seal;
> Since this in turn is sealed by Vajrasattva,
> It cannot be a concrete independent thing.
> Pure experience alone
> Does not allow us to speak of Vajrasattva:
> Since time without beginning no thing has had a place,
> All that is imagined can be turned to nothingness.

'In this way the stumbling-block of some existing stuff has been removed, and the axiom of the Mādhyamika school of thought remains vindicated—this axiom is that Being which by its very nature is nowhere localized, self-authentic, coincident, and non-dual, is the noetic act in itself.'[2]

It will have been observed that wherever 'seals' are spoken of, the semantic meaning of this term does not relate to entities to which some ontological status can be assigned, but to the act of sealing. Not only does this emphasize the fact that philosophy is a task and not a mechanical system to be taken up and played around with at leisure, but it also abolishes any philosophical atomism which conceives of relations as coupling-rods lying in between the terms from which they are quite distinct. 'To seal', therefore, means that relations are pervasive from their foundational source to their termini. In this sense, the Akṣobhya-seal is the task of seeing everything from a viewpoint of pure sensation, and the Vajrasattva-seal becomes the task of achieving complete spiritual awareness and of being without that partiality which always attaches to every univocal

[1] The similarity of this branch of the Vijñānavāda doctrine with William James's philosophy is remarkable. According to the latter, a given undivided portion of experience which has 'no inner duplicity', can be in one context a knower, and in another something known.

[2] The Tantric analysis of this term is that it means noetic action by itself; the Mādhyamikas analysed it as meaning the noetic act directed towards itself as object. It remains doubtful whether this interpretation was correct and whether the Mādhyamikas did not willfully misunderstand and misrepresent the Vijñānavāda conception.

abstraction. The fulfilment of these tasks is in a certain sense a rediscovery of the source from which we grew and which we allowed to disappear under the tangle of ideological claims and other immature opinions. At the same time every attempt to fulfil these tasks that are ahead of us is a step towards integration which means that the multifarious traits of human nature are organized into a well-knit whole so that the whole functions as a unity.[1]

It is important to note that the noetic capacity is also a mood, because every noetic act is accompanied by a certain mood in such a way that the cognitive aspect coincides with the feeling-tone aspect. Moreover, noetic capacity refers to the patterns of being-in-the-world, communication and situationality which are broader horizons of the individual's acts, words, and thoughts, and in the ultimate world of reality form an indivisible whole, while the three worlds of desire, form, and formlessness (or possible form) are man's limitations, his specifically human characteristics as manifest in his bodily acts, his speech, and the intentional scope of his thoughts.[2] The wider horizons which, though unfathomable because they have not been devised by us, enter into the finite nature of man, impel him to transcend his finitude by becoming aware of their transcendent reality. In proportion to our success in relating our finite existence to the transcendent, the meaning of life deepens and in enlightenment is revealed to be something unchanging and unified rather than a mere succession of passing instants. In no way does the fulfilment of this task, to find meaning, end in the Hegelian delusion of an absolute spirit which simply swallows up human finitude. The task remains an eminently and distinctly human enterprise. It addresses itself to the individual and not to an abstraction. Awareness, which is, according to Buddhist Tantrism, at the core of human nature, is ever ready to unite with and be filled by a term. If this potency is actualized we become aware of the intentional phases and limits of our relational being as interacting with-others in-the-world by body, speech, and mind, and since all awareness is revealing and manifesting we are aware both of our finitude and of our infinite potentialities.

[1] For the meaning of the term Vajrasattva see above pp. 133 sqq.

[2] This is expressly stated in the *Pratipatti-sāra-śataka-vivaraṇa*, 295*a*.

So far we have discussed the meaning of 'seal' as 'sealing', in particular by bliss and nothingness, which makes it possible for man to find contentment and knowledge so that he can live in-the-world without becoming entangled in it and that he can find freedom in all his limitations. In this sense 'seal' corresponds to what we may call some basic pattern or unity theme which serves as an integrating focus for a wide range of specific activities all related to the developmental process leading up to spiritual maturity. Although integration, which essentially means unity between mentality and behaviour, is a feature of development, development itself does not guarantee integration. Therefore, in order to attain integration or spiritual maturity it becomes necessary not to go beyond the values and principles through which we hope to reach those goals which will impart meaning to our existence and to our way of life. This is the second meaning of 'seal', namely 'not to go beyond'. This character is clearly reflected in the statement:[1]

'"Seal" has the meaning of sealing and of not going beyond. It means to seal the patterns of body, speech and mind with co-emergence;[2] to seal with unoriginatedness all entities which pass away in the process of their appearance; to seal experience with non-mentation; and intentionality with resolution and compassion. It means not to go beyond the unity of bliss-nothingness and noetic potency.'

Or, as Mi-la-ras-pa says:

> '*Phyag:* the indivisibility of bliss and nothingness;
> Not to go beyond it: *rGya.*'[3]

It is this latter aspect that has been most lucidly elaborated by sGam-po-pa. He explains the term Mahāmudrā (*phyag-rgya-chen-po*) as follows: '*Phyag* is the intuitive understanding that all

[1] *Caturmudrāvyākaraṇa*, 315*b*.

[2] Although we can easily distinguish between bodily, verbal, and mental processes, it would be dangerous to consider them as separate operations. Such a conception would only facilitate complete disintegration. In order to avoid this and to achieve integration it is imperative to understand that the different processes which owe their separateness to their descriptive analysis occur within a unity. This unity, however, is not achieved by mere addition. It is the all-encompassing and undifferentiated 'field factor'. Co-emergence always refers to this character.

[3] Quoted in Phgdz 25*b*; Sphyd 90*b*.

that appears and is possible, Saṃsāra and Nirvāṇa, do not go beyond the sphere of the ultimate which is unoriginated. *rGya* means that all that appears as something and can become something does not go beyond that which alone is genuine. *Chen-po* means that this happens because of the intuitive understanding that the ultimate is free in itself.'[1]

Philosophically speaking, Mahāmudrā teaches the absolute unity of reality. But if reality is one, we can only know it when we merge with it; when we cease to separate and to step beyond what reality offers, thereby impoverishing ourselves by losing all contact with reality. On the practical side, the Mahāmudrā teaching aims at securing an inner immunity which cannot be assailed by doubts, hopes, and fears, and sGam-po-pa throughout his works declares that this must be a genuine fact of character, not a pose.

12. THE INTERMEDIATE STATE

The intermediate state is one of the most important topics in Tantric Buddhism. Generally speaking, man's life is something between birth and death and, on a smaller scale, a passage between sleeping (dreaming) and waking. But it would be wrong to conceive of the intermediate state as a now, separating the past from the future. In the previous chapter it has been pointed out that Mahāmudrā is not an event in time but rather time itself and in experiencing it man feels that time is close to his inner being. To bring this temporality of his being to the foreground is the aim of the instruction on the intermediate state as the unique means of taking over the past and its unfinished possibilities and linking it with the future as the guiding phase of his being in an integrated structure which will hold from beginning to end. Thus knowing himself not to be merely an object in time but to be temporality, man is called upon to make a choice as to authenticity or unauthenticity, as the existentialists would say. In Buddhist terms unauthenticity would be the disruption of a unitary reality into the events of Saṃsāra and Nirvāṇa, the one succeeding the other in a meaningless flux. It is the moment of decision that holds man's past and

[1] sGam-po-pa, xxv. 2*a*.

future together in an order of wholeness and integrity. Here, as so often before, the terminology and the penetrating analysis of human existence by the existentialist philosophers becomes extremely helpful. To make this decision is the advice which Mi-la-ras-pa gives to the lady bKra-śis tshe-riṅ-ma, thereby revealing his conception of the intermediate state:

> In the intermediate state of Saṃsāra-Nirvāṇa,
> In order to penetrate to Being, Mahāmudrā,
> Try to decide on it as the ground by an act of philosophical insight.[1]

Mi-la-ras-pa discusses seven types of an intermediate state, of which three are of primary importance.[2] They are those mentioned in the body of the text. The intermediate state between birth and death or, as the texts define it, the period after birth and before death,[3] is dominated by the human body 'consisting of flesh and blood'. Although the text emphasizes this aspect, 'body' is here not contrasted with 'mind'. In Tantric terminology 'body' is always a short term for body-mind; it includes what we call mind, and is at best contrasted with spirituality as the all-encompassing reality.[4] Moreover, the present body-mind is a carry-over of the unfinished possibilities of the past. It is thus in the fullest sense of the word a 'path', not in the sense of a link between a past which is no more and a future which is not-yet-now, but in the sense of an unfolding of man's temporality. Hence the two other intermediate states which the texts mention and which will be explained in due course, are not isolated events but aspects of this temporality.

The aim of all instructions has been goal-achievement through man's own efforts. So also the intermediate state is not something ready-made, but a task. Preliminary to a solution is the realization

[1] Bargd 3*a*.
[2] Ibid. 3*b*.
[3] sGam-po-pa, xxxii. 10*a*.
[4] Tilopa, op. cit.; Sphžg; Sphkh; sGam-po-pa, xxx. However, spirituality is not separated from and contrasted with body-mind in an absolute manner. It reaches into the latter and is accessible through mentality. This makes it possible that the same term may also be used for that which approximates to our usage of 'mind'. Once we get rid of our entitative thinking and develop the idea of a field character many apparently unresolvable contradictions will disappear.

of the whole of reality as being of the nature of radiant light, which is equated with the philosophical insight of Mahāmudrā as ground, path, and goal with particular emphasis on the path. The task is a process of attunement as a sort of meditational activity, where meditation must not be understood as discursiveness. In our physical existence, the body consisting of flesh and blood, we are to a large extent governed by passion, lust, and covetousness, and this disruptive power must be attuned to and transformed into the unitive bliss which comes after a complete de-objectification. The moment when these two apparently opposed features become linked is the 'third confirmation' (of transcending awareness through discrimination and appreciation) which 'brings about unsullied bliss'[1] and which is felt in connexion with the Karmamudrā[2] when the idea of the other as object has completely disappeared. Thus again sex, which is never mere sense gratification, is a unique means in the realization of the real. 'Discrimination-appreciation' as a transcending function enables man to become aware of and immediately experience and live by transcending awareness which is the fount of his being. As sGam-po-pa explains: 'transcending awareness through discrimination-appreciation is nothing concrete but is radiancy, non-conceptualization, and bliss. It is the really real of reality.'[3]

In this process of attunement the practices of the Developing and Fulfilment Stages are particularly significant. It is through the former that one relinquishes one's 'matter of fact' status and opens oneself to a world of values. One learns to see the whole of one's environment as a divine mansion of infinite beauty and every man and woman as a god or goddess.[4] This practice, however, serves still another purpose. It makes man see his possibilities for realization. It is as if life is spread out before him as it takes shape in birth, continues in a limited presence, and then in death breaks through its boundaries. Therefore it is said that in conceiving of himself in his whole being (not as being a divine soul in a mortal body) as a god or goddess man purifies himself of the mistaken idea that

[1] sGam-po-pa, xxviii. 3*b*.

[2] See above, pp. 212 sqq.

[3] sGam-po-pa, xxvii. 9*a*.

[4] Dchb 17*b*; Dchlsp 41*a*; sGam-po-pa, xxx. 11*a*.

birth, which is the miracle of creativity or, to use one of Alfred North Whitehead's terms, 'the entry into a world of facts', is something to be held in contempt.[1] The importance attached to the human body in this instance makes it clear that the human body focalizes all degrees of creative activity, including that which soars up to the ultimate. On the other hand, this idea of the intrinsic value of the human body as a whole, the organ of and the means for experience, effectively destroys the notion that spirituality is in fact equivalent to a contempt of the body, such as is displayed in the ascetic habits of 'saints'.[2]

Since men vary in their ability to practise the Developing Stage, the value of the experience gained thereby varies accordingly. In any case, attachment to the ordinary 'objects' is abolished. sGam-po-pa says about the function of this practice: 'by the Developing Stage the intuitive understanding of the coincidence (of spirituality and materiality, of transcendence and appearance) is attained. The mediocre and lower types of those who practise this Stage turn away from ordinary craving. The superior type sees himself as a god, that is, he sees himself as (being of the nature of) the five Buddhas,[3] four goddesses,[4] and sixteen Bodhisattvas.[5] The mediocre type becomes convinced about the apparitional nature of his reality and the inferior type develops an interest for higher things.'[6]

However, it is not that the Developing Stage is absolutely apart from the Fulfilment Stage. They are related to each other in such a way that the Developing Stage is more the 'objective' imagery of the process, while the Fulfilment Stage is the inherent understanding of it. Thus, sGam-po-pa declares: 'to see oneself in meditation as a god is the Developing Stage, to know this god to

[1] Dchb 8*a*; Dchlsp 33*a*, 41*a*; Tshk 9*a*.

[2] William Pepperell Montague, op. cit., p. 61. Howard W. Haggard, *Devils, Drugs and Doctors*, p. 284.

[3] See note 2, p. 231.

[4] The four goddesses Locanā, Māmakī, Pāṇḍaravāsinī, and Tārā symbolize the four materiality functions of solidification, cohesion, temperature, and motion.

[5] They symbolize the interactional fields of sensory perceptions of which twelve belong to the ordinary world of consciousness and four to meditational experiences.

[6] sGam-po-pa, vi. 5*a*.

be like a reflection of the moon in water, like an apparition or like a rainbow, is the Fulfilment Stage'.[1] This can be understood only individually, and hence such references as that it is 'the direct seeing of the radiant light or nothingness'[2] must be understood as imperfect verbalizations or as mere indexes.

The Fulfilment Stage is referred to in a double manner, by a simile and its significance. sGam-po-pa says: 'In Tibet there is a highway connecting the provinces of dbUs and gTsaṅ. To the right of this highway lives a wild boar, to the left a snake, and in the middle of the road an elephant roams. These three animals kill and devour anyone who ventures on this road. They make traffic on it for men impracticable. But these three animals are enemies of each other. If the elephant sets out the snake comes and kills it; if the snake sets out the boar kills it; and if the boar sets out the elephant kills it. Through fear of each other these three cannot move, and in seven days they will die of starvation. The significance of this simile is that the spirituality of man, like a highway, is encompassed by Buddhahood, non-dual transcending awareness. As is stated in the first chapter of the rTags-pa daṅ-po (Hevajratantra):

> There is supreme transcending awareness in the body,
> Though staying in the body it is not of the body.

'Thus, to the right and left and in the middle of the road there are three vital forces, and just as the three animals make any traffic for man impracticable, these three forces within man's spirituality, passion-lust which is like an elephant, aversion which is like a snake, and bewilderment which is like a boar, prevent the birth of transcending awareness which is in his spirituality. Similarly as the three animals die of starvation, these three poisons become non-dichotomic[3] when one has meditated upon the Guru's instruction for seven days.'[4]

[1] sGam-po-pa, vii. 13*b*.
[2] sGam-po-pa, xi. 9*a*.
[3] 'Non-dichotomy' (*mi-rtog, nirvikalpa*) is not merely epistemological, as usually understood by Western scholars. It refers much more to a state where man is no longer divided against himself. Although *rtog-pa* ((*vi*)*kalpa*) 'dichotomy' has to be overcome it is never held to be something bad. It is best understood as a kind of conflict that urges man on toward a solution. Tantrism is

Footnotes 3 and 4 continued overleaf.

Conceiving of oneself as a god or a goddess, as awe-inspiring and as elusive as an apparition, is, in a sense. a preliminary step to the second intermediate state, that of dreaming. As has been pointed out before,[1] a dream is not a passive surrender to a stream of images. It is as much a reality as is the waking state and offers even greater possibilities than the latter with its rigidity of well-defined objects. Hence the dream-'body' is not one of flesh and blood, but one of potentialities, whch are in C. D. Broad's words: 'relatively permanent *after-effects* of actual experiences'[2] and 'relatively permanent *cause-factors* in producing and modifying subsequent experiences,'[3] in brief, 'experientially initiated potentialities of experience.'[4]

It is a well-known fact that most dreams occur shortly before waking up and after a period of deep sleep which, as the texts say, precedes dreaming. For this reason the dream intermediate state is more narrowly circumscribed as the period after the onset of the bewildering play of dream images and before the waking up from sleep. Just as the technique of the intermediate state between

definitely against any attempts to deaden mind. On the contrary it aims at letting mind come to real life. When Karl Jaspers, op. cit., pp. 29–30 says: 'The subject-object dichotomy has many facets: Being-there is within its world which is the environment; consciousness as such is confronted by objects; the mind lives in ideas. Existence stands in relation to transcendence. But environment, ideas, transcendence become objects of cognition only in consciousness through the objectivization in schemata and symbols.—What I know is therefore always object consciousness and hence limited; but though finite, it is a possible springboard toward transcendence,' the same line of thought is developed by sGam-po-pa who stresses the springboard character of knowledge. He says: 'When we lump everything together we can speak of dichotomy and non-dichotomy, but dichotomy itself is Dharmakāya' (x. 34*a*; xxxi. 23*a*). The statement that dichotomy is Dharmakāya must again be understood in the light of the field character of reality. sGam-po-pa continues and says: 'By recognizing dichotomy as a benefactor one makes it the path' (xxxi. 15*a*). Here 'to make it the path' is clearly Jaspers's 'springboard'. The consequence is that only a person who does not use dichotomy as a springboard, but remains with it as if it were unalterable and final, is inextricably involved in the dichotomy and has to bear its pangs. As sGam-po-pa says: 'For those whose outlook is not changed by a philosophical endeavour, there is dichotomy' (xi. 9*b*) and 'those who use dichotomy do not despair over Saṃsāra' (x. 45*a*).

[4] sGam-po-pa, xxxii. 11*ab*.

---

[1] See above, p. 183.

[2] C. D. Broad, *Religion, Philosophy and Psychical Research*, p. 65.

[3] Ibid., p. 63.

[4] Ibid., p. 66. See also sGam-po-pa, xxxii. 13*b*.

birth and death is destined to open man's eyes to wider horizons and to purify him from his objectifying tendencies, because man is not an object, a thing, so also the dream techniques are meant to make man realize his potentialities and possibilities. Thus sGam-po-pa says: 'when today one has seen a spectacle at night one dreams of horses racing (along the course), of conch shells being blown, and of flags being waved and so on, similarly through the power of one's previous firm resolutions at the time of dreaming one recognizes the dream as a dream. One thinks that when one dreams of dogs, women, and other encounters, these are dream dogs, dream women, dream encounters.'[1] In this experience one is led to that realm in which the 'experientially initiated potentialities of experience' are located. Of course, to say that the potentialities are located somewhere is to speak metaphorically. All that one can possibly say is that these experientially initiated potentialities of experience as cause-factors can be subsumed under the designation 'bewilderment', and that they are mainly responsible for the fact that man is divided against himself and finds himself in a world of opposing forces. But just as passion-lust can be overcome and attuned to a feeling of bliss, so also bewilderment, our dividedness against ourselves, can and must be overcome in an attunement to 'non-dichotomy'. The dream state seems to be particularly favourable in this respect, because in dreams the inhibitions of the waking state are largely eliminated and this makes it easier for man to fulfil his existence. This statement becomes more intelligible when we take the following into account. By experiencing whatever appears to him as a dream or a magic spell—dreams and the magic of an apparition are very often mentioned together as being on the same level—man purifies himself of the habit of taking his presence, which is the richness of enjoyment through communication, as something ultimate and solidly reliable.[2] This serves to free him also from his self-deception as to taking his presence and being-in-the-world for granted. It induces him to search for that from which this spell has sprung. To take it for something ultimate would mean to run foul of what Alfred North Whitehead calls 'the fallacy of misplaced concreteness'.

[1] sGam-po-pa, xxxii. 13*b*.

[2] Dchb 8*a*. Tshk 9*a*.

Finally, learning to see in deep sleep the entry into the primordial radiant light out of which man lives and draws his strength, rather than as a passing away into a (merely postulated) nothingness, he loses his terror of death, which is the shining forth of his ultimate nature, because he no longer has any false conceptions about it.[1] Death is certainly not the mere biological stoppage observed from outside. It is, as the following account of the intermediate state of possibilities will show, and as the existentialist thinkers in the West have pointed out with great cogency, much more an inner phenomenon, open only to philosophical analysis and description. In death we become free from our self-imposed shackles, the unauthentic structure of our being-in-the-world. And so the moment we strive and philosophize in the Tantric sense, we die. In death we gain the life of pure transcendence.[2] In this connexion it may be pointed out again that Nirmāṇakāya, Sambhogakāya, and Dharmakāya are not three mysterious entities. Rather they are existential norms. Such norms, as John Wild points out, 'are not determinate traits or properties. They are existential norms, ways of being that are active and dynamic, and must be maintained throughout the whole of life. Furthermore, these norms are not invented or constructed by man. They are grounded on human existence itself, its necessary modes and limits. This existence is authentic when it really is itself. It is unauthentic when warped or deprived.'[3] The same author continues: 'it is noteworthy that each of these norms includes a theoretical as well as a practical component, a way of understanding as well as a way of acting.'[4] This leads to the conclusion that the better I understand myself, the more humane my actions become, the most humane form being benevolence and compassion. And so sGam-po-pa states: 'attention to the radiant light is Dharmakāya, attention to godliness as merely apparitional is Sambhogakāya, and attention to benevolence, compassion, and the striving for enlightenment together with altruism in deeds, speech, and thought is Nirmāṇakāya.'[5]

[1] Dchb 8*a*. Tshk 9*a*.
[2] Sphžg 195*a*, 183*a*.
[3] John Wild, op. cit., p. 262.
[4] Ibid.
[5] sGam-po-pa, xix. 5*b*.

Not only is dreaming as existence fulfilment intimately related to the waking state of the individual—actually the two cannot be legitimately separated from each other as independent entities—it also forms an integral part of sleep. Sleep is often called the younger brother of death, and the similarity between the two has also been pointed out by sGam-po-pa.[1] This has important consequences. For if dream and sleep are modes of existing, death also becomes an existential phenomenon. Death as a mode of existing is connected with the third intermediate state, the one of potentialities and possibilities and the form in which man exists here is termed 'the mind-body'. While the translation of the technical term in this way may be said to be philologically correct, like most similar translations it completely fails to convey a meaning. *yid* (*manas*) is a term capable of multiple definition and being a concept by intuition rather than by postulation, it is a denotatively given particular, not a syntactically designated universal. But although, as F. S. C. Northrop says, 'no amount of syntactical discourse can convey what such a concept means unless one has immediately apprehended and experienced that to which it refers,'[2] the abortive attempt to clarify it has to be made. Thus Padma dkar-po explaining this term which Tilopa has called the most subtle in man, says that 'it is the three types of light which assuming the nature of dichotomy, emotionality, and activity, create Saṃsāra. This creation is not like that of a jar which may exist independently after it has been formed by a potter, it is rather like the clay turning into a jar.'[3] He then explains that to the status of these three types of light when they are about to develop into the action patterns of body, speech, and mind, the term *yid-kyi lus* (*manomaya-kāya*) is applied.[4] This certainly cannot be called a mind in any sense of the word. I therefore suggest that it be called 'the human constant' in so far as it underlies all human activity. But at the same time this 'constant' is not an invariable. In a certain sense it is a carry-over of past experiences and according to the varying degrees of intensity the 'human constant' is varyingly charged.

[1] sGam-po-pa, x. 43*a*.
[2] F. S. C. Northrop, op. cit., p. 448.
[3] Sphžg 10*b*.
[4] Ibid. 15*ab*.

Hence Padma dkar-po points out that 'if any of the three types of light becomes predominant, the two remaining are its attendants.'[1] In actual life this accounts for the differences in temperament. Padma dkar-po makes another statement which is highly significant. He declares that the human constant is 'the actuality of spirituality or the radiant light mixed with the experientially initiated potentialities of experience.'[2] Put more positively, what he is saying is that the human constant is composed of two components, one a determinable field component which in course of time will distinguish one individual from another, and the other an indeterminate and all-encompassing one. Philosophically speaking this means that the human constant is transcendence though simultaneously present in the given and existential. It is precisely because of this field character of the human constant that man is able to turn his eyes either to the indeterminate and all-encompassing field, which leads to the realization of Buddhahood, transcendence, or the radiant light, or to the determinate field with its differentiations being transitory events in time, which in due course will lead to suffering and entanglement in a multiform world. Hence the experience of the human constant is a unique opportunity for attaining enlightenment. sGam-po-pa expressly states that the purpose of this existential phenomenon is to awaken to Buddhahood.[3]

Now every differentiation comes out of something undifferentiated in birth, and fades back into death. Hence the undifferentiated factor is not only prior to all differentiations but even needed by them for their existence. sGam-po-pa confirms this by saying that the radiant light, which appears at the moment of death, is prior to the existential phenomenon of the human constant.[4] This priority, it must be understood, is not something entitatively given, it is an integral part of the human constant, and only the failure on the part of the individual to grasp and understand its total character is responsible for making this distinction between priority and posteriority which is a disruption of something unitary.

[1] Sphžg 15*b*.
[2] Ibid. 10*b*.
[3] sGam-po-pa, xvii. 4*b*.
[4] sGam-po-pa, xxxii. 10*a*.

To regain the unitary character of human existence is the main task of this intermediate state. Just as in the intermediate state between birth and death passion-lust had to be attuned to bliss, thus becoming disentangled from objects and the futile attempt to possess them, and just as in the intermediate state of dreaming bewilderment-errancy had to be attuned to non-dichotomy, both types of attunement being facilitated through certain practices, so also in this third intermediate state aversion-hatred has to be attuned to lucidity. Now it is of the utmost importance that we should understand properly what is meant by passion-lust, aversion-hatred, and bewilderment-errancy, terms with which every student of Buddhism is familiar. Most students will consider these emotionally disturbing forces as inherent in human nature. After all man covets, hates, and is bewildered. They would consider these forces as instincts or appetites which assert themselves in all circumstances, like hunger, in response to internal processes. Tantrism does not share this view. It considers them as potentialities evoked by almost inevitable circumstances. They are completely contingent upon environmental stimuli. This makes a big difference both as to theory and practice. Theoretically it means that passion-lust, bewilderment-errancy, and aversion-hatred, need never have been evoked at all and thereby authentic being could have been preserved. In practice it means that these three forces are capable of sublimation in the true sense of the word as refinement. But what the majority of the psycho-analysts understand by sublimation can never be called so by any stretch of imagination. To divert unavoidable hatred and violence to socially harmless targets is assuredly not sublimation.[1]

The occasion for the sublimation of passion-lust was the practice of the Developing Stage and that of bewilderment-errancy was dreaming, when in the one case passion-lust could be attuned to and fused with bliss and in the other bewilderment-errancy with non-dividedness. The unique occasion for aversion-hatred becoming sublimated and attuned to and fused with the primordial radiant light or the indeterminate field character of the human

[1] See the critique of the Freudian conception in Ian D. Suttie, *The Origins of Love and Hate*, pp. 16 sqq.

constant, is the moment when man temporalizes himself into a concrete human being. This is the moment when, physically speaking, man is about to be conceived in a womb, or as the Buddhist Tantric texts say, when this 'intermediate being' (Gandharva) sees his prospective parents in the act of copulation. At this moment the being to be conceived develops attachment to the mother and aversion to the father if it is going to become a male, and vice versa, if a female. In this case 'aversion-hatred', operating in the third intermediate state, must be taken in a wider sense, covering all modes of response, although the antagonistic element is predominant. However, since this intermediate state is part of man's existence-fulfilment, we need not consider the moment of conception, which as far as the exact biological sciences are concerned is still shrouded in mystery. We find this 'aversion' as sex antagonism in daily life and in particular in dealing with the Karmamudrā. But inasmuch as aversion-antagonism disrupts the unitary existence of man, sGam-po-pa expressly warns us that 'one must not show antagonism or jealousy towards the Karmamudrā, that one has to take an interest in all the entities of reality as apparitions, and that one must not become attached to any object which one may encounter.'[1]

It is now obvious that the three intermediate states—the one between birth and death, the one of dreams, and the one of potentialities and possibilities after death and before birth—are not separate entities. They all are aspects of one and the same existence. Failing to see them as a unity we tend to take them as independent entities; in this way we find ourselves in a state of un-authenticness. In order to regain authentic being an essential task is to attune the various intermediate states to each other. Thus sGam-po-pa expressly states: 'the intermediate state of birth-death has to be attuned to the intermediate state of dreaming, and the latter must be attuned to the former, and both must be attuned to the intermediate state of potentialities.'[2] In otherwords, each intermediate state is an aspect of man's total being and no single one of them can be considered as independent of the other, although each

[1] sGam-po-pa, xvii. 4*b*. See also xxix. 2*a*; xxxii. 28*a*; and xv. 19*b*.
[2] sGam-po-pa, xvii. 4*b*.

aspect seems to be governed by laws applicable only to the level on which the aspect seems to be found.

We have seen that the human constant has a field character, which in its transcendent aspect is likened to the light of a cloudless sky just before sunrise,[1] and which in its determinate aspect is composed of the reaction potentialities of passion-lust, aversion-hatred, and bewilderment-errancy. As potentialities they have an ambivalent character. Being allowed to develop unchecked they become the cause-factors of certain forms of life. Passion generates the unhappy status of spirits, beings insatiable in their greed but always frustrated in the attainment of their desires. Aversion creates the state of hell, a life of suffering, and the infliction of suffering. Bewilderment leads to brute animality. In this triad bewilderment is of a more persistent nature, while aversion and passion have more of a passing quality. Man may recover from his frustration or from his suffering with perhaps little effort, but it needs almost superhuman strength to break through the darkness of bewilderment and out of a state of unknowing to enter the radiant light of transcendence. As Padma dkar-po declares, the latter is only possible for the philosopher who, instructed by his Guru, has made this task the content of his striving throughout life.[2]

But even if sublimated these potentialities are cause-factors of certain pitfalls. Passion creates the status of a god of the world of sensuality, aversion that of a god of pure forms, and bewilderment that of a god of formlessness. Each type is a fragmentation, positive or negative, we may say, and a disavowal of the unitary character of man's existence. Stated otherwise, man's experience of himself as, say, a brute or a god, is a neglect of the transcendent in his total nature. It is only in and through transcendence that what is termed bliss, radiance, and non-dividedness, can have any meaning and thereby become a norm up to which man has to live. These considerations will help us to understand sGam-po-pa's short summary:[3]

'In our being we find passion, aversion, and bewilderment. Through passion we become spirits, through aversion denizens of

[1] Sphžg 187*b*; Bargd 14*b*.

[2] Sphžg 187*b*.

[3] sGam-po-pa, xxxii. 30*a*.

hell, and through bewilderment brute animals. While through these three poisons we are bound to wander endlessly in Saṃsāra, by making them a path according to the teaching of Nāropa, there will be no birth for us (in Saṃsāra). Passion must be sublimated into bliss, aversion into radiance, and bewilderment into non-dividedness. However, by clinging to bliss (i.e. by taking it as something ultimate instead of seeing it as an index) we become gods of the sensual world, to radiance gods of the world of forms, and to non-dividedness gods of the world of formlessness. By understanding this from our Guru we realize that this or that experience is our own spirituality (i.e. an aspect of it); and by understanding our spirituality as unoriginated we do not develop a yearning for a (specific) experience (which always has an origin and hence must end). Then bliss is present (in its own right) and we speak of Sambhogakāya, radiancy is present as Nirmāṇakāya, and non-dividedness as Dharmakāya. The indivisibility of these three patterns or existential norms is Great Bliss.'

The process of dying, not so much as a passage into nothingness, but rather as a change or shift in perspective, has been elaborated in all texts dealing with the intermediate state. It is a sort of home-coming after a spell of alienation and vagrancy. In the symbolic language of the Tantras it is called 'the meeting of mother and child', the 'mother' being the all-encompassing radiant light that shines at the moment of death, ready to receive, as it were, the light freed from the distorting impurities of determinate reactions which had their origin in the reaction potentialities of the human constant. This latter light, though in nothing different from the light with which it may fuse under favourable conditions, is called the 'child'. This symbolism is of tremendous significance. It immediately relates to what is inadequately described as the emotional factor in the nature of man. Buddhahood or the radiant light is characterized as Great Compassion, thus differentiating it from ordinary compassion as a mere sentimentality. It is not of a calculating type, but stretches out boundlessly and spontaneously. The mother also goes on living in the child, however little the child may recognize it. It is for this reason that man, the 'child', can be compassionate and thus is given the chance to live up to the existential norm called Nirmāṇakāya, which consummation is only possible if the other norms are attended to as well.[1]

[1] If in spite of all instructions man cannot awaken to Buddhahood, but will relapse into worldliness, certain instructions are given for avoiding unfavourable forms of birth. These have since become known through W. Y. Evans-Wentz, *The Tibetan Book of the Dead.*

APPENDIX

In the following pages the complete text of the twelve instructions contained only in B is given, while in Note K, pp. 273 sqq., three specimens of text A, a calligraphic copy of which was used by A. Grünwedel for his edition and translation, and of text B, a complete translation of which is contained in this book, are given for comparison.

Tibetan calligraphies abound in orthographic mistakes. Moreover, the letters *ṅ* and *d* are, even in print, easily mistaken for each other. Wherever this occurs it does not mean that there is a *varia lectio.* Anybody who is familiar with the subject-matter also knows the correct spelling. For this reason the many misreadings of A. Grünwedel's transliteration of the text have not been listed. However, two examples of his translation, due to actual or intentional misreadings, are given in substantiation of the harsh verdict that he did not understand this text and that, for other reasons as well, his translation must be characterised as pure fancy.

The blockprint of text B, apart from being difficult to decipher in places, abounds in orthographic inconsistencies. As a rule, I have given these inconsistencies as they occur in the text but have corrected such technical terms as *bskyed-rim* instead of *skyed-rims*, *zuṅ-'jug* instead of *gzuṅ-'jug*, *mṅon-du 'gyur-ba* instead of *sṅon-du 'gyur-ba*, *žu-ba glus bskul-ba* instead of *ži-ba glu bskul-ba*, &c., on the basis of other, orthographically correct, texts.

'The Ordinary Wish-Fulfilling Gem'

(19*a*) gdams-ṅag-gi sṅon-'gro blon-po rigs-gsum las-byed ni/ sdig-sgrib sbyoṅ-ba rdo-rje-sems-dpa'i bsgom-bzlas/ tshogs sog-pa bla-ma'i rnal-'byor/ smin-byed tiṅ-ṅe-'dzin-gyi dbaṅ blaṅ-ba'o// dṅos-gži-la rgyal-po chos-ñid mi 'gyur-ba ni/ thun-moṅs yid-bžin-nor-bu žes-bya-ba bskyed-rim-gyi mtshan yin-la/ bskyed-rim/ cho-ga rnam-pa bži'i sgo-nas/ srid-pa gsum-gyi skye-gnas rnam bži sbyoṅ/ sbyoṅ-tshul ni/ mṅon-byaṅ lṅa skyed-kyi cho-gas mṅal-skyes sbyoṅ/ žu-ba glus bskul-gyi cho-gas sgoṅ-skyes sbyoṅ/ cho-ga gsum skyed-kyis drod-gśer-skyes sbyoṅ skad-cig dran rdzogs-kyi cho-gas rdzus-skyes sbyoṅ-ṅo// de yaṅ skyed-pa'i rim-pas/ skye śi bar-do gsum daṅ rnam-pa 'thun-pa'i sgo-nas/ skye śi bar-do gsum sbyoṅ-ba yin-la/sbyoṅ-tshul-gyi ñams-len dṅos ni/ des-na me-ris dur-khrod daṅ bcas-pa'i gžal-yas-khaṅ gru-bži/ sgo bži/ rgyan rta-babs mtshan-ñid thams-(19*b*) cad yoṅs-su rdzogs-pa'i naṅ sku gsuṅ thugs-kyi 'khor-lo'i lte-ba/ bde-chen 'khor-lo'i dbus-su/ pad ñi 'jigs-byed dus-mtshan gñis snol-ba'i gdan-gy steṅ-du/ drug-bcu-rtsa-gñis-kyi gtso-bo raṅ he-ru-ka sku-mdog mthiṅ-kha/ žal bži phyag bcu-gñis-pa yum daṅ bcas-pa'i skur bžeṅs-pa/ g-yas rkyaṅ-gi stabs-kyis bžugs-pa/ sgeg-pa la-sogs-pa gar dgu'i ñams daṅ ldan-pa/ dur-khrod-kyi chas brgyad-las gos-pa'i rgyan sna-tshogs-kyis spas-pa'i dam-tshig-par bskyed/ yab-yum raṅ-raṅ-gi go bgo/ thun-moṅ-du sku gsuṅ thugs byin-gyis brlabs-la/ skye-srid sbyoṅ/ ye-śes-pa bžag/ rgyas btab/ mchod bstod yab-yum-gyi sñiṅ-po bzlas-pa sogs-kyis bar-srid sbyoṅ/ raṅ-gi sñiṅ-kha'i 'od-zer-gyis snod-bcud rten daṅ brten-par bcas-pa-rnams raṅ-la bsdus-te/ mthar nā-da yaṅ 'od-gsal-du bcug-pa-la/ yun-riṅ-du mñam-par bžag-pas 'chi-ba sbyoṅ/ 'od-gsal-las bžens-pa'i lha'i skur snaṅ-la raṅ-bžin-med-pa-la/ ṅa-rgyal brtan-pa ni/ bskyed-rim-pa'i ñams-len-gyi gdan dam-par bžed-do// žar-la rdzogs-rim-pas skye śi bar-do gsum dṅos-su sbyoṅ-tshul ni/ gnas-pa rtsa'i 'khor-lo/ g-yo-ba rluṅ-gi rgyu-tshul/ bkod-pa byaṅ-chub-kyi thig-le-rnams gsal btab ste/ gtum-mo 'bar-'dzag/ rluṅ-gi rdor-bzlas/ rig-ma 'du-byed-pa la-sogs-pa'i spros-bcas rdzogs-rim-gyis skye-srid dṅos-su syboṅ/ sgom-stobs-kyi rluṅ dbu-mar žugs gnas thim-pa'i rtags bži daṅ steṅ-pa'i 'od-gsal ṅos-zin-pa'i spros-med/ rdzogs-rim-gyi 'chi-srid dṅos-su sbyoṅ/ 'od-gsal-gyi rluṅ sems dbyer-med de ñid phuṅ-po rñiṅ-pa-las logs-su phye ste/ rten daṅ brten-par bcas-pa'i mtshan-dpe gsal rdzogs-kyis spras-pa'i lha'i skur bžeṅs-pa/ bar-do dṅos-su sbyoṅ-byed yin-no// des-na gtum-mo 'bar-'dzag-gi ñams-len-la gnad-du bsnun-pa ni/ rdzogs-rim-(20*a*) pa'i gnad mthar thug-tu bžed-do// skye śi bar-do gsum sbyoṅ-byed/ bskyed rdzogs-kyi ñams-len 'dis/ yab bka' rgyas bsdus/ yum bka' rgyas bsdus/ gaṅ ñams-su len kyaṅ śes-par bya'o// gsum-pa ni/ sbyor-lam rnam bžir 'jug-pa'i tshe/ bza'-ba zas-kyi rnal-'byor/ bgo-ba gos-kyi rnal-'byor/ bkru-ba khrus-kyi . . ./ mchod-sbyin gtor-ma'i . . ./ smra-brjod bzlas-pa'i . . ./ 'gro-'dug bskor-ba'i . . ./ ñal-ba gñid-kyi rnal-'byor bdun-gyis ñams-len-la brtson-pa gal-che-ba yin-no//

'One-Valueness'

(20*a*) bsre-ba ro-sñoms-kyi gdams-pa-la gñis/ bsre-ba daṅ ro-sñoms-so// daṅ-po ni/ spyir bsre-ba 'di-la smin-byed dbaṅ bži daṅ bsre-ba/ bsruṅ-bya'i dam-tshig bži/ grol-byed-kyi lam bži/ 'bras-bu sku bži daṅ bsre-ba ste/ bcu-drug-go// yas-babs-kyi dga'-ba bži/ mas-brtan-(20*b*) gyi dga'-ba bži/ 'bras-bu'i dga'-ba bži daṅ bsre ste bcu-gñis/ 'chi-dus-kyi sku gsum daṅ bsre-ba/ gñid-dus-kyi sku gsum daṅ bsre-ba/ sad-dus-kyi sku gsum daṅ bsre-ba ste bskor dgu/ yaṅ 'dod-chags gtum-mo daṅ bsre/ že-sdaṅ sgyu-lus daṅ/ gti-mug 'od-gsal daṅ/ ṅa-rgyal bskyed-rim daṅ/ phrag-dog dag-snaṅ daṅ bsre ste lṅa/ 'chi-ba chos-sku daṅ bsre/ bar-do loṅs-sku daṅ/ skye-ba sprul-sku daṅ bsre ste gsum-mo// ñams-len dṅos ni/ gnas-lugs-kyi don yin-pa yin thog-tu ṅo 'phrod-pa'i/ blo-bral-gyi śes-pa so-ma yeṅs-med-du skyoṅ-ba 'di-la bžed// gñis-pa ro-sñoms ni spyod-pa'i miṅ yin-la/ de yaṅ bsre-ba ro-sñoms byas kyaṅ bzaṅ-ṅan-gyi chos tha-dad-pa cig bsres-nas 'dres-pa'am ro-sñoms-pa ni ma yin-gyi/ gnas-lugs-kyi don yin-pa yin thog-tu ṅo-sprod-pa-la bsre-ba žes kyaṅ bya/ ro-sñoms-pa žes kyaṅ bya/ yin-lugs-kyi don ṅo-'phrod-pa-la 'dres-pa žes kyaṅ bya'o// ro-sñoms tshul ni/ de yaṅ mig-gi gzugs lta-bu cig-la mtshon-na/ mig-yul-du gzugs cig mthoṅ-ba'i mod-la mdzes-sdug-gi 'dzin-pa cig 'byuṅ/ de-ñid-kyis raṅ-žal-la gcer ltas-pas/ gzugs snaṅ-stoṅ-du 'char-ba spyi'i skad yin ciṅ/ phra-žib-tu phyin de dus phyir yul snaṅ-stoṅ/ naṅ-du śes-pa 'dzin-bral/ zuṅ-'jug blo-'das snaṅ-la ma ṅes-pa gsum cig-char-du 'char/ de-bžin-du rna-ba'i yul-du sgra grag-stoṅ/ sna'i yul-du dri/ lce'i yul-du ro/ lus-kyi yul-du reg-bya reg-stoṅ/ yid-kyi yul-du 'gyu-ba-stoṅ 'gyu-ba-rnams khams-gsum phrugs-su 'char-ba ni/ ro-sñoms tshul drug daṅ/ de-rnams cig-char-du ñams-su len-pa ni/ tshe 'di blos btaṅ 'chi-ba sñiṅ-la cug/ 'gro drug-gi sdug-bsṅal sems/ ci mdzad legs-par mthoṅ-ba'i bla-ma'i mos-gus daṅ ldan-pa des 'du-'dzi daṅ g-yeṅ-ba spaṅs te/ dmigs-med-kyi ṅaṅ-la yeṅs-med-du skyoṅ-ba 'di bsre-ba'i ñams-(21*a*) gyi gnad dam-par bžed-do//

'Commitment'

(21*b*) gdams-ṅag-la gñis/ yid-ches-ba'i myoṅ-ba daṅ/ ñams-su len tshul-lo// daṅ-po ni/ spyir skyabs-'gro'i sdom-pa blaṅs-tsam yin-gyis/ khas-blaṅs-nas dam-bcas-pa'i tshig daṅ mi 'gal-bar byed-pas-na/ dam-tshig sruṅ-ba žes-bya-la/ khyad-par gsaṅ-bsṅags-kyi skyabs-su grags-che žin bye-brag-tu gsaṅ-sṅags bla-na-med-pa'i bum-dbaṅ thob-nas/ snod thams-cad gžal-yas-khaṅ daṅ/ bcud thams-cad lha daṅ lha-mo'i raṅ-bžin-du lta-bar khas-blaṅs-śiṅ dam-bcas-pa'i tshig mi ñams-par byed-pa yin/ de-la rgya-che-ba sku'i dam-tshig-gi rtsa-ba bum-dbaṅ-gi ñams-len/ thuṅ-moṅs yid-bžin-nor-bu/ gñis-su med-pa gsuṅ-gi dam-tshig rtsa-ba gsaṅ-dbaṅ-gi ñams-len steṅ-sgo rnam-par grol-ba'i chos drug/ zab-pa thugs-kyi dam-tshig-gi rtsa-ba śer-dbaṅ-gi ñams-len/ 'og-sgo bde-chen mkha'-'phro'i gsaṅ-sgrogs/ ches-śin-tu zab-pa sku gsuṅ thugs dbyer-med-kyi dam-tshig-gi rtsa-ba tshig-dbaṅ-gi ñams-len/ phyag-rgya chen-po ye-śes gsal-byed-rnams sgom-žiṅ/ de-rnams-kyi yan-lag-tu mi bsag-pa/ sgrub-pa mi 'bral-ba/ bza'-ba/ gsaṅ-ba bsruṅ-ba'i dam-tshig-rnams-kyi ñams-len-la rtson-par bya'o// rgya-che-ba'i dam-tshig-la gsum/ gži tiṅ-ṅe-'dzin (chos)-sku lhan-skyes-kyi sgo-nas bsruṅ/ ñams-myoṅ bde-ba chen-po'i tiṅ-ṅe-'dzin loṅs- sku rtogs-tshul-gyi sgo-nas bsruṅ/ grogs tiṅ-ṅe-'dzin sprul-sku ṅos-'dziṅ-gyi sgo-nas bsruṅ-ba'o// gñis-su med-pa'i dam-tshig-la gsum ste/ gži ṅos-gzuṅ-ba'i dam-tshig daṅ/ lam ñams-su blaṅ-ba'i dam-tshig daṅ/ 'bras-bu ñams-pa bśags-pa'i dam-tshig-go// gži ṅos-bzuṅ-ba ni/ sems rig-stoṅ gñis-med cir yaṅ mi 'dzin-pa-la (*22a*) snaṅ-ba 'gag-med sems-ñid-kyi rol-par śar-ba'o// des-na snaṅ-ba sems-ñid/ sems chos-ñid/ chos-ñid chos-sku daṅ dbyer-med-pas/ gaṅ-du'aṅ mi bsam-pa'o// gñis-pa lam ñams-su blaṅ-ba ni/ sems-ñid 'gro 'oṅ gnas gsum-gyi/ dam-tshig yid-bžin-nor-bu'i sruṅ-'tshams śes-par byas-nas ñams-su blaṅ-bar bya/ 'bras-bu ñams-pa bśags-pa ni/ bla-ma'i sku gsuṅ thugs-kyi dam-tshig ñams-na ltuṅ-ba chen-pos phog-pa yin-pas/ bla-ma dṅos-su bžugs-na/ thog-mar rdo-rje-sems-dpa'i sgom-zlas rtags nam byuṅ-gi bar-du bya žiṅ dbaṅ-bskur-la žu/ mi bžugs-na de'i brgyud-pa-la dbaṅ-bskur bdun-nam/ gsum la-sogs-pa bskyar-te žus-la bśags/ de-bžin-du rdo-rje-spun-la khros-pa la-sogs rtsa-ltuṅ phog-na/ tshogs-'khor-la brten-te dṅos-su bśags/ gžan yaṅ sdom-pa daṅ ñes-byas la-sogs-pa'i ltuṅ-ba byuṅ-na/ yan-lag tshaṅ-ba'i sgo-nas bśags-pa bya'o// bye-brag-tu bla-ma'i sku gsuṅ thugs-kyi dam-tshig-rnams ma ñams-par bsruṅs-na/ dam-tshig kun bsruṅs-par 'gyur-te/ de yaṅ bla-ma daṅ yi-dam yab-yum dbyer-med-pa'i rnal-'byor sgoms-pas/ bla-ma raṅ ni dṅos-bstan/ yum ni rdo-rje-rnal-'byor-ma de/ bla-ma daṅ yi-dam dbyer-med-du bžugs-pa'o// dkon-mchog gsum yaṅ bla-ma'i sku gsuṅ thugs-la thus-te/ bla-ma'i sku dge-'dun dkon-mchog /mkha'-'phro chos-skyoṅ rdo-rje-spun-rnams dge-'dun yin-pas bla-ma'i sku-la thus/ gsuṅ dam-chos/ thugs saṅs-rgyas-su bžugs-so// ñams-su len tshul ni/ des-na bla-ma'i sku gsuṅ thugs-kyi dam-tshig-rnams/ raṅ-gis raṅ-la mkhrel-ba yeṅs-med-du bsruṅ-ba ni gnad dam-po'a// mdor-na dge-bar śes-pa bde-ba'i rgyu phra-žiṅ-phra-ba-nas sgrub-pa daṅ/ mi-dge-bar śes-pa sdig-pa'i rgyu phra-žiṅ-phra-ba-nas spaṅs-pas/ gnod-'gyoṅ med ciṅ dga'-(*22b*) spro gdeṅ daṅ ldan-pa yin-no//

'The Mystic Heat'

(*22b*) gtum-mo'i gdams-pa-la gñis/ go-myoṅ-la yid-ches-bya-ba daṅ/ lam-du 'khyer tshul-lo// daṅ-po-la gsum/ gži dṅos-po lus sems 'thun-moṅ-ba'i gnas-tshul/ lam sgrod-pa gtum-mo ñams-len-gyi rim-pa/ 'bras-bu bde-stoṅ chos-sku mṅon-du 'gyur-tshul-lo// de yaṅ paṇ-chen Nā-ro-pas/

> dṅos-po'i gnas-tshul lam daṅ ni/
> 'bras-bu skye-ba'i rim-pa'o//

ces gsuṅ/ daṅ-po-la gsum/ lus-kyi gnas-tshul/ sems-kyi gnas-tshul/ lus sems 'thun-moṅ-ba'i gnas-tshul dṅos-so// daṅ-po-la gsum/ (*23a*) gnas-pa rtsa bśad-pa/ g-yo-ba rluṅ bśad-pa/ bkod-pa byaṅ-chub-kyi thig-le bśad-pa/ Nā-ro-pas/

gnas-pa rtsa-la g-yo-ba rluṅ/
bkod-pa byaṅ-chub-sems-su śes/

ces gsuṅs/ daṅ-po gnas-pa rtsa bśad-pa-la gsum/ rtsa rags-pa daṅ phra-ba śín-tu phra-ba'o// rtsa rags-pa ni/ rdo-rje-lus mchod-rten lta-bu'i dbus-na/rtsa dbu-ma srog-śiṅ-gi tshul-du yas-sna spyi-bo tshaṅs-pa'i bu-kha-nas/ mas-sna gsaṅ-gnas-su zug ciṅ/ khyad-chos bži daṅ ldan-pa/ de'i g-yas-na ro-ma dmar-mo dmar-la dkar-ba'i mdaṅs chags/ mas-sna lte-'og sor bži-nas dbu-ma-la skyes-te/ yas-sna sna-bug g-yas-la zug/ g-yon-na rkyaṅ-ma dkar-mo dkar-la dmar-ba'i mdaṅs chags/ mas-sna lte-'og sor bži-nas dbu-ma-la skyes-te/ yas-sna sna-bug g-yon-la zug-pa'o// ro rkyaṅ gñis-la yal-ka maṅ-du yod-pa'i/ yas-sna'i rags-pa gñis spyi-bo dkar-cha smin-mtsams-su dbu-ma-la zug-nas rtsa maṅ-du bcas/ de 'og-gi rags-pa gñis mig gñis daṅ sna-bug gñis-la zug-nas las yed/ gžan brla rtsa gñis ma gtogs/ yan-lag-gi 'phar-rtsa-rnams yin/ rtsa dbu-ma-la spyi-bo-na spyi-bo bde-chen-gyi 'khor-lo rtsa-'dab sum-bcu-rtsa-gñis/ kha-dog sna-tshogs-pa'am/ dkar-po chu-khams-pa cuṅ-zad kha 'thur-du lta/ mgrin-pa-na mgrin-la loṅs-spyod-kyi 'khor-lo rtsa-'dab bcu-drug/ dmar-po me-khams-pa kha gyeṅ-du bstan/ nu phrag-gi thaṅ-na'aṅ sñin-kha-na sñiṅ-kha chos-kyi 'khor-lo rtsa-'dab brgyad/ rluṅ-khams-(pa) nag-po kha 'thur-du lta/ lte-ba-na lte-ba sprul-pa'i 'khor-lo rtsa-'dab drug-bcu-rtsa-bži/ ser-po sa-khams-pa kha gyeṅ-du bstan te/ rags-pa brgya ñi-śu/ rtsa phra-ba ni/ sñiṅ-kha'i rtsa-'dab brgyad-kyi rtse-mo re re'aṅ/ gsum gsum-du gyes-pa/ yul ñi-śu-bži'i rtsa/ de'i rtse-mo re'aṅ gsum (23*b*) gsum-du gyes-pas bdun-bcu-rtsa-gñis padma padma-gdan-can-gyi rtsa/ de'i rtse-mo re re'aṅ stoṅ stoṅ-du gyes-pas/ stoṅ phrag bdun-bcu-rtsa-gñis te phra-ba'o/ śin-tu phra-ba ni/ ba-spu'i graṅs daṅ mñam-pa'i bye-ba phrag phyed daṅ bži yod// g-yo-ba rluṅ bśad-pa-la gñis/ ṅo-bo daṅ dbye-ba'o// daṅ-po ni/ lus sems mi 'bral-ba'i rten byed-pa'i (lus) yaṅ žiṅ g-yo-ba de/ skabs 'dir bstan-gyis rluṅ-gi ṅo-bo yin// gñis-pa ni/ rtsa-ba'i rluṅ lṅa'i sgo-nas dbye-na/ thur-sel don-grub rluṅ-gi rluṅ ljaṅ-khu 'dos-na gnas/ gsaṅ-lci 'phen sdom-gyi las byed/ me-mñam rin-'byuṅ sa'i rluṅ ser-po lte-ba-na gnas/ zas 'ju-ba'i las byed/ srog-'dzin mi-skyod-pa chu'i rluṅ sṅon-po sñiṅ-kha-na gnas/ srog 'dzin ciṅ dbugs phyi naṅ-du rgyu-ba'i las byed/ gyeṅ-rgyu 'od-dpag-med me'i rluṅ dmar-po mgrin-pa-na gnas/ mchil-snabs 'dor-ba sogs-kyi las byed/ khyab-byed rnam-snaṅ nam-mkha'i rluṅ 'dkar-po spyi-bo daṅ sor tshigs kun-la gnas/ 'gro 'dug la-sogs-pa'i las byed/ yan-lag-gi rluṅ lṅa'i sgo-nas dbye-na/ me-mñam-gyi yan-lag rgyu-ba mig-gi dbaṅ-po zar-ma'i me-tog kha-phye-ba lta-bu-la gnas/ gzugs mthoṅ-ba'i las byed/ srog-'dzin-gyi yan-lag yaṅ-dag-par rgyu-ba/ rna-ba'i dbaṅ-po gro-ga bcus-pa lta-bu-la gnas/ sgra thos-pa'i las byed/ gyeṅ-rgyu'i yan-lag mṅon-par rgyu-ba sna'i dban-po zaṅs-mo khab-žib-pa lta-bu-la gnas/ dri tshor-ba'i las byed/ 'thur-sel-gyi yan-lag rab-tu rgyu-ba lce'i dbaṅ-po zla-ba bkas-pa lta-bu-la gnas/ ro myoṅ-ba'i las byed/ khyab-byed-kyi yan-lag śin-tu rgyu-ba lus-kyi dbaṅ-po reg-bya-na bde'i spu lta-bu pags-pa kun daṅ/ gsaṅ-gnas-na gnas/ reg-bya tshor-ba'i las byed/ byed-las-kyi sgo-nas dbye-na/ las-rluṅ daṅ/ ye-śes-kyi rluṅ gñis/ sgom-thsul-gyi sgo-nas (24*a*) dbye-na/ pho-rluṅ/ mo-rluṅ/ ma-niṅ-gi rluṅ daṅ gsum te/ re re-la yaṅ gsum gsum-du yod-do// rgyu-tshul-gyi sgo-nas dbye-na/ skye-bu rgan-gžon-daṅ nad-kyi skyon med ciṅ lus ṅal-dub-kyi dus ma yin-par ṅal-bar gnas-pa cig-gis/ rluṅ 'jug 'byuṅ gnas gsum-la khug-pa gcig-tu byas-pa'i ñin-žag phrugs-gcig-la rluṅ ni-khri-chig-stoṅ-drug-brgya re rgyu/ de dbu-mas bdag byed/ de-bžin-du ñin-mtshan mñam-pa'i ñin-mtshan re-la rluṅ khri-brgyad-brgya re rgyu te ro rkyaṅ gñis-kyis bdag byed/ thun-chen bži'i rluṅ-la lṅa-stoṅ bži-brgya re rgyu/ de rdo-rje-nor-bu'i rtsa-'khor-gyi bdag byed/ thun-phran brgyad-la rluṅ ñis-stoṅ bdun-brgya re rgyu/ de sñiṅ-kha'i rtsa-'khor-gyi bdag byed/ 'pho-ba bcu-drug-gi rluṅ-la stoṅ-phyed-daṅ-bži-brgya re rgyu/ de mgrin-pa loṅs-spyod-kyi rtsa-'khor-gyi bdag byed/ chu-tshod gsum-bcu-rtsa-gñis-la rluṅ drug-brgya bdun-bcu-rtsa-lṅa re rgyu/ de spyi-bo bde-chen-gyi 'khor-los bdag byed/ dbyug-gu drug-bcu-rtsa-bži-la rluṅ gsum-brgya so-phyed daṅ brgyad re rgyu/ de lte-ba sprul-pa'i rtsa-'khor-gyi bdag byed/ 'pho-chen bcu-gñis-la rluṅ stoṅ daṅ brgyad-brgya re rgyu/ de 'khor-lo bži-kas bdag byed/yaṅ gsaṅ-gnas bde skyoṅ-gi 'khor-lo/ rtsa-'dab bcu-gñis-la 'pho-chen-gyi rluṅ stoṅ-brgyad-brgya re rgyu/ rtsa bcu-gñis-kyi rtse-mo re re lṅa lṅar gyes-pa'i drug-bcu re la rluṅ sum-brgya drug-bcu re rgyu-ba'i 'pho-'tshams-su ye-śes-kyi rluṅ bcu-gcig bži-cha re dbu-ma-nas rgyu/rtsa chen bcu-gñis-kyi 'pho-'tshams-su ye-śes-kyi rluṅ lṅa-bcu-ṅa-drug bži-cha re dbu-ma-nas rgyu/ sdoms-pas ñin-žag phrugs-gcig-la dbu-ma-nas ye-śes-kyi rluṅ drug-brgya bdun-bcu-rtsa-lṅa re cuṅ-zad mi-mṅon-pa'i tshul-gyi rgyu-bar bžed/ sgo lṅa'i dbaṅ-śes-pa daṅ sñam-du las-byed-pa'i rluṅ ni (24*b*) rags-pa/ raṅ-bžin brgyad-bcu'i rtog-pa daṅ sñam-du las-byed-pa'i rluṅ ni phra-ba/ snaṅ-ba gsum daṅ sñam-du las-yed-pa'i ye-śes-kyi rluṅ ni śin-tu phra-ba'o// thig-le bśad-pa ni/ rags-pa/ a-haṃ gñis-la zer/ phra-ba ni sñiṅ-kha'i mi-śigs-pa'i thig-le/ śin-tu phra-ba ni thog-ma med-pa-nas (pha-ma gñis-)kyi thig-le dkar dmar-gyi daṅs-ma-la zer-ro// sems-kyi gnas-tshul-la/ rags-pa ni sgo lṅa'i dbaṅ-śes/ phra-ba ni raṅ-bžin brgyad-bcu'i rtog-pa/ śin-tu phra-ba ni snaṅ-ba gsum-gyi ye-śes-so// lus sems thun-moṅ-ba'i gnas-tshul ni/ rluṅ phra-ba daṅ/ sems snaṅ-ba gñis thog-ma med-nas chu-la chu žugs-pa bžin dbyer-med-du 'dres-nas 'khor-'das kun-gyi bya-ba rdzogs-par byed-pa/ rgyud rdo-rje-'phreṅ-ba-nas gsuṅs-so// gñis-pa lam ñams-len-gyi rim-pa-la/ gtum-mo'i ṅes-tshig ni/ spaṅ-cha mi-mthun-pa'i phyogs mtha'-dag btsan-thabs-su gžom-par byed-pas-na gtum thob-cha yon-tan-gyi dge-legs-rnams thod-rgal-du skyed-par byed-pa'i ma yin-pas-na mo žes-bya/ ṅo bo ni/ raṅ-byun 'bar-'dzag-la brten-nas skyes-pa'i bde-stoṅ-gi ye-śes de yin/ dbye-na/ phyi'i gtum-mo/ naṅ-gi gtum-mo/ gsaṅ-ba'i gtum-mo/ de-kho-na-ñid-kyi gtum-mo'o// chos-mtshuṅs-ni/ phyi'i gtum-mo/ me daṅ chos-mtshuṅs/ naṅ-gi gtum-mo sman daṅ chos-mtshuns/gsaṅ-ba'i gtum-mo seṅ-ge daṅ chos-mtshuṅs/ de-kho-na-ñid-kyi gtum-mo/ me-loṅ dan chos-mtshuṅs-so// byed-las mi/ phyi'i gtum-mo'i bgegs-rigs stoṅ-phrag brgyad-bcu 'joms śiṅ lus-la drod skyed-par byed/ naṅ-gi gtum-mo'i nad bži-brgya-rtsa-bži ži žiṅ lus-la bde-ba skyed/ gsaṅ-ba'i gtum-mo'i ñon-moṅs-pa brgyad-khri-bži-stoṅ 'joms śiṅ/ lus-la bde-stoṅ-gi ye-śes skyed/ de-kho-na-ñid-kyi (25*a*) gtum-mo'i ma-rig-pa'i mun-pa 'joms-pas gtum/ raṅ-rig-gi ye-śes skyed-par byed-pa'i ma yin-pas-na mo žes-bya/ gnad-sgrim-ni/ phyi'i gtum-mo'i lus-gnad li-khri ltar sgrim-pa/ naṅ-gi gtum-mo'i dmigs-gnad gžu-gduṅs-pa'i rgyud ltar sgrim-pa/ gsaṅ-ba'i gtum-mo'i rluṅ-gnad rtsal-po che'i mda'-'phan-pa ltar sgrim-pa/ de-kho-na-ñid-kyi sems-gnad/ rluṅ-bseb-tu mar-me 'dzin-pa ltar sgrim-pa'o// sbar thabs ni/ steṅ raṅ-byuṅ ye-śes-su sbar te/ steṅ-sgo'i lam ston/ 'og zad-med-kyi bde-chen-du sbar te 'og-sgo'i bcud ston/ bar 'khor-ba rgyun-chags-su sbar te rtsa-rluṅ-gi chiṅs ston-pa yin/ dbye-ba'i skyes-tshad ni/ phyi'i gtum-mo/ skyes-pa'i tshad/ gnas-skabs-su rluṅ rtsol žan yaṅ lus-kyi drod mi 'chor/ naṅ-gi skyes-pa'i tshad/ lus-la nad blo-bur-ba mi 'byuṅ/ gsaṅ-ba'i tshad ni/ las-rluṅ-gi 'gyu-ba chad thub/ de-kho-na-ñid-kyi tshad ni/ rnam-rtog ye-śes-su 'char thub/ rtags bcu ni/ zin-pa thun-moṅ-ba'i rtags lṅa/ brtan-pa khyad-par-ba'i rtags lṅa'o// daṅ-po ni/ sa-rluṅ zin-pas du-ba/ chu-rluṅ zin-pas mig-rgyu/ me-rluṅ zin-pas me-khyer/ rluṅ-gi rluṅ zin-pas mar-me ltar 'bar-ba/ nam-mka'i rluṅ zin-pas nam-mkha' sprin-med 'byuṅ-ba yin te/ ti-lo-pas

'byuṅ-ba lṅa'i rluṅ zin-pas ni/
du-ba mig-rgyu me-khyer mar-me sprin-med nam-mkha' 'byuṅ//

ces gsuṅs-so// gñis-pa ni/ sa-rluṅ brtan-pas lus 'dug tshugs/ ñi-ma'i zer mthoṅ/ chu-rluṅ brtan-pas lus rṅul žiṅ graṅ zla-baṅ zla-ba'i zer/ me-rluṅ brtan-pas lus drod che glog-gi zer/ rluṅ-gi rluṅ brtan-pas lus stobs che 'gro mgyogs 'ja'-tshon/ nam-mkha'i rluṅ brtan-pas lus žan žiṅ bde yod-du mi tshor/ ñi-zla 'dres-pa-rnams rab dṅos/ 'briṅ ñams/ tha-ma rmi-lam-du mthoṅ te/ (25*b*) Ti-lo-pas brtan-pa'i rtags-su ñi-zer zla-zer glog-gi zer daṅ/ 'ja'-tshon ñi-zla-'dres-pa dṅos-su mthoṅ/ yon-tan brgyad ni/ 'thun-moṅ-ba'i 'du-ba bži daṅ/ mchog-gyur-gyi yon-tan bži'o// daṅ-po ni/ rtsa'i nor 'du/rluṅ-gis mi 'du/ thig-les ma-mo 'du/ cha-mñam-gyis khams-gsum-gyi tshe-dpal 'du-ba'o// gñis-pa ni/ 'thur-sel daṅ gyeṅ-rgyu'i rluṅ-la dbaṅ thob-pas/ ñi zla stoṅ-la gnod ciṅ bskal-pa'i thor-rluṅ-gyi kyaṅ gžom mi nus/ srog-'dzin-gyi rluṅ-la dbaṅ thob-pas/ chu-bo chen-po gyeṅ-la zlog nus/ khyab-byed-kyi rluṅ-la dbaṅ thob-pas/ nam-mkhar 'gro 'chag ñal sogs nus-so//

'Apparition'

(25*b*) sgyu-lus-kyi gdams-ṅag-la gñis/ grub-mtha' spyi bžed-kyi sgyu-ma daṅ/ bye-brag rdo-rje-theg-pa'i sgyu-lus bśad-pa'o// daṅ-po ni/ sgyu-ma-mkhan-gyi rde'u śiṅ-bu-la sṅags btab-pas/ skyes-pa bud-med rta glaṅ boṅ dre khaṅ khyim sogs 'khrul-pa mi-bden bžin snaṅ-ba'i dṅos-po-(26*a*) rnams-la bya/ de-lta-bu de mig sṅags-rdzas-kyis slad-pa'i lta-mig-rnams-la bden-grub-tu snaṅ žiṅ zen-pas chags sdaṅ skye/ sgyu-ma-mkhan raṅ-la rta glaṅ-du snaṅ yaṅ žen-pa med/ sṅags-rdzas-kyis ma slad-pa'i mi-la/ rta glaṅ-gi 'khrul-pa'i snaṅ-ba med ciṅ/ rde śiṅ raṅ-sar snaṅ-ba ltar/ snaṅ-srid 'khor-ba'i chos thams-cad so-skye-rnams-la bden-grub snaṅ žiṅ žen-pas las sog ciṅ/ rnam-smin myoṅ-ba byed/ stoṅ-nid mṅon-sum-du rtogs-pa'i/ ñan-raṅ daṅ byaṅ-'phags-rnams-la/ bden-par snaṅ-ba yod-kyi žen-pa med/ saṅs-rgyas 'phags-pa-rnams-la 'khrul-pa'i snaṅ žen gñis-ka med-par/ dag-pa'i snaṅ-ba 'ba'-žig-tu 'char-ro// des-na chos thams-cad sgyu-ma'i dpe bcu-gñis-kyis gtan-la 'babs te/ Nā-ro-pas/

sgyu-ma rmi-lam mig-sgyu daṅ/
gzugs-brñan glog daṅ brag-cha daṅ/
'ja'-tshon chu-zla dri-za'i groṅ/
mig-yor sprin daṅ sprul-pa ste/
bcu-gñis dpe yin don daṅ mtshuṅs/

ces gsuṅs-so// mdor-na 'khor-ba sdug-bsṅal-gyi raṅ-bžin-du śes/ nam 'chi ṅes med sñiṅ-khoṅ-du bcug-nas/ sgo lṅa'i yul-gyi snaṅ-ba gaṅ śar-gyi ṅo thog-tu bžag/ ṅag-tu rmi-lam yin sgyu-ma yin nar mar thol-thol-du smra žiṅ/ yid-kyis mdaṅ-gi rmi-lam gaṅ gsal-ba cig daṅ sres te/ sgo gsum yeṅs-med-du sgyu-lus-kyi dran-pa-la 'bad-par bya'o// bye-brag sbas-don-gyi sgyu-lus ni/ spyir sems-can-gyi lus ni gñis yin te/gnas-skabs-pa'i lus daṅ/ gñug-ma'i lus gñis-so// daṅ-po ni/ rigs drug-tu skye-ba'i/ bag-chags bgos-pa'i 'byuṅ-lus/ gñis-pa ni/

rluṅ-sems-tsam-las grub-pa'i lus-so// gñug- ma'i lus ni gnas-skabs-pa'i lus de thams-cad-du mi 'dor žiṅ 'bral mi ruṅ yin-la/ 'byuṅ-lus rags-pa dor-ba'i tshe-na'aṅ sems-can-gyi gnas-skabs-pa'i lus med-pa ma yin te/ dbaṅ-po kun tshaṅ-gi bar-(26*b*) do'i yid-lus de-ga gnas-skabs-pa'i lus-so// yid-lus de gñug-ma'i lus ni ma yin te/ dper-na chu daṅ tsha-ba bžin-no// gñug-ma'i lus ni rluṅ-sems-tsam-gyi lus te/ dper-na chu daṅ gśer bžin-no// da lta 'byuṅ-lus rags-pa'i dus-na'aṅ gnas-skabs-pa'i lus ni 'gron-khaṅ daṅ 'dra-la/ gñug-ma'i lus ni 'gron-po daṅ 'dra'o// des-na phra-ba gñug-ma'i rluṅ-sems de-ñid rten daṅ brten-par bcas-pa'i/ sgyu-lus sgrub-pa'i gži yin-no// gñis-pa ñams-len-gyi rim-dṅos ni/ rluṅ rtsub-mo steṅ 'og bar gsum-gyi gtum-mo srog-rtsol-gyi lam-gyis gži bzuṅ/ rluṅ 'jam-po yi-ge rluṅ rtsa'i rdor-zlas gsum-gyis sna-draṅs/ ril-'dzin daṅ rjes-gžig bsam-gtan gñis-kyis sdud rim-gyis lus-la gnad-du bsnun ciṅ/ phyag-rgya srog-rtsol-gyi lam-gyi mdaṅs-bkrag ston te/ ñams-su blaṅs-pas sgom-stobs-kyis las-rluṅ-gi 'gyu-ba chad-nas rluṅ dbu-mar žugs gnas thim gsum 'byuṅ te/ žugs-pa'i rtags-su rluṅ mñam-rgyu byed/ gnas-pa'i rtags-su lto-ba mi 'gyu-la/ thim-pa'i rtags-su/ sa chu-la thim-pas mig-rgyu/ chu me-la thim-pas du-ba/ me rluṅ thim-pas srin-bu me-khyer/ rluṅ rnam-śes-la thim-pas mar-me ltar 'bar-ba ste/ rtags bži daṅ/ haṃ-las bdud-rtsi'i rgyun sñiṅ-khar babs-pas snaṅ-ba'i ye-śes/ a-śad-las rakta'i me gyeṅ-du 'bar-ba sñiṅ-khar sleb-pas mched-pa'i ye-śes/ ñi-mas zla-ba gtums-pas ñer-thob śar-ba'i mthar/ thams-cad-stoṅ-pa'i 'od-gsal chos-kyi sku rjen-pa mṅon-sum-pa cig 'char te/ de-na'aṅ thams-cad-stoṅ-pa'i 'od-gsal-las rluṅ g-yos-pa daṅ lugs-zlog-gi ñer-thob grub-pa'i tshe/ 'od-gsal-gyi žon-pa'i rluṅ sems dbyer-med de-ñid raṅ-gi phuṅ-po rñiṅ-pa-las logs-su dbye ste/ mtshuṅs-pa lṅa khyad-chos lṅa daṅ ldan-pa'i mtshan-dpe gsal rdzogs-kyis spras-pa'i rluṅ lus bžin lag-gi rnam-pa-can-gyis/ rten daṅ brten-par bcas-par śin-tu dkar žiṅ 'tsher-ba'i sgyu-ma'i skur bžeṅs-pa yin ciṅ/ de yaṅ thog-mar yid-ṅo daṅ mthar dṅos-gnas-su bžeṅs-so// (27*a*) 'di'i dus-su rjes-śes-kyi snaṅ-ba bde-stoṅ-gi ye-śes rten daṅ brten-par bcas-pa'i sgyu-mar 'char-ro// de-la g-yo-med-du gñis-snaṅ nub-pa'i tshul-gyis 'jogs-pa ñams-len-gyi gnad yin-no// de-lta-bu'i gñug-ma'i lha-sku rten daṅ brten-par bcas-pa ñid/ slar yaṅ phuṅ-po rñiṅ-pa dam-tshig-pa-la ye-śes-pa'i tshul-gyi žugs-nas lugs-zlog-gi snaṅ rtags-rnams rim-par śar-ba'i mig-rgyu'i tshe/ gaṅ snaṅ stoṅ pa/ stoṅ-pa bde-ba/ bde-ba lha daṅ lha-mo'i rnam-rol-du 'char-ba yin-no// gsum-pa 'bras-bu zuṅ-'jug mṅon-du 'gyur tshul ni/ de-lta-bu'i sgyu-ma'i sku de-ñid ri-rab-kyi rdul phra-rab-kyi graṅs daṅ mñam-pa'i phyag-rgya daṅ sñoms-par sbyar te/ 'od-gsal-du yaṅ-yaṅ žugs-pa'i mthus naṅ-du ye śes ran-sgrib-kyi dri-ma zad-pas śes-bya ji-lta-bu'i chos-rnams mṅon du gyur/ phyir śes-bya zad-pas/ chos phra žiṅ phra-ba rnams-la mkhyen pa'i ye-śes rgyas te/ chos-kyi dbyiṅs dan ye-śes gñis-su med-pa'i lam daṅ 'bras-bu'i 'od-gsal gcig-tu 'dres te/ kha-sbyor bdun ldan-gyi loṅs-spyod rdzogs-pa'i sku tshe 'dir mṅon-du byed-do//

'Dream'

(27*b*) rmi-lam-gyi gdams-pa-la gñis/ rmi-lam 'dun-pa'i stobs-kyis sbyoṅ-ba daṅ/ rluṅ-stobs-kyis sbyoṅ-ba daṅ// daṅ-po ni/ mdo sṅags gñis-ka yaṅ chos thams-cad rmi-lam daṅ 'dra-ba bžed-la/ de-lta-bu'i ñams-len-gyi sgo-nas bdag-'dzin-gyi 'khrul-pa bśigs-par byed/ 'di-la yaṅ gñid-nas rmi-lam ma byuṅ-gi bar/ 'chi-ba 'khyer rmi-lam śar-nas ma sad-kyi bar/ bar-do lam-'khyer/ sad-pa sprul-sku lam 'khyer yin-no// des-na ñin snaṅ-gi a-'thas-kyi bden-'dzin gśigs-pa-la sgyu-ma'i dpe bcu-gñis-kyi naṅ-nas rmi-lam mchog-tu gyur-pa yin-no// sbyoṅ-tshul ni/ tshe 'di blos btaṅ/ sgyu-lus-kyi dran-pa yeṅs-med-du skyoṅ-ba'i gaṅ-zag de/ mtshan dus sogs gñid-du 'gro-bar rtsom-pa-na/ mgrin-pa'i rtsa-'khor-gyis dbus-su ñams-len-la gnad-du bsnun-pas/ gñid-kyi rtags snaṅ phra žiṅ myur-ba/ sñiṅ-khar snaṅ-med 'od-gsal 'thug-po śin-tu rtogs dka'-ba cig 'char-ro// 'od-gsal-la rluṅ g-yos ma-thag mgrin-par rmi-lam-gyi snaṅ-ba śar-ba'i tshe/ sgo lṅa'i yul-du gaṅ śar-gyi snaṅ-ba cig raṅ-la yun-riṅ-du gnas-par sbyaṅ-ba/ 'byoṅs-nas du-mar spel-ba/ 'phel-ba'i rnam-pa bzaṅ-por sgyur-ba/ sgyur-ba'i rnam-pa 'jigs-skrag-(28*a*) gi gñen-por sprul-pa/ žiṅ-khams lta-ba sogs-kyi rmi-lam-gyi rdzu-'phrul-la sbyaṅs-pas/ ñin snaṅ bden-'dzin-gyi 'khrul-pa-'jig'go// rluṅ-stobs-kyi bzuṅ-ba ni/ gtum-mo 'bar-'dzag-gi ñams-len daṅ/ srog-rtsol gsum-gyi rdor-zlas la-sogs-pa'i rnal-'byor-pa de/ mtshan dus sogs gñid-du 'gro-bar rtsom-pa na/ goṅ ltar ñams-su blaṅs-pas/ rmi-lam-gyi snaṅ-ba śar-ba'i tshe/ rmi-lam-gyi lus khyad-par bde/ raṅ he-ru-ka rten daṅ brten-par bcas-pa'i skur bžeṅs-pa-la sems yun-riṅ-du gnas-par 'byaṅ-ba/ 'byoṅs-nas bcu-phrag sogs du-mar spel-ba/ 'phel-ba'i rnam-pa dag-pa'i žiṅ sogs-su sgyur-ba/ sbyar-ba sna-tshogs-su sprul te/ kha-cig rigs drug-gi gnas-su sṅon-las sbyoṅ/ 'ga'-žig tiṅ-ṅe-'dzin-gyi rnam-graṅs maṅ-po-la sñoms-par 'jug ldaṅ byed/ la-la žiṅ-khams mi-'dra-ba maṅ-por saṅs-rgyas-la chos ñan-pa sogs/ rmi-lam-gyis rtsol-'byoṅs-par byas-pas/ gñid sad dus ñin snaṅ-la phyi-rol-du bden-snaṅ-gi 'khrul-pa 'dzin ciṅ/ naṅ-du rtsa-mdud-rnams 'grol-bar byed-do//

'The Radiant Light'

(28*b*) 'od-gsal-gyi gdams-pa-la gsum/ gži'i gnas-tshul/ 'od-gsal-gyi rnam-graṅs/ lam ñams-len dpe'i 'od-gsal-gyi rim-pa/ 'bras-bu don-gyi 'od-gsal mṅon-du 'gyur tshul-lo// daṅ-po ni/ gži'i 'od-gsal/ don-gyi 'od-gsal/ dpe'i 'od-gsal/ rtogs-pa'i 'od-gsal/ snaṅ-byas 'od-gsal/ snaṅ-med 'od-gsal/ ñams-kyi 'od-gsal/ de-la gži'i 'od-gsal ni/ 'khor-'das-kyi bde-sdug-la loṅs-spyod-pa'i da-ltar-gyi rig-pa gsal-la ma 'gags-pa 'di yin/ don-gyi 'od-gsal ni/ rog-cig chen-po rgyud-la skyes-pa yan-chad-kyi bde-stoṅ-gi ye-śes-la zer/ dpe'i 'od-gsal ni/ rtse-cig chen-po-nas/ ro-cig chuṅ-ṅu'i bar-gyi mñam-gžag-gi ye-śes-la zer/ rtogs-pa'i 'od-gsal ni/ spros-bral chuṅ-ṅu rgyud-la skyes-pa yan-chad-kyi mñam-gžag-gi ye-śes-la 'dod/ snaṅ-byas 'od-gsal ni/ spros-bral chen-po yan-chad-kyi rnam-par grol-ba'i ye-śes de yin/ snaṅ-med 'od-gsal ni/ rtse-cig-nas spros-bral 'briṅ-po man-chad-kyi gnas-pa'i tiṅ-ṅe-'dzin-la bžed/ ñams-kyi 'od-gsal ni/ gtso che-bar rtse-cig chuṅ 'briṅ che gsum-gyi tiṅ-ṅe-'dzin-la bžed-do// gñis-pa lam ñams-su blaṅ-ba ni/ lam-pa'i gaṅ-zag-la ñin dus sgom-stobs-kyis 'od-gsal 'char-ba cig daṅ/ mtshan dus gñid-kyi rkyen-gyi 'od-gsal btsan-thabs-su 'char-ba gñis yod-pa-las/ 'dir ni gñid dus-kyi 'od-gsal-lo// de yaṅ spyir khams drug ldan-gyi gaṅ-zag/ khyad-par 'dzam-bu-gliṅ-pa'i mi-rnams gñid-du (29*a*) 'gro-bar rtsom-pa-na/ 'byuṅ-ba bži'i thim-rim śar-ba'i mthar/ sñiṅ-khar sems-ñid nam gnas-kyi bar-la/ snaṅ-med 'od-gsal 'char-ba ni khyad-chos yin-la/ de-ñid man-ṅag zab-mo'i gnad-kyis ṅos-zin-na/ ṇaṅ snaṅ-gi 'khrul-pa tiṅ-ṅe-'dzin-gyi ñams-su 'char žiṅ/ sñiṅ-kha'i rtsa-mdud 'grol-bar byed-pa'i gnad zab-mo cig yin-no// dbaṅ bži thob/ dam-tshig daṅ ldan žiṅ/ bskyed rdzogs-la myoṅ-ba thon/ sdug-bsṅal-gyi raṅ-bžin śes śiṅ/ yeṅs-med dran-pa daṅ ldan-pa'i rnal-'byor-pa de/ sna-bži'i dkor zas spaṅs te/ dben-pa'i gnas-su/ bu-su-ku gsum ldan-gyi sñiṅ-kha'i mi-śigs-pa'i thig-le-la/zla drug chig ril-du byed-pa zab-mo'i gnad-do// gsum-pa 'bras-bu ni/ de-ltar spros-byas spros-med śin-tu spros-med-kyi spyod-pa rnam gsum ñin mtshan-du yeṅs-med bskyaṅs-pas/ me-lces 'khyag-rom btsam-thabs-su chu-ru byed-pa ltar rtsa-rnams-kyi mdud-pa žig-nas dhū-tīr gyur/ las-rluṅ-rgyun-chad-nas ñon-moṅs-pa ye-śes-su dag/ thig-le dkar dmar mi-śigs-pa'i thig-ler gyur te/ lus 'ja'-lus sems 'od-gsal bde-stoṅ chos-kyi sku mṅon-du byed-do//

'Transference'

(29*b*) gdams-pa-la gži'i gnas-tshul/ 'pho-ba'i bžed-pa/ lam 'pho-tshul ñams-len-gyi rim-pa/ 'bras-bu 'pho-ba'i sa-'tshams mṅon-du 'gyur tshul-lo// daṅ-po ni/ spyi-bar pho-ba 'di mdo sṅags kun-gyi bžed-pa yin ciṅ/ de yaṅ rgyud-sde 'og-ma gsum daṅ/ mdo-lugs gñis-kas/ 'dug gnas daṅ raṅ lus dman-pa cig-nas/ sems-ñid 'di lam spyi-bo tshaṅs-pa'i bu-kha-nas/ hig-gis 'phaṅs te dag-pa'i žiṅ-du rdzus te skyes-nas/ raṅ rigs daṅ 'thun-pa'i chos-la spyod-par 'dod-do// bla-med-kyi bskyed-rim-pas/ rten daṅ brten-par bcas-pa'i lhar gsal-ba/ 'od-gsal-du sñiṅ-khar 'dus te/ hūṃ yig ye-śes lṅa ldan de-ñid/ tshaṅs pa'i bu-kha-nas rluṅ-gis 'phaṅs te/ 'og-min nam/ u-rgyan-du skyes-nas gsaṅ-sṅags-kyi chos-la spyod-par 'dod/ rdzogs-rim-pa dbaṅ-rnon tshe 'dir 'ja'-lus 'grub-pa-la ni 'chi-ba med/ 'briṅ 'chi-kha'i 'od-gsal ṅos-zin-pa-la ni bar-do med/ rdzogs-rim-pa tha-ma de-la bar-do 'char te/ dbaṅ-po rno-rtul gñis-su yod-pa'i dbaṅ-rnon de bar-do'i snaṅ-ba śar ma-thag/ bsam-gtan gñis-kyis 'od-gsal-du bsdus te lhar ldaṅ-ba'am/ bdun-phrag daṅ-po'i 'chi chuṅ-gi tshe/ 'od-gsal ṅos-zin-nas 'ja'-lus 'grub/ gal-te skye-srịd 'byuṅ-ba'i pho mo'i khrig-sbyor byed-pa mthoṅ-pas/ pha-la sdaṅ žiṅ ma-la chags-pa'i tshe/ pho mo gñis yid-dam gaṅ-run-du gsal btab/ ma'i mṅal-gnas rten daṅ brten-par bcas-pa'i dam-tshig-par bskyed/ raṅ ye-śes-sems-dpa'i tshul-gyis pha'i kha sna gaṅ-run-nas žugs (30*a*) 'dzam-bu-gliṅ-pa'i mi'i lus gsaṅ-sṅags spyod-pa'i rten khyad-par-can-du bsam žiṅ skye-ba blaṅs-nas 'ja'-lus mṅon-du byed-do// dbaṅ-rtul de pho mo 'khrig-sbyor byed-pa'i tshe/ mṅal-gnas-la 'jigs-skrag skyes te/ 'og-min nam/ u-rgyan-du 'phos-nas gsaṅ-sṅags-kyi chos-la spyod-par byed/ sñiṅ-po bla-na-med-pa'i bžed-pa-la/ gnas-lugs-kyi don ṅo ma 'phrod-pa-la 'khrul-pa'am/ 'khor-ba'am/ ma-rig-pa žes-bya/ des-na dbaṅ bži bskyed-rdzogs la-sogs-pa'i sgo-nas gnas-lugs-kyi don yin thog-tu ṅo-sprod-pa'i gdams-pa-rnams-la 'pho-ba žes-bya'o// raṅ ṅo-phrod-pa-rnams-la 'phos-pa žes-bya-bar 'dod-kyi/ ṅan-pa cig spaṅs-nas bzaṅ-po cig sṅar med-par gsar-du sgrub-pa'am/ yaṅ-na ṅan-pa'i chos-rnams bzaṅ-po yaṅ-dag-gi chos-su bsgyur-bar 'dod-pa ni/ gnas-lugs rig thog-gi chos skad-du gtan-nas mi bžed-do// mdor-na ñams-len dṅos ni/ gcig-car-ba'i gaṅ-zag-gi/ bla-ma riṅ-du mñes-par byas phyi-ma 'ba'-žig don-du gñer 'du-'dzi g-yeṅ-bas dben-pa'i gnas-su/ gaṅ snaṅ-gi raṅ žal yeṅs-med-du tshe gaṅ lta-ba 'pho-ba'i gnad zab-mor mthoṅ-ṅo// rim-skyes-pa'i 'pho tshul ni/ sṅon-'gro rtsal chen-gyi dpa'o chas-su gžug-pa/ dṅos-gži rnam-śes-kyi dpag chen-gyi mda' smon-yul-gyi 'ben-la 'phaṅs/ rjes 'ben ṅos-bzuṅ-ba daṅ gsum-gyi sgo-nas/ sku gsum-du 'pho tshul ni gaṅ-zag-gi blo daṅ sbyar te 'pho'o//

'Resurrection'

(30*b*) groṅ-'jug-gi gdams-pa-la phal-pa daṅ mchog gñis yod-pa'i/ daṅ-po-la/ rten-'brel rdzas-la brten-nas 'jug-pa daṅ/ nus bsṅags-la brten-nas 'jug-pa gñis yod-pa'i daṅ-po ni/ rgya-gar-na rig-pa 'dzin-pa'i gaṅ-zag phal-pas kyaṅ/ ro-la bkud-pa'i rdzas/ raṅ-ñid za-ba'i sman/ gñis-ka-la khoṅ-du gtoṅ-ba'i sṅags chu-la brten-nas groṅ-du 'jug-par byed/ sṅags-kyis 'jug-pa ni dbaṅ-phyug-gi bden-tshig bor-ba'i ṅan-sṅags-kyi nus-pa-la brten-nas 'jug-pa'o// mchog sgom-stobs-kyis 'jug-pa-la bskyed-rdzogs gñis yod-pa'i/ bskyed-rim-pas/ phra-mo-la reg-mthoṅ-gi mtshan-ma rñed-pa-nas/ raṅ-gi sdig-sgrib sbyoṅ žiṅ rdzogs-rim-gyi rtogs-pa khyad-par-can thob-pa'i thabs-su tiṅ-ṅe-'dzin-gyi mus-pas 'jug/ rdzogs-rim-pas rluṅ dbu-mar žugs gnas thim gsum byuṅ ste/rtags bži śar-ba'i 'tshams-nas rluṅ sems-la dbaṅ bsgyur-ba'i mthus gžan-don-du 'jug-la/ de-ltar groṅ-du 'jug tshul du-ma yod kyaṅ/ 'dir ni lam zab-mo bskyed-rdzogs-kyi mthus gžan-don-du groṅ-du 'jug-pa'i ñams-len cig ston-pa yin-no// (31*a*) ñams-su len tshul cig-car daṅ rim-gyis-pa gñis yod-pa'i gcig-car-bas/ bla-ma'i mos-gus-la thaṅ-lhod-med-par gtum-mo 'bar-'dzag-gi ñams-len-la myoṅ-ba thon ciṅ/ 'ja'-lus mṅon-du byed tshul-la/ go-ba legs-par chags-pa'i gaṅ-zag de/ ñin dus sgyu-lus-kyi dran-pa yeṅs-med daṅ/ gñid dus rmi-lam-gyi lus khyad-par-ba de/ rten daṅ brten-par bcas-pa'i lha-skur ldaṅ-ba-la gnad-du bsnun-pa ni śin-tu zab-pa'i gdams-pa'o// rim-gyis-pa'i sbyoṅ tshul ni/ rnam 'jug-pa dus-kyi gnad/ gaṅ-la 'jug-pa yul-gyi gnad/ phuṅ-po gsar-pa-la 'jug dus daṅ/ žugs-nas ñams-pa gso-ba rdzas-kyi gnad/ blo brtan žiṅ ñams-myoṅ daṅ ldan-pa/ grogs-kyi gnad-rnams-kyi sgo-nas ñams-len bya'o//

'Eternal Delight'

(31*a*) gdams-pa-la gsum/ gži gaṅ-la ñams-su blaṅ-ba rig-ma'i gnas tshul/ lam dga' bži'i ñams-len-gyi (31*b*) rim-pa/ 'bras-bu zag-med-kyi bde-ba mṅon-du 'gyur tshul-lo// daṅ-po ni/ padma glaṅ-po ri-dags sna-tshogs-can bži/ rigs mchog tshaṅ žiṅ/ sgo gsum phyi naṅ gsaṅ-ba'i mtshan rtags daṅ ldan-pa/ padma'i skyon bži daṅ bral te/ zag/ rul/ nad-med-pa/ 'dod-pas myos žiṅ rnal-'byor-pa-la ṅo-tsha'i rdul daṅ bral-ba/ bcu-drug ñer-lṅa'i bar-gyi na-tshod daṅ ldan-pa cig dgos/ gñis-pa ni/ spyir gsaṅ-sṅags bla-na-med-pa de'i bskyed-rdzogs gñis-kyi naṅ-nas/ rdzogs-rim-pa rluṅ dbu-mar žugs-nas thim rtags śar ciṅ/ tshe 'dir 'ja'-lus mṅon-du byed-par 'dod-pa de/ raṅ-lus gžan-lus gñis-kyi ñams-len-la brtson ciṅ/ de gñis-kyi sgra-bśad ni/ raṅ-ñid-kyi khams mi ñams žiṅ goṅ-nas goṅ-du 'phel-bas-na/ raṅ-lus žes bya'o// gžan phyag-rgya'i rluṅ-gi daṅs-ma raṅ-gi lus-la draṅs-nas/ bde-stoṅ rgyun-chags-su skye-bar byed-pas na/ gžan-lus žes-bya'o// ñams-len dṅos ni/ mkhas-pa bži-la bslab ste/ 'babs-pa-la mkhas-pa mgar-bas me-loṅ brduṅs-pa bžin-du/ rus-sbal-gyi 'gros-kyis dal-bos dbab ste lugs-'byuṅ-gi dga' bži ṅos-gzuṅ/ bskyil-ba-la mkhas-pa rluṅ-bseb-tu mar-me 'dzin-pa ltar/ lta-staṅs drag-gis grims-par bskyil-nas lhan-skyes-kyi raṅ žal lta/ bzlog-pa-la mkhas-pa glaṅ-po-che chu 'thuṅ-ba bžin-du dud-'gro'i 'gyur bžis bzlog-nas lugs-bzlog-gi dga' bži brtan-par bya/ 'grems-pa-la mkhas-pa žiṅ-pa 'bru chu gtoṅ-ba bžin-du bag-yod yaṅs-kyis rtsa-dmig kun-tu khyab-par bkram-nas 'bras-bu'i dga' bži mṅon-du byed/ gsum-pa ni tshogs-drug snaṅ-grags-kyi chos thams-cad zag-med-kyi bde-ba chen-por rgyun chags-su śar-bas phuṅ-po lhag-med-du 'ja'-lus mṅon-du byed-do//

(32*a*) gdams-pa ni/ snaṅ-ba'i dṅos-po 'di thams-cad/ rig-pa tha-mal-gyi śes-pa'i raṅ-rtsal/ lhan-cig-skyes-pa bde-stoṅ-gi rol-rtsed-du gnas-pa yin kyaṅ/ naṅ-du ye-śes raṅ-grib-kyi dri-mas sgribs-nas/ lhan-skyes-kyi ma-rig-pa byuṅ/ phyir gñis-su snaṅ-ba'i kun-btags-kyi ma-rig-pa/ gñis-su gzuṅ-bas las-'bras-la rmoṅs-pas ma-rig-pa ste/ ma-rig-pa'i rkyen-gyis 'du-byed la-sogs-pa rten-'brel bcu-gñis-kyis bsdus-pa'i/ rnam-smin sgyu-lus blaṅs-nas dug gsum-gyi rkyen-gyis/ rigs drug 'khrul-pa'i groṅ-khyer-du/ sdug-bsṅal-gyis mnar žiṅ loṅs-spyod byed-pa'i 'khrul-pa 'di-dag/ bla-ma dam-pa'i žal-gyi gdams-pas ṅo-sprad/ raṅ-rig-pa'i ye-śes-kyi bžugs tshul. raṅ ṅo śes śiṅ/ yeṅs-med-du bskyaṅs-pas tshogs-drug-gi snaṅ-ba thams-cad /lhan-skyes-kyi bde-ba'i rol-par 'char-ro// mdor-na bya-spu rluṅ-gis bskyod-pa bžin-du yul ṅes-med-du 'khyam žiṅ/ rkyen phra rags sbom gsum lus thog-turo-sñoms-pa ni zab-mo'i gnad-do//

'Mahāmudrā'

(32*b*) gdams-pa-la gsum/ mñam-bžag-gi sgo-nas/ skye-med gži-phyag-rgya-chen-po gtan-la dbab-pa/ rjes-thob-kyi sgo-nas/ 'gag-med lam-phyag-rgya-chen-por ṅo-sprad-pa/ zuṅ-'jug-gi sgo-nas/ rjod-bral 'bras-bu-phyag-rgya-chen-po mṅon-du 'gyur tshul-lo// daṅ-po ni/ tha-mal-gyi śes-pa so-ma blo-'das 'di/ gśis ci yaṅ ma yin-pa-la/ rkyen-gyis cir yaṅ byar btub-pa/ gśis don-dam-du bden-par med ciṅ gdaṅs kun-rdzob-tu-rdzun-par med-pa/ dṅos-po'i phyogs-su ma skyes/ dṅos-med-kyi phyogs-su ma 'gags/ tha-dad-kyi phyogs-su mi gnas/ mtha' brgyad raṅ-grol/ yeṅs 'khrul-gyi gol-sa gsum daṅ bral-ba'i/ rnam kun mchog ldan-gyi stoṅ-pa de/ sems raṅ ṅo śes-pa'i mñam-gžag-gi dus-na mṅon-du 'gyur// gñis-pa ni/ stoṅ-nid 'gag-med śar-ba-la rig-pa byuṅ (33*a*) rig-pa 'gag-med-du śar-ba'i raṅ-gdaṅs-la/ ñon-moṅs-pa-can-gyi yid-kyi kha naṅ-du bltas-nas bdag-tu gzuṅ/ yid-śes-kyi sgo lṅa phyir bltas-nas ris-su bcad de 'khor 'das-su miṅ btags-pa'i gzuṅ-'dzin-gyi chos gñis-snaṅ-gi 'khrul-pa 'di-dag kyaṅ/ bden-par snaṅ-tsam-nas snaṅ ma myoṅ-ba/ rmi-lam 'khrul-pa'i snaṅ bas dpes ston te/ rjes-śes sgyu-ma lta-bu cig 'char-ba'am/ stoṅ-par 'char-ba'i dus-na mṅon-du 'gyur// gsum-pa ni/ smra-bsam-brjod-bral-gyi rig-pa gsal-stoṅ 'di/ rkyen gsum daṅ bral-ba/ dga'-ba bži-las 'das-pa/ 'od-gsal-las khyad-par-du 'phags-pa/ blo-'das 'gro-ba'i don-la/ stoṅ-ñid sñiṅ-rje'i sñiṅ-po-can 'char-ba de-ñid/ zuṅ 'jug ro-cig chen-po'i dus-na mṅon-du gyur/ ñams-len dṅos ni/ gnas-na gnas-mkhan-gyi raṅ-žal lta/nam-mkha' daṅs-pa'i skyil ltar/ spros-pa'i mtha' thams-cad daṅ bral-ba'i rig-stoṅ rjen-pa cig 'char/ sgo lṅa'i yul-du snaṅ-na snaṅ mkhan-gyi raṅ žal lta/ a-'thas bden-grub-kyi snaṅ-ba/ ro-cig bde-stoṅ sgyu-ma lta-bur 'char/ 'phro-na 'phro-mkhan-gyi raṅ-žal lta/ 'phro-ba yul-med-du mñam-gžag-gi rtogs-pa'i gdaṅs/ dmigs-med-kyi sñiṅ-rje/ 'khrul-pa'i sems-can-gyi don byed-pa/ sgom-med chuṅ-ṅuyan-chad-la mṅon 'gyur-pas/ gnas 'gyu'i raṅ-žal lta-ba'i gnad śin-tu zab-mo// sgom-med dpa'o rtag-tu mñam-gžag kho-na yin kyaṅ/ rjes-śes 'jig-rten-las 'das-pa'i lam sñiṅ-rjer 'char-ba mi 'gal te/ sdud-pa-las/

phuṅ-po 'di-dag gdod-nas stoṅ žiṅ bdag-med śes/
mñam-par ma gžag sems-can khams-la sñoms-par 'jug/
bar-skabs der yaṅ saṅs-rgyas chos-la yoṅs mi dma'/

ces gsuṅs-so//

'The Intermediate State'

(33*b*) gdams-ṅag-la lṅa/ sbyaṅ-bya lus ldan-gyi bar-do ṅos-gzuṅ-ba/ sbyaṅ-gži chos-ñid mtshan-ma'i bar-do 'od-gsal ma-yi gnas-tshul bstan-pa/ sbyaṅ-bya dri-ma-can chos-can chos-ñid-kyi bar-do/ sbyaṅ byed sre-ba lam-gyi gdams-pas 'od-gsal bu'i 'char thabs sbyaṅ/ (34*a*) 'bras mṅon-du 'gyur tshul-lo// daṅ-po ni skye śi bar-do rnam-smin sa-khrag-gi lus/ rmi-lam bar-do phra-ba rluṅ sems dbyer-med-kyi lus/ srid-pa bar-do dri-za yid-kyi lus-so// gñis-pa ni/ gliṅ bži-pa'i mi-rnams 'chi-bar rtsom-pa-na/ 'byuṅ-ba bži'i thim-rim 'char ciṅ'/ snaṅ mched thob gsum śar-ba'i mthar/ thams-cad-stoṅ-pa'i 'od-gsal ston-dus-kyi tho-raṅs nam-mkha' g-ya'-dag-pa lta-bu/ skye 'gro kun-la 'char-ba ni 'od-gsal ma yin-no// gsum-pa ni chos-can chos-ñid-kyi bar-do byas kyaṅ/ gnas 'gyu gñis yin lags/ gnas-pa ñid gti-mug-gi dri-ma-can-gyis 'dud-'gro'i rgyu byed/ 'gyu-ba chags-sdaṅ-gi dri-ma-can-gyis yi-dags daṅ dmyal-ba'i rgyu byed-pas/ dug gsum-gyi rtog-pa dri-ma-can ni sbyaṅ-bya'o// bži-pa ni lam sgom-pa-po'i gaṅ-zag-gi sgom-stobs-kyis rluṅ dbu-mar žugs gnas thim gsum byuṅ-nas/ rtags bži daṅ stoṅ-pa gsum-gyi mthar/ thams-cad-stoṅ-pa'i 'od-gsal 'char-ba ni/ 'od gsal bu te/ skye śi bar-do gsum daṅ sre byed dṅos-so// lṅa-pa ni/ rdzogs-rim-pa 'chi-ba-la sṅon-du phyogs-pa'i gaṅ-zag-la/ dbaṅ-po rno-brtul gñis yod-pa'i/ dbaṅ-rnon de rtags snaṅ-rnams śar-ba'i mthar/ 'od-gsal-las rluṅ g-yos ma-thag śin-tu phra-ba'i rluṅ sems dbyer-med de-ñid/ ṅes-pa lṅa ldan mtshuṅs-pa lṅa ldan-gyi skur bzeṅs te/ loṅs-spyod-rdzogs-skur saṅ-rgya/ gaṅ-zag dbaṅ-rtul de/ 'od-gsal-las rluṅ g-yos ma-thag/ ṅes ma-ṅes-kyi rtags drug daṅ ldan-pa'i bar-do 'grub-la/ yon-tan bdun ldan-gyi bar-do de ñams-len-gyi gnad-kyi phuṅ-po 'od-gsal-du yaṅ-yaṅ bžus-pa'i mthus/ bdun-phrag gñis-pa'i 'chi chuṅ-gi 'od-gsal-las rluṅ g-yos-pa'i tshe/ 'ja'-lus grub te rten de-las saṅ-rgya/

gal-srid ma grub-na/ 'dzam-bu-gliṅ-pa'i mi (34*b*) pho mo 'khrig-pa spyod-pa mthoṅ-ba'i tshe'ma-la chags-pa'i mṅal-du gsaṅ-sṅags-spyod-pa'i rten khyad-par-can-du bsam žiṅ skye-ba blaṅs-nas/ rten de-las 'ja'-lus mṅon-du byed-do//

NOTES

NOTE A. The Three Kāyas, Dharmakāya, Sambhogakāya, and Nirmāṇakāya, can be subsumed under Dharmakāya and Rūpakāya, both of which form an integral unity. Dharmakāya is an abbreviation for Jñāna-dharmakāya and signifies the noetic mode in man when it is divested of all bias and presupposition. This cognitive mode is always in union with the operational mode (Rūpakāya) which manifests itself as communication-with-others (Sambhogakāya) and significant being-in-the-world (Nirmāṇakāya). In a certain sense, the operational mode presupposes the cognitive mode; on the other hand, the cognitive mode needs the operational one in order to express itself. In symbol representations Dharmakāya becomes rDo-rje-'chaṅ and Sambhogakāya the five so-called Dhyānibuddhas (*rgyal-ba rigs-lṅa*). Because of the intimate connexion between Dharmakāya and Sambhogakāya, rDo-rje-'chaṅ is not some divine personality apart from the Dhyānibuddhas, but is merely *primus inter pares*. This is indicated by the term *dbaṅ*, which is a short expression for *bdag-por gyur-pa* 'having become the lord (amongst others)'. Each Sambhogakāya represents an integral unity of the noetic and communicative. This is indicated by the term *rdo-rje rnal-'byor* (*vajrayoga*). In Buddhism, *yoga* never means to become swallowed up by an Absolute, it always indicates the union of the noetic (*prajñā*) and the communicative (*upāya*) and thus insists on the harmony between action, speech, and thought, which are called *vajra* because in this realm of discourse there is unbiased perspective (*thugs*), not opinionatedness; authentic communication (*gsuṅ*), not empty verbiage; and significant being-in-the-world (*sku*), not the anonymity of the mass man. Significant being-in-the-world is not restricted to any determinate form. In Nāropa's case it refers to the various forms in which he saw his teacher Tilopa who also was known as Prajñābhadra. The relation between Nāropa and Tilopa is to be understood dialectically. What appears to be the activity of Nāropa is that of Tilopa and through him of Vajradhara, and vice versa. The equation of space and Dharmakāya is frequently found in bKa'-brgyud-pa works. The dGe-lugs-pas object to it on the ground that in view of the fact that Reality can be considered as consisting of that which is real and exists and that which is real but does not exist, Dharmakāya would have to be classified as something that is real and exists and hence is transitory, while space is real, but does not exist and hence is eternal.

NOTE B. That which is termed *śūnyatā* is so different from all that we think and feel and to which we are attached that in comparison it is just 'nothing'. On the other hand, our words 'empty' and 'void' mean that which has nothing in it and is absolutely empty as far as the senses can discover. Now *śūnyatā* hardly ever means something which has nothing in it, it denies the existence of the thing under consideration. When Saṃsāra and Nirvāṇa are said to be *śūnya*, this does not mean that they are like some empty container. Saṃsāra and Nirvāṇa exist as interpretations of experience, not as a thing in itself. The following distinction should be borne in mind. There are times when we have the sickening feeling that everything recedes from us and we are utterly lost in emptiness, when there is nothing to which we can cling. After such an experience has passed we are apt to say, ‘Oh, it was nothing’. But this nothing, far from soothing, is on later reflection the object of dread, for which the term ‘emptiness’ or ‘void’ should be reserved. It is this type of nothingness to which existentialists have given special attention. Martin Heidegger seems to have divined something of the Buddhist *śūnyatā* when in his *Sein und Zeit*, p. 187, he declares this ‘nothingness revealed by dread’ to be a pathway to a ‘total nothingness’. *śūnyatā* is a positive factor that can be indicated only negatively, that it is not this, not that, no thing, nothing. The indiscriminate translation of *śūnyatā* by ‘void’ or ‘emptiness’ by the linguistic specialists serves to blur the philosophical distinction between that which is called *raṅ-stoṅ* and *gžan-stoṅ*. The latter expresses the notion that ultimate reality is ‘void’ of everything relative. There remains something after it has been emptied. Here the translation by ‘void’ would be permissible. *raṅ-stoṅ* means that ultimate reality is ‘void’ of itself, it is nothing in itself. This is the view of Nāgārjuna and the Mādhyamikas. See my *Three Essentials*, p. 103. Shinichi Hisamatsu, *The Characteristics of Oriental Nothingness*, pp. 65 sqq.

NOTE C. In the bsTan-’gyur (Derge edition) the following works of Nāropa have been preserved:

Śrīhevajrasādhana	(dPal dGyes-pa rdo-rje’i sgrub-thabs)
Ratnaprabhā	(Rin-po-che’i ’od)
Paramārthasangraha-nāma-sekoddeśaṭīkā	(dbaṅ mdor bstan-pa’i ’grel-bśad don-dam-pa bsdus-pa)
Ekavīraherukasādhana	(dPa’-bo gcig-pa He-ru-ka’i sgrub-thabs)
Śrīguhyaratnacintāmaṇi	(dPal gsaṅ-ba rin-po-che’i yid-bžin nor-bu)
Vajrayoginīsādhana	(rDo-rje rnal-’byor-ma’i sgrub-thabs)
Dharmābhiṣekamārgasantati	(dBaṅ-chos rten-’brel ’gro-ldog)
Śridevīkālīsādhana	(dPal lHa-mo nag.mo’i sgrub-thabs)
Vajragīti	(rDo-rje’i glu) (two poems bearing the same name)
Pañcakramasangrahaprakāśa	(Rim-pa lṅa bsdus-pa gsal-ba)
Śrīcakrasaṃvaropadeśamukha-karṇaparamparācintāmaṇi	(dPal ’Khor-lo sdom-pa’i man-ṅag žal-nas sñan-du brgyud-pa’i yid-bžin nor-bu)
Karṇatantra vajrapada	(sÑan-brgyud rdo-rje tshig-rkaṅ)
Śatākṣarabhaṭṭārakasattva-trayabhāvana	(rJe-btsun yi-ge brgya-pa’i sems-dpa’ gsum-gyi bsgom-pa’i thabs)
Nā-ro paṇḍi-ta’i glu	(no Sanskrit title)

NOTE D. A discussion of all four confirmations which also serve as empowerments, on the whole agreeing with the one given here, is found in Dchlsp 41*a* sq.; Sphžg 68*b* sqq.; sGam-po-pa, x. 18*a*; xvii. 3*b* sq.; xxvii. 9*a*; and xxviii. 3b. sGam-po-pa gives an explanation of *dbaṅ* (*abhiṣeka*) which is characteristic of his philosophy, but which I have not found elsewhere. In xxxi. 27*b*, he defines *dbaṅ* as 'man's dividedness against himself coming under control, and making Reality exert control'. This is precisely that which is aimed at by what is termed *dbaṅ* 'confirmation', 'empowerment'.

The name 'jar'-confirmation is taken from the Eastern habit of pouring water from a jar over oneself while bathing. Just as in so doing all dirt is washed away and one feels a different man afterwards, so Padma dkar-po combines both phenomena in explaining 'confirmation'. Loc. cit. 68*b*, he says: '*abhisiñc* means to wash off, that is to wash away the dirt of body, speech, mind and awareness which makes man unsuitable for realization. *abhiṣeka* means to found, that is the power to refine impure body, speech, mind, and awareness so that man is made suitable'.

The purpose is to ennoble man, to release him from the feeling of being merely a thing, and to make him realize his inherent divine quality. In the language of existentialist philosophy, man is changed from a status of unauthentic being-in-the-world to that of an authentic being-in-the-world. Here man sees himself as a god (*lha*, *deva*), not as a miserable creature at the mercy of dark powers, and the world around him as a divine mansion (*gžal-yas-khaṅ*, *vimāna*) rather than as a valley of tears. Seeing oneself and others as gods does not mean deification, it points to a feeling of transfiguration.

The peculiar philosophical viewpoint that is connected with this confirmation and change of attitude is according to Padma dkar-po, op. cit. 70*a*, the mentalistic thesis that sensa are veridical (*sems-tsam rnam bden*).

NOTE E. According to sGam-po-pa, xxvii. 9*a*, this confirmation is the realization of transcending awareness (*ye-śes*, *jñāna*) through union with the Karmamudrā (*śes-rab*, *prajñā*). Similarly Padma dkar-po, op. cit. 69*a* sqq., states: 'discriminative-appreciative awareness (*śes-rab*, *prajñā*) is Karmamudrā. When in uniting with her, in the contacting of the two organs (male and female), the individualistic attitude (lit.: the materiality producing forces (*khams*, *dhātu*)) is dissolved and a feeling of flowing vitality passing through the whole body is experienced, sixteen varieties of joyfulness are felt. This joyfulness is the quintessence of transcending awareness (*ye-śes*). The unity of the process is this transcending awareness together with and through discrimination-appreciation (*śes-rab ye-śes*)'.

According to Nāropa the Karmamudrā is a real woman. This is stated by Padma dkar-po clearly in Phgdz 20*b*. This must not be understood as implying that the relation a man has with a woman is merely biological, a release of tensions, the easing of a locally circumscribed urge. It is much more 'projective', outlining possible ways to a larger world. The relation is not purely genital, it involves the whole individual, body and mind. The determination of the Karmamudrā as 'discrimination-appreciation' (*śes-rab*, *prajñā*), emphasizing the cognitive mode of man's relation with her, marks it off from the *thing*-Karmamudrā, the object of our desires and intentions, so predominant in our ordinary object thinking, from which we should be liberated by a proper understanding of the relation that holds between man and woman. Another designation which clearly brings out that the Karmamudrā is more than a physical tension release, is 'messenger' (*pho-ña*). This psychological phenomenon has been recognized in Western psychology and been described by C. G. Jung as the 'anima'. The term 'messenger' is used in a purely psychological context and is a sort of inspiratory force. This shows what is aimed at by the confirmation under discussion here. Man always finds himself in a situation which he attempts to solve. This has been clearly recognized by existentialist thinkers who, however, unlike the Tantric sages, make no reference to that power of discrimination by which we can meet the various situations successfully. Just as the two preceding confirmations aimed at authentic being-in-the-world and communicating with-others, the one being concerned, as it were, with the body (*lus*) (which is always body-mind), and the other with speech (*ṅag*) (as the readiest means of communication), this third confirmation deals with 'mind' (*yid*), man's cognitive power of feeling and practical reason. This confirmation thus corrects the existentialist thinkers' omission and comprises all that which John Wild in his critique of existentialist thought, *The Challenge of Existentialism*, p. 218, so aptly describes as: 'the human person is always in a situation, striving to fulfil his tendencies amidst a nexus of surrounding persons and forces, which is at least confusedly revealed to him by mood and feeling. He may devise clever schemes for meeting a given situation, but no sooner is he out of one than he finds himself in another. Like all other ultimate limits, this situationality of human existence reveals the finiteness and fragility of human nature, surrounded as it is by alien and disruptive forces. In addition to this, however, it shows that the individual exists in an imperfect and tendential way, always seeking to fulfil a need or lack in the same stream of temporal succession which sweeps along all other entities of nature. It also shows that he naturally possesses cognitive powers of feeling and practical reason which can manifest his own existence, and that of other agencies around him. What is chiefly omitted from the existentialist accounts is any explicit reference to that power of theoretical insight, which they themselves exemplify, by which we can describe, classify, and illumine these situations as they come, and by which, if we take them seriously, we may guide ourselves toward authentic action'.

NOTE F. The current translation of this technical term by 'vital air' or 'vital breath' is inadequate. In Sphžg 38*a* it is defined as 'to set the whole of reality into motion' (*g'yo-bar byed-pa*), and this meaning is present wherever the word *rluṅ* is used. Since it is of theoretical importance—Tantric Buddhism has two aspects, its metaphysics and its way of life, its theory and its practice—I translate it by 'motility', a term implying the capability of motion irrespective of actual movement. In a sense, motility is an aspect of the ultimate which is referred to by such terms as 'radiant light' (*'od-gsal*, *prabhāsvara*), 'transcending awareness' (*ye-śes*, *jñāna*) or 'spirituality' (*sems-ñid*, *citta eva*). See for instance sGam-po-pa, v. 38*b*; 40*ab*; vi. 6*b*, 11*b*; viii. 13*a*; x. 31*b*, 46*b*, &c. Zmnd 63*b*. These terms, it must be understood, are not names for entities, but mere indexes, operational counters, as is made quite clear by sGam-po-pa, xxi. 3*a*. The ultimate viewed as motility is also designated by the term 'non-dichotomic motility' (*rnam-par rtog-pa med-pa'i rluṅ*) and as such it is the vehicle of the three reaction possibilities (*snaṅ-ba gsum*) which preconsciously determine the overt responses. They are passion (*'dod-chags*, *rāga*), aversion (*že-sdaṅ*, *dveṣa*), and bewilderment (*gti-mug*, *moha*), not in their manifest forms but as diffuse patterns. This non-dichotomic motility becomes more and more specialized and in its specialization is known as 'dichotomic motility (*rnam-par rtog-pa'i rluṅ*) and is the vehicle of the distinct reaction patterns in overt behaviour informed by the diffuse patterns. In modern terms this means that conscious behaviour evolves in the course of motor activity.

Another distinction is that 'transcending awareness' which is at the core of human existence and moves along the central pathway (*dbu-ma*, *avadhūti*) in its creative-arranging activity. In this function it is known as 'awareness-motility' (*ye-śes-kyi rluṅ*, *jñānavāyu*), and operates both in the human sphere and on a cosmic level where it is known as sGra-can (Rāhu, a term belonging to Indian astrology). Similarly as non-dichotomic motility becomes dichotomic motility, awareness-motility spreads along the right and left pathways (*rkyaṅ-ma*, *lalanā*, and *ro-ma*, *rasanā*) and in this movement becomes known as 'action-motility' (*las-kyi rluṅ*, *karmavāyu*). Through its activity the split into subject and object appears. Passing along the right path (*ro-ma*) it sets up the objective pole. In this activity it is known as 'the object-creating motility' (*gzuṅ bskyed-kyi rluṅ*), also symbolically referred to as the sun. Passing along the left way (*rkyaṅ-ma*) it sets up the subjective pole and is symbolically called the moon. It is also termed 'subject motility' (*'dzin-gyi rluṅ*). From these three aspects, Rāhu, sun, and moon, there emerge the five primary forms of motor activity, forming the co-ordinating and sustaining physiological systems. They are: *srog-'dzin* (*prāṇa*) or vitality in general, *thur-sel* (*apāna*) corresponding to the eliminative and reproductive system, *rgyen-rgyu* (*udāna*) forming what T. Burrow, *Science and Man's Behavior*, p. 407, calls the 'semiotic system' (facilitating speech and communication), *mñam-rgyu* (*samāna*) corresponding to the digestive system, and *khyab-byed* (*vyāpin*) the muscular system enabling movement in space. From these five systems the five sensory perceptions as motor acts derive. The above is the gist of the lengthy discussion by Padma dkar-po in Sphžg 38*a* sqq. and Zmnd 71*a* sqq., 95*a* and elsewhere. It is interesting to note that the Buddhist conception greatly coincides with the findings of psychobiology. Sense perception is possible through motor equipment, or as Judson C. Herrick, *The Evolution of Human Nature*, p. 340, puts it; 'sensitivity and motility are equally essential components of the perceptive process. The amount and quality of perceptual knowledge which it is possible for an individual to acquire depend on the sensory and motor equipment available'. 'Consciousness emerges within behavior, and motility is the seedbed of mind' (p. 262). Or we may quote Sir Charles Sherrington, *Man on His Nature*, p. 213: 'Mind, recognizable mind, seems to have arisen in connexion with the motor act. Where motor integration progressed and where motor behaviour progressively evolved, mind progressively evolved.' 'The motor act as conative would seem to have been the earliest nurse of infant mind' (p. 193). 'Motor behaviour would seem to be the cradle of recognizable mind' (p. 324). Another point to note is that when *rluṅ* (*vāyu*) is used in connexion with the breathing technique, it never stands for the actual breathing, but for the perceptions and excitation of sensations in a real or imagined part of the body. (sGam-po-pa, xiii. 6*a*; xvii. 2*a*.)

NOTE G. The text has *śes-rab, prajñā*. The account oscillates between the 'physical' and 'spiritual' world. Here the meaning of *śes-rab* as a transcending function (*Überleitungsfunktion*) is most obvious. The current translation of this important term by 'wisdom' reveals a sovereign disregard of its position within the framework of Buddhist psychology. The noetic (*śes-pa*) reveals two features; one is what may be called higher order acts (*raṅ-rig*), the other is its intentionality, which means that all awareness is intentional or relational, from a subjective pole to an object of some sort (*gžan-rig*). This latter aspect of the noetic consists of the readiness to respond (*sems*), and psychological processes (*sems-byuṅ*) which determine the readiness to respond in various ways. Much attention has been given to the psychological processes. Some described a total of forty-six, others noted fifty-one, and still others seventy-one such processes. There is no reason to deride this tendency to give numerical lists, because the numerical list of instincts in Western psychologies is in no way less grotesque. Among the psychological processes which determine the readiness to respond there are five which are ever-present and fulfil the functions of mood, imagining, motivation, coordination, and discursiveness. Five others are object-determined, and the last among them is *śes-rab, prajñā*. Although a small psychological function, *śes-rab* mediates between two frames of reference. Following W. T. Stace, *Religion and the Modern Mind*, p. 274, these two frames of reference may be said to refer to the natural or temporal order and the eternal order. Inasmuch as *śes-rab* is discriminative and appreciative it can choose between the two orders and either become entangled in Saṃsāra or liberated in Nirvāṇa and beyond Nirvāṇa. For the structure of the noetic in Buddhism see Srph and Sgg.

NOTE H. The same statement is found in Tshk 7*b* sq. The analysis there, however, is different from the one given here. There the topic is as follows:

'I. Through mystic illumination to determine the unoriginated or ground (Being) Mahāmudrā; by
 (i) relaxing the tensional patterns of the senses;
 (ii) recognizing spirituality-mentality as basic to philosophical insight;
 (iii) arriving at pure sensation;

(iv) having self-confidence and
(v) thereby determining the 'ground' in its ever-present actuality as
(*a*) uncreated,
(*b*) unchanging, and
(*c*) without beginning or end (birth or death).

'II. Through subsequent presentational knowledge to recognize the unceasing or the path Mahāmudrā by comprehending that

(i) all the entities of an outer objective world are both appearance and nothingness and hence 'mind' and thus
(*a*) will have to be understood as having a relational character and
(*b*) can be used without affirmation or negation.

(ii) spirituality-mentality is the self-authenticity of the Three Kāyas (existential norms) and thus realizing that
(*a*) the actuality of spirituality being without origin is Dharmakāya (authentic being as such),
(*b*) the incessant flux of appearance in its luminosity is Nirmāṇakāya (authentic being-in-the-world) and
(*c*) the coincidence (of relativeness and absoluteness) being unlocalized is Sambhogakāya (authentic being-with-others), which means that
(1) Saṃsāra and Nirvāṇa forever inseparable are the 'ground' (Being), which is the meaning of *phyag*,
(2) by knowing that this can never be reduced to the subject-object dichotomy there is freedom from Saṃsāra or the path, which is the meaning of *rgya*,
(3) by knowing that appearance and nothingness coincide there is victory over ignorance or the goal, which is the meaning of *chen-po*,
(4) one comprehends that all of them are beyond conditional existence and freedom as such.

'III. Through coincidence to attain the ineffable or the goal Mahāmudrā (which means that)

(i) what is ordinarily said to be something that has to be renounced is ultimately pure,
(ii) particularizing mind and its constructs have been overcome, and
(iii) all the virtues that are ordinarily said to be something that should be attained are present in all perfection in spirituality, and hence this constitutes self-originated Buddhahood.'

As to the relaxation of the tensional patterns of the senses relevant material is found in Trigant Burrow, op. cit., s.v.

NOTE I. The development of the final structure is discussed in Dnz 47*b* sq.: 'when the organism begins to develop after the noetic capacity has united with the generating powers of father and mother, in the middle of the potential being (*thig-le*) the central structure pathway develops first. From this two pathways (*ro-ma* and *rkyaṅ-ma*) branch off. From these three structural pathways a four-petaled net derives, of which one pathway called Sum-skor-ma (*traivṛttā*) extends to the east, another 'Dod-ma (*kāminī*) to the south, still another Khyim-ma (*gehā*) to the west, and lastly one, gTum-mo (*caṇḍālī*), to the north. Each pathway separates into two and the result is known as the eight-petaled network of the heart. Each of these divides into three pathways called *rdul* (and forming the object polarity), *sñiṅ-stobs* (forming the subject polarity) and *mun* (holding the polarities together). Thus there are twenty-four pathways. Each of these divides into the possibilities of being-in-the-world (*sku*), communicating with-others (*gsuṅ*), and dealing with situations (*thugs*), so that there are seventy-two pathways. Each of these divides into a thousand pathways, so that there is a total of 72,000 structural pathways. From these the three and a half million subtler pathways derive. Wherever the two main branches (*ro-ma* and *rkyaṅ-ma*) meet there is in the central pathway a focal point, the one in the head has thirty-two petals, the one in the throat sixteen, the one in the heart eight, and the one in the navel sixty-four. These are the four (main) focal points of experience. Then there are still one in the sex region with thirty-two petals and another one in the glans penis with eight, so that there are six focal points in all. In the heart, in the centre of the materiality producing forces, symbolized as white and red streams (white for the male and red for the female), motility (*rluṅ*) and mentality (*sems*) form a unit and are held together by the network of the pathways. From here the white stream passes upwards and is present mostly in the head. It produces semen, bones, and marrow. The red stream passes downwards and is found mostly in the navel. It produces flesh, blood, and skin. In this way the total organism is gradually completed.'

Special attention should be directed towards the statement that the subject and object polarities permeate the whole organism. This shows that the subject-object dichotomy is not restricted to a mind and that we do not live in a world of 'pure reason' in the Kantian or any other sense. Similarly the fact that *sku*, *gsuṅ*, and *thugs* operate before there is a body or speech or a mind, shows that the current translation of these terms by Body, Speech, and Mind is utterly inadequate. The fact that they too permeate the whole organism shows that, in the words of C. Judson Herrick, op. cit., p. 92: 'they are "field" functions which can be served by any tissue which has the requisite plasticity or flexibility without a high degree of specialization for a particular function'.

NOTE J. 'Quadruple potency' is a descriptive term of the manner in which the creative potentiality unfolds itself. It will be helpful if again for the moment we conceive of this potentiality as having a field character, one indeterminate, the other determinate or rather becoming determinate. The indeterminate field factor is in philosophical language pure transcendence. In the original texts it is referred to by such terms as 'transcendence' (*blo-las 'das-pa*, *matyatīta*), 'radiant light' (*'od-gsal*, *prabhāsvara*) or 'complete nothingness' (*thams-cad stoṅ-pa*, *sarvaśūnya*). The first term belongs to the line of thought developed by Saraha, the remaining ones to that by sGam-po-pa, Padma dkar-po, and others, and these have superseded the earlier terminology. The process of unfolding and of becoming determinate is that in pure transcendence, as it were, a phase begins to operate, which, according to the two lines of thought mentioned above, is either called 'the unoriginated', 'that which has no origin' (*skye-med, anutpāda*) or 'great nothingness' (*stoṅ-pa chen-po, mahāśūnya*). Because of its luminous character it is also called 'inner glow' (*ñer-thob, upalabdha*) and in a purely psychological framework 'unknowing' (or as commonly translated 'ignorance') (*ma-rig-pa, avidyā*). This is the onset of the differentiating process, the field factor that is to develop. The next phase is 'non-memory' (*dran-med, vismaraṇa*) or 'intense nothingness' (*śin-tu stoṅ-pa, atiśūnya*) or 'intense spread of light' (*mched-pa, ālokābhāsa*). The final stage is 'memory' (*dran-pa, smṛti*) which is always considered as a power, not as an act, or 'plain nothingness' (*stoṅ-pa, śūnya*) or 'light' (*snaṅ-ba, āloka*). Graphically this is:

blo-las 'das-pa	*'od-gsal*	*thams-cad stoṅ-pa*	transcendence
skye-med	*ñer-thob*	*stoṅ-pa chen-po*	unknowing
dran-med	*mched-pa*	*śin-tu stoṅ-pa*	experientially initiated potentialities of experience
dran-pa	*snaṅ-ba*	*stoṅ-pa*	the above potentialities in a state of actualization.

It is important to note that the whole process is pre-conscious. Further, although we are inclined to say that the differentiations come out of something undifferentiated, 'out' does not mean coming out of a container. The four aspects form a unit. Hence everything determinate has the flavour of the indeterminate. Appearance is pervaded and encompassed by transcendence. This is termed 'co-emergence' (*lhan-cig-skyes-pa, sahaja*).

NOTE K. Specimens of text A, a calligraphic copy of which was used by A. Grünwedel, and of text B, a complete translation of which is contained in this book.

THE INTRODUCTORY VERSES

A

mKhas-grub mñam-med dpal-ldan Nā-ro-pa'i rnam-par thar-pa dri-med legs-bśad bde-chen 'brug-sgra žes-bya-ba bžugs-so.

Na-mo gu-ru bud-dha-dhotstsha-ye.

chos-dbyiṅs-žiṅ-na chos-sku Kun-tu-bzaṅ/
'og-min-žiṅ-na loṅs-sku rDo-rje-'chaṅ/
'mi-mjed-žiṅ-na sprul-sku Thub-dbaṅ-rje/
sku-gsum dbyer-med rje-btsun Nā-ro-pa/
blo-'das bciṅs-grol-bral-ba 'khor-ba'i gśis/
de-ñid raṅ-tshaṅ rig-pa myaṅ-'das-lam/

raṅ-śar raṅ-grol śar-grol dus-mñam-pa'i/
'od-gsal phyag-chen ṅaṅ-nas brkyaṅs phyag-'tshal//
(2*a*) sṅon-tshe bde-gśegs Padma'i bla-mar grags/
bar-du sprul-sku Me-tog-zla-mdzes žes/
thub-pa'i bstan-la mkhas-grub Nā-ror grags/
bstan-pa'i srog-śiṅ 'Jigs-med-grags-pa-la/
sprin-med mkha'-la 'ja'-'od śar-ba ltar/
snaṅ-stoṅ zuṅ-'brel yon-tan-gyis bskrun-pa'i
rnam-dag bskyed-rims gsal-ba'i ṅaṅ-ñid-nas/
sgyu-ma sprul-pa'i kun-bzaṅ (2*b*) mchod-sprin 'bul//
phyogs-bcu dus-gsum rgyal-sras ma-lus-pa'i/
sku-gsuṅ-thugs-kyi yon-tan rab-rdzogs te/
'phrin-las raṅ-gzugs kun-mkhyen gñis-par grags/
thams-cad-mkhyen-pa Nā-ro-ta-pa-la/
bdag-gis thogs-med dus-nas da-lta'i bar/
'khor-'das dbyer-med du-ma ro-gcig-la/
gñis-su bzuṅ-nas sdig-sgrib graṅs-med bsags/
bde-chen khyab-brdal ṅaṅ-nas bśags-pa 'bul//
rig-pa'i gnas lṅa gyes-pa yal-ga'i tshogs/
'chad rtsod rtsom-pa'i chu-skyes mdaṅs-bkra žin/
ji-lta ji-sñed mkhyen. (3*a*) pa'i 'bras-bus dud/
yoṅs-'du'i dpag-bsam mkhas-mchog Nā-ro-yis/
sprul bsgyur bkod-pa rnam-thar graṅs-med-las/
rig-pa'i yon-tan bye-ba phrag brgya mthoṅ/
blo-'das chos-sku dag-pa'i snaṅ-bar bžeṅs/
nam-mkha'i skar mtshuṅs rjes-su yid-raṅ 'phel//*
gdoṅ-bži mig-stoṅ gdeṅs-ldan rgyal-pos mchod/
gnas-lṅa rig-pa'i paṇ-chen 'bum phrag-gis/
žabs-rdul spyi-bos len-pa'i skyes-bu mchog/
rnal-'byor dbaṅ-phyug chen-po Nā-ro-pa/
yun-riṅ-dus-la mi ltos tshe-gcig-la/
mchog-gi dṅos. (3*b*) grub ster-ba sṅags-kyi lam/
myur-mgyogs lam-mchog rtsa rluṅ thig-le'i gnad/
bla-med chos-'khor rgyun-du skor-du gsol//
luṅ rigs gnam-lcags 'khor-lo'i rdzu-'phrul-gyis/
phyi-rol mu-stegs grub-mtha' rdul-du brlags/
lhan-skyes-ye-śes phyag-chen raṅ-'gros-kyis/
'khor-ba doṅ dkrugs mdzad-pa'i Nā-ro-pa/
rje-btsun khyed-la gśegs bžugs gñis mi mṅa'/
gñis-med gñis-su 'dzin-pa'i gdul-bya'i ṅor/
khams-gsum 'khor-ba'i miṅ 'di ma stoṅs bar/
mya-ṅan mi 'da' rtag-par bžugs-su gsol//**
ñi-ma'i gñen-mchog Bu-ram-śiṅ-pa'i gduṅ/
gaṅs-ri'i khrod-kyi skal-bzaṅ gdul-bya-rnams/
brtse-ba'i thugs-rjes bu bžin skyoṅs mdzad-pa/
Nā-ro'i rnam-thar 'khyoṅs-par byin-gyis rlobs/
mchod ciṅ bstod-pa'i rlabs-chen dge-ba'i mthus/
rnal-'byor bdag daṅ 'gro kun pha ma-yis/

bsod-nams ye-śes tshogs gñis mthar phyin-nas/
bcu-gsum rdo-rje (4*a*) 'dzin-pa'i sa thob śog/
bde-chen rgyal-po mkhas-grub Nā-ro-pa'i/
rnam-par thar-pa zab rgyas chu-gter-las/
zab bsdus cuṅ-zad-tsam žig bśad-par bya/
bla-ma yi-dam mkha-'gro'i lha tshogs-kyis/
thugs-mchog dgyes-bžin bka'-yis gnaṅ-du gsol//

Specimen II: A passage which is identical in A and B except for the literary style.

A

(fol. 24*b*) *(Grünwedel, 26*a*–26*b*) . . . da ni khyer-ka bskyed-la bla-ma tshol-du 'gro dgoṅs-nas/śar-phyogs-su tshol-du byon-pas luṅ-pa ṅam-nag-pa / brag rṅam-la tsoṅ-roṅ-du soṅ-ba lce-spyaṅ-gis rol-śal byed-pa / rmugs-pa 'thib-pa yid mi dga'-ba cig-gi naṅ-du byon tsa-na khyi-skad lhaṅ-lhaṅ grags tsa-na / śa-ba cig byuṅ-ba'i phyi-nas śa khyi thod kha dmar chag-ge-ba maṅ-po byuṅ / de'i phyi-nas mi nag-po skra spyi-bor bciṅs-pa mda' gžu thogs-pa cig byuṅ-ba-la / dpal 'Jigs-med-grags-pas rje-btsun Tai-lo-pa mthoṅ-ṅam gsuṅs-pas / kho na-re / śa-ba 'di gsod grogs-gyis-daṅ de-nas bstan-gyis zer-nas mda' gžu gtad byuṅ-bas / ṅas rṅon-pa'i grogs mi yoṅ sñam-pa daṅ / mi de na-re /

sgyu-lus žen-pa-med-kyi mda'/
'od-gsal ñams-kyi gžu bkaṅ-nas/
ṅar-'dzin lus-kyi ri-bo-la/
gzuṅ-'dzin ri-dvags rgyu-ba de/
gsod-la mos-pa'i rṅon-pa bdag/
saṅ-ni ña-pa rgya-mtshor sñeg

zer nas spraṅ-po de-ñid mi snaṅ-bar gyur-to// . . .

Specimen III: Text A giving merely the name of the instruction, text B giving the contents of the instruction.

A

(fol. 38*a*–38*b*) *(Grünwedel, 40*b*–41*a*) . . . de-nas yaṅ rje-bstun Tai-lo-pa de-ñid lo-gcig-tu spyod-lam sṅar-ltar bžugs-nas gsuṅ chos ma gnaṅ / skabs-cig-tu tiṅ-ṅe-'dzin de-las bžeṅs byuṅ-ba-las / maṇḍal phyag mchod sogs sṅon-du btaṅ-nas / gsol-ba btab-pas / ṅa'i phyi-nar 'deṅ gsuṅs byon-pas / thaṅ stoṅ cig-na mi khred-po khur-ba gcig 'gro-ba-la rje-bstun Tai-lo-pas mi pha-gis khyod-la sdug-cig rañ btaṅ-bas pha-gi ded gsuṅ ded-pa-las / smig-rgyu ltar je-riṅ-la soṅ-nas ma zin yaṅ da-duṅ ded gsuṅ ded pas thaṅ-chad 'gyel-ba-la rtsa-ru byon-nas / Nā-ro-pa (38*b*) khyod ci ñes gsuṅs/

ri-dvags mig-rgyu sñog-pa ltar/
med snaṅ riṅ soṅ bdag sug-bsṅal/

žus-pas/

khams-gsum 'khor-ba'i rgyun-thag 'di/
chad kyaṅ ruṅ-gi Nā-ro-pa/

mkha'-'gro-ma-yi gsaṅ-ba'i gnas/
rmi-lam sems-kyi me-loṅ ltos/

gsuṅ phyag-gis byin-brlabs mdzad-pas sku-sñel bsos-pa'i rjes-la / rmi-lam 'khrul-pa raṅ-saṅs-kyi gdams-nag mtha'-dag gnaṅ-ṅo// de-nas yaṅ rje-btsun Tai-lo-pa de-ñid lo-gcig spyod-lam sṅar ltar bžugs-nas gsuṅ chos ma gnaṅ/. . .

Specimen I:

B

mKhas-grub kun-gyi gtsug-brgyan / paṇ-chen Nā-ro-pa'i rnam-thar/
ṅo-mtshar rmad-byuṅ bžugs-so.

Na-mo gu-ru de-wa ḍa-ki-ni.
rDo-rje-'chaṅ-dbaṅ chos-sku lha-lam mtha'-bral kloṅ-yaṅs-na/
rdo-rje rnal-'byor loṅs-sku lṅa ldan nam-mkha'i nor-bu rgyas/
śes-rab bzaṅ-po mchog-gi sprul-sku 'od stoṅ zer 'phros-pas/
sku gsum gdul-bya Nā-ro'i blo-gros pad-mo'i kha phye ste/
mdo rgyud sñiṅ-po sñan-rgyud sbraṅ-rtsi phyogs-mthar rgyas-la 'dud/
mi-'jigs seṅ-khri pad-ma ñi zla'i gdan steṅs-na/
dri-med nam-mkha'i sñiṅ-po nor-bu rtsa-bśad-pa/
sñan-grags bzaṅ-po mchog-gi ye-śes dṅos-grub brñes/
kun-tu-bzaṅ-po chos-kyi rgyal-mtshan bstan-pa 'dzin/
saṅs-rgyas-rnams sprul Nā-ro'i žabs-la phyag-'tshal-lo//
rtsibs stoṅ rgyan mdzes skabs gsum dbaṅ-po pad-mo'i gñen/
dbaṅ-po'i dgra daṅ dri-za gdeṅs-can tshogs-kyi bdag/
dbaṅ-phyug 'jug-dgu mi daṅ mi-min-rnams-kyis ni/
gus mchod ci gsuṅ bka' sgrub 'gro-ba'i skyabs-mchog rje/
rigs-sad lha'i btsun- (2*a*) pa'i spyi-gtsug-rgyan bžugs cig/
Nā-ro la-sogs dṅos daṅ rgyud-par bcas-rnams-la/
lus ṅag yid gsum mos-gus sñiṅ-nas phyag-'tshal-lo//
bdag lus loṅs-spyod phyi naṅ gsaṅ gsum mchod-par 'bul//
thog-med dus-nas bsags daṅ sog-'gyur sdig-rnams bśags//
'phags daṅ so-skye'i dge-rtsa-rnams-la rjes-yi-raṅ//
ji-srid 'khor-ba ma stoṅs de-srid chos-'khor bskor//
mya-ṅan mi 'da' srid-mtha'i bar-du bžugs-su gsol//
bdag gžan dge-rtsa phra rags byaṅ-chub chen-por bsṅo//
lhag-bsam gžan-phan kho-nas 'jigs-med-grags-pa-yi/
rnam-thar ṅo-mtshar rmad-byuṅ chu-thigs tsam žig brjod/
bla-ma yi-dam mkha'-'phro'i tshogs-kyis gnaṅ-du gsol/
phyi-ma don-gñer ṅes-'byuṅ-can-rnams sñan-gsan 'tshal//

Specimen II:

B

(fol. 14*b*) . . . yaṅ laṅs te gsol-ba 'debs bžin phyin-pas / sṅon-na mar khyis śā-ba ded-pa'i phyi-nas mi nag-po mda' gžu thogs-pa cig byuṅ-bas/ Ti-lo-pa mthoṅ-nam dris-pas / mthoṅ zer / ṅa-la ston byas-pas / mda' gžu gtad-nas ri-dags 'di sod zer-ba-la ma bsad-pas / kho na-re/

sgyu-lus žen-pa-med-kyis mda'/
'od-gsal ñams-kyi gžu bkaṅ-nas/
ṅar-'dzin lus-kyi ri-bo-la/
gzuṅ-'dzin ri-dags rgyug-pa de/
bsod-la mos-pa'i rṅon-pa bdag/
saṅ-ni ña-pa rgya-mtshor sñog

zer mi snaṅ-bar gyur-to// . . .

Specimen III:

B

(fol. 27*a*) . . . yaṅ Ti-lo-pa de-ñid lo-gcig spyod-lam gsum-gyis bžugs-pa-la / Nā-ro-pas maṇḍal phul phyag daṅ skor-ba byed ciṅ gsol-ba btab-pas / skabs-cig-tu spyan hur byuṅ-ba-la / gdams-ṅag žu žus-pas / gdams-ṅag 'dod-na ṅa'i phyi-nar 'deṅ gsuṅ phyin-pas / thaṅ chen-po cig-gi guṅ-na mi khres-po khur-ba cig soṅ-ba / de ded gsuṅ-nas ded-pas / mig-rgyu ltar je-riṅ-la soṅ-nas (27*b*) ma non / da-duṅ ded gsuṅ ded-pas ma non-par/ chad-nas 'gyel te 'gul ma nus-pa-la / Ti-lo-pa byon-nas / Nā-ro-pa khyod ci ñes gsuṅ / Nā-ro-pas/

ri-dags mig-rgyu sñog-pa bžin/
med snaṅ riṅ soṅ bdag sdug-bsṅal/

ces žus-pas / Ti-lo-pas/

khams-gsum 'khor-ba'i rgyun-thag 'di/
chad kyaṅ ruṅ-gi Nā-ro-pa/
mkha'-'phro-ma-yi gsaṅ-ba'i gnas/
rmi-lam sems-kyi me-loṅ ltos/

gsuṅ-nas / phyag-gis byis byas-pas / lus sṅa-ma ltar sos-pa-la / rmi-lam 'khrul-pa raṅ-saṅs-kyi gdams-ṅag-rnams rdzogs-par ghaṅ-ṅo // rmi-lam-gyi gdams-pa-la gñis / rmi-lam 'dun-pa'i stobs-kyis sbyoṅ-ba daṅ / rluṅ-stobs-kyis sbyoṅ-ba daṅ // daṅ-po ni / mdo sṅags gñis-ka yaṅ chos thams-cad rmi-lam daṅ 'dra-ba / bžed-la / de-lta-bu'i ñams-len-gyi sgo-nas bdag-'dzin-gyi 'khrul-pa bśigs-par byed / 'di-la yaṅ gñid-nas rmi-lam ma byuṅ-gi bar / 'chi-ba lam-'khyer / rmi-lam śar-nas ma sad-kyi bar / bar-do lam-'khyer / sad-pa sprul-sku lam-'khyer yin-no // des-na ñin snaṅ-gi a-'thas-kyi bden-'dzin gśigs-pa-la sgyu-ma'i dpe bcu-gñis-kyi naṅ-nas rmi-lam mchog-tu gyur-pa yin-no // sbyoṅ-tshul ni / tshe 'di blos btaṅ / sgyu-lus-kyi dran-pa yeṅs-med-du skyoṅ-ba'i gaṅ-zag de / mtshan-dus sogs gñid-du 'gro-bar rtsom-pa-na / mgrin-pa'i rtsa-'khor-gyis dbus-su ñams-len-la gnad-du bsñun-pas / gñid-kyi rtags snaṅ phra žiṅ myur-ba / sñiṅ-khar snaṅ-med 'od-gsal 'thug-po śin-tu rtogs dka'-ba cig 'char-ro // 'od-gsal-la rluṅ gyos ma-thag mgrin-par rmi-lam-gyi snaṅ-ba śar-ba'i tshe / sgo lṅa'i yul-du gaṅ śar-gyi snaṅ-ba cig raṅ-la yun-riṅ-du gnas-par sbyaṅ-ba / 'byoṅs-nas du-mar spel-ba / 'phel-ba'i rnam-pa bzaṅ-por sgyur-ba / sgyur-ba'i rnam-pa 'jigs-skrag- (28*a*) gi gñen-por sprul-pa /..

* Grünwedel gives the following translation:

'A lotus flower offers a beautiful sight as it employs all its strength to uphold the shrubs of hanging-down branches of the five sciences. As this infinite work of deliverance is a statement about the development of the magic forms of the Great Master Nāropa, the all-gathering tree of paradise with the buds for the fruit of knowledge, as and as far it obtains, one hundred times ten million virtues of corporeality being visible, the pure Dharmakāya, unfathomable by reason, is thereby declared to have appeared. One's own soul is lifted up to a trace which resembles the stars of the sky.'

The verse, however, is to be rendered as follows:

'Out of the countless biographies (*rnam-thar*) in which is recorded the coming and the working of Nāropa, the greatest scholar, (comparable to) the tree of paradise weighed down by the fruits of the double knowledge, the awareness which sees Reality as it is and the awareness of Reality as it becomes manifest, with far-spreading branches, the five sciences, embellished by the flowers of explanation, debates and writings, a hundred times ten million qualities of mind are to be seen and the Dharmakāya, transcending mind, manifests itself in pure appearance. May my joy spread like the stars over the sky.'

** Grünwedel translates:

'Venerable One, in order to come to you there is no need of the pair; you without copulation, let those who are in need of conversion, yoked in, enter eternity where there is no more misery, so that the praise of the name "round of births (*saṃsāra*) of the triple world" ceases.'

The text says:

Venerable One, for you there is neither passing into Nirvāṇa nor staying on in Saṃsāra;
Yet from the standpoint of the trainees, who believe in the duality of the non-dual,
I pray that you may not pass into Nirvāṇa but stay on
Until the triple world, known by the name of Saṃsāra, has become empty of beings.'

BIBLIOGRAPHY

ONLY books referred to in the text are listed here.

A

BOLLNOW, O. F., *Existenzphilosophie* (4th ed.), W. Kohlhammer Verlag, Stuttgart, n.d.

BOSS, MEDARD, *The Analysis of Dreams*, Rider, London.

BROAD, C. D., *The Mind and Its Place in Nature* (6th impr.), Routledge & Kegan Paul Ltd., London, 1951.

—— *Religion, Philosophy and Psychical Research*: Selected Essays, Routledge & Kegan Paul Ltd., London, 1953.

BROSS, THÉRÈSE, 'Altruism and Creativity as Biological Factors of Human Evolution' in Pitirim A. Sorokin, *Explorations in Altruistic Love and Behavior*, Beacon Press, Boston 1950.

BURROW, TRIGANT, *Science and Man's Behavior*: The Contribution of Phylobiology, ed. by W. E. Galt, Philosophical Library, New York, 1953.

CARNAP, R., *Philosophy and Logical Syntax*, Routledge & Kegan Paul Ltd., London, 1935.

DREVER, J., *A Dictionary of Psychology*, Penguin Books, Harmondsworth-Middlesex, 1952.

ELLIS, HAVELOCK, *Psychology of Sex*: A Manual for Students (Mentor Book), The New American Library, New York, 1957.

EVANS-WENTZ, W. Y., *The Tibetan Book of the Dead* (2nd ed.), Oxford University Press, London, 1951.

FERRARI, A., *mK'yen brtse's Guide to the Holy Places of Central Tibet*, completed and edited by Luciano Petech with the collaboration of Hugh Richardson, Serie Orientale Roma XVI, Rome, 1958.

FLÜGEL, J. C., *Man, Morals and Society*: A Psycho-analytical Study (Penguin Books), Harmondsworth-Middlesex, 1955.

FROMM, E., *The Art of Loving*, George Allen & Unwin Ltd., London, 1957.

GRÜNWEDEL, A., *Die Legenden des Nā-ro-pa*, Otto Harrassowitz, Leipzig, 1933.

GUENTHER, H. V., *Jewel Ornament of Liberation*, Rider, London, 1959.

—— 'The Philosophical Background of Buddhist Tantrism', *Journal of Oriental Studies*, vol. v, University of Hong Kong, Hong Kong, 1959–60.

—— 'Three Essentials', *The Middle Way*: Journal of the Buddhist Society, vol. xxxvi, London, 1961.

HAAS, W. S., *The Destiny of the Mind*: East and West, Faber & Faber, London, 1956.

HAGGARD, H. W., *Devils, Drugs and Doctor* (Cardinal Edition), Pocke Books, Inc., New York, 1953.

HEIDEGGER, M., *Sein und Zeit* (3rd ed.), Max Niemeyer Verlag, Halle, 1931.

—— *What is Philosophy?* Vision Books, Farrar, Straus & Cudahy, New York, 1958.

HERRICK, C. J., *The Evolution of Human Nature*, University of Texas Press, Austin, 1956.

HISAMATSU, SHIN-ICHI, 'The Characteristics of Oriental Nothingness', *Philosophical Studies of Japan*, vol. ii, Japan Society for the Promotion of Science, Tokyo, 1960.

HOCKING, W. E., *The Coming World Civilisation*, George Allen & Unwin Ltd., London, 1958.

—— *Types of Philosophy* (3rd ed.), Charles Scribner's Sons, New York, 1959.

HOSPERS, J., *An Introduction to Philosophical Analysis*, Routledge & Kegan Paul Ltd., London, 1956.

JAQUIN, N., *The Theory of Metaphysical Influence*: A Study of Human Attunements, Perception, Intelligence and Motivation, Rockliff, London, 1958.

JASPERS, K., *The Perennial Scope of Philosophy*, Routledge & Kegan Paul London, 1950.

—— *Die geistige Situation der Zeit* (8th ed.), W. de Gruyter & Co., Berlin, 1955.

—— *Philosophie* (3 vols., 3rd ed.), Springer Verlag, Heidelberg-Berlin, 1956.

KAUFMANN, W., *Critique of Religion and Philosophy*, Faber & Faber, London, 1959.

KINSEY, A. C. and others, *Sexual Behavior in the Human Female*, W. B. Launders & Co., Philadelphia, 1953.

LANGER, S. K., *Philosophy in a New Key*: A Study in the Symbolism of Reason, Rite, and Art (Mentor Book, 6th impr.), The New American Library, New York, 1954.

MONTAGUE, W. P., *The Ways of Knowing*: or the Methods of Philosophy; George Allen & Unwin Ltd., London, 1953. (4th impr.).

NORTHROP, F. S. C., *The Meeting of East and West*: An Inquiry concerning World Understanding, Macmillan, New York, 1949.

—— *The Logic of the Sciences and the Humanities*, Meridian Books Inc., New York, 1959.

RAGHU VIRA and LOKESH CHANDRA, *A New Tibeto-Mongol Pantheon*, part 1, International Academy of Indian Culture, New Delhi, 1961.

RICHARDS, I. A., *Mencius on the Mind*: Experiments in Multiple Definition, Kegan Paul, Trench, Trübner & Co., London, 1932.

ROERICH, G., *The Blue Annals* (2 vols.), Asiatic Society, Calcutta 1949, 1953.

RUSSELL, B., *History of Western Philosophy* and its Connection with Political and Social Circumstances from the Earliest Times to the Present Day (4th impr.), George Allen & Unwin Ltd., London, 1954.

SHELDON, W. H., 'On the Nature of Mind', *Journal of Philosophy*, vol. 38, New York 1941.

SHERRINGTON, SIR CHARLES, *Man on his Nature* (2nd ed.), Cambridge University Press, London, 1952.

SNELLGROVE, D. L., *The Hevajra Tantra*: A Critical Study (2 vols.), Oxford University Press, London, 1959.

STACE, W. T., *Religion and the Modern Mind*, J. B. Lippincott Company, Philadelphia–New York, 1960.

STOUT, G. F., *A Manual of Psychology* (5th ed.), University Tutorial Press Ltd., London, 1935 (reprint 1949).

SUTTIE, I. D., *The Origins of Love and Hate*, Kegan Paul, Trench, Trübner & Co., London, 1935 (4th impr. 1948).

TYRRELL, G. N. M., *Apparitions*, Pantheon Books, New York, 1953.

WHITEHEAD, A. N., *Science and the Modern World*, Cambridge University Press, London, 1926.

—— *Modes of Thought*, Cambridge University Press, London, 1938.

WHYTE, L. L., *Accent on Form*: An Anticipation of the Science of Tomorrow, Routledge & Kegan Paul Ltd., London, 1955.

WILD, J., *The Challenge of Existentialism*, Indiana University Press, Bloomington, 1955.

YOUNG, K., *Personality and Problems of Adjustment* (2nd ed.), Routledge & Kegan Paul Ltd., London, 1952.

B

A	mKhas-grub mñam-med dpal-ldan Nā-ro-pa'i rnam-par thar-pa dri-med legs-bśad bde-chen 'brug-sgra
B	mKhas-grub kun-gyi gtsug-rgyan paṇ-chen Nā-ro-pa'i rnam-thar ṅo-mtshar rmad-byuṅ
sGam-po-pa	The Collected Works of sGam-po-pa (38 volumes)
mKhas-grub	The Collected Works of mKhas-grub dge-legs bzaṅ-po (10 volumes, Tashilhunpo Ed.)
Thkv	The Collected Works of bLo-bzan chos-kyi ñi-ma dpal bzaṅ-po (Thu'u kvan Lama, 10 volumes, Lhasa Ed.)
Tsoṅ-kha-pa	The Collected Works of Tsoṅ-kha-pa (18 volumes, Tashilhunpo Ed.)
Barb	Bar-do'i chos-bśad mi-rtag sgyu-ma'i baṅ-chen daṅ-po
Bargd	Bar-do gsol-'debs-kyi dgoṅs-don mdo-tsam bkral-ba myur-dam zab-mo'i them-skas
Dc	sDom-pa bcu-ma' bsñen-thabs gsal-byed grol-ba mchog ster
Dchb	bDe-mchog mkha'-'gro sñan-rgyud-kyi bum-dbaṅ daṅ 'brel-ba ñams-len-gyi gtso-bor bskyed-rim ston-pa thun-moṅs yid-bžin nor-bu

Dchlsp	bDe-mchog mkha'-'gro sñan-rgyud-kyi naṅ loṅs-spyod rdzogs-pa sku'i gdams-pa smin-lam yid-bžin-gyi nor-bu
Dchkh	Nā-ro-lugs-kyi bde-mchog bcu-gsum-gyi 'khor-lo'i khrid
Dchog	dpal bde-mchog sñan-rgyud-kyi chos-skor-las 'og-sgo bde-chen mkha'-'gro'i sñiṅ-khrag
Dchžr	mDe-mchog 'khor-lo'i bsñen-pa'i sa-bcad mun-pa'i zla-ris
Dkt	Doha skor-gsum-gyi ṭīkā
Dnz	rje-btsun rdo-rje rnal-'byor-ma'i bskyed-rdzogs-kyi zin-bris mkha'-spyod bgrod-pa'i gsaṅ-lam sñiṅ-gi thig-le
Khd	dpal mkha'-'gro sñan-rgyud-las 'khor-lo sdom-pa'i sgrub-thabs 'briṅ-po rnal-'byor bži-pa 'dod-dgu'i char 'bebs
Khsg	Khrid-kyi sṅon-'gro'i cho-ga khrigs-dag 'don-du bkod-pa rdo-rje'i groṅ-du 'dren-pa'i śiṅ-rta
Kylg	Kye-rdo-rje lha-dgu'i mṅon-rtogs dkyil-'khor-gyi cho-ga daṅ bcas-pa dṅos-grub-kyi gter-mdzod
Lzph	sñan-rgyud gsaṅ-ba mthar-thug lam-zab 'pho-ba'i gdams-pa sñiṅ-gi thig-le
Lzzl	Lam-zab-kyi rnam-par bśad-pa zab-lam-gyi sñe-ma
Nbydztsh	rnal-'byor bži'i bśad-pa don-dam mdzub-tshugs-su bstan-pa
Phgdz	Phyag-rgya-chen-po'i man-ṅag-gi bśad-sbyar rgyal-ba'i gan-mdzod
Phntm	Phyag-rgya-chen-po rnal-'byor bži'i bśad-pa ṅes-don lta-ba'i mig
Phzb	Phyag-chen zin-bris
Rzd	Ri-chos mtshams-kyi žal-gdams
Sphkh	Jo-bo Nā-ro-pa'i khyad-chos bsre-'pho'i khrid rdo-rje'i theg-par bgrod-pa'i śiṅ-rta
Sphyd	bsre-'pho'i lam-skor-gyi thog-mar lam dbye-bsdu
Sphžg	Jo-bo Nā-ro-pa'i khyad-chos bsre-'pho'i gžuṅ-'grel rdo-rje-'chaṅ-gi dgoṅs-pa gsal-bar byed-pa
Sgg	Sems daṅ sems-byuṅ-gyi tshul gsal-bar ston-pa blo gsal mgul-rgyan
Srph	Sems daṅ sems-byuṅ-gi tshul rnam-par bśad-pa'i sdom-tshig rin-po-che'i phreṅ-ba
Ssrdz	gsaṅ-sṅags rig-pa 'dzin-pa'i sde-snod-las byuṅ-ba'i miṅ-gi (rnam-)graṅs
Tbr	rten-'brel kho-bo lugs-kyi khrid chos thams-cad-kyi sñiṅ-po len-pa
Tshk	sñan-rgyud rdo-rje tshig-rkaṅ-gi sa-bcad ma-rig mun sel žib-mo bkod-pa

Zmnd Zab-mo nan-don-gyi rnam-bśad sñiṅ-po gsal-bar byed-pa'i ñin-byed 'od-kyi 'phreṅ-ba

Zl Byaṅ-chub lam-gyi rim-pa'i 'khrid-yig 'jam-pa'i žal-luṅ

C

(Unless specified otherwise the following works are available only in their Tibetan translations in the bKa'-'gyur and bsTan-'gyur)

Abhidharmakośa *L'Abhidharmakośa de Vasubandhu.* Traduit et annoté par Louis de la Vallée Poussin, Paul Geuthner—Paris, J.-B. Istas—Louvain, 1923–31.

Āhapramāṇa-samyak-nāma-ḍākinī-upadeśa

Guhyasamājatantra ed. Benoytosh Bhattacharyya, Oriental Institute, Baroda, 1931.

Dohākośa-nāma-mahāmudrā-upadeśa

Dohākośa-nāma-caryāgīti-arthapradīpa-nāma-ṭīkā

Mudrācatura-ṭīkā-ratnahṛdaya-nāma

Pañcakrama Études et textes tantriques. Pañcakrama. Par L. de la Vallée Poussin. Université de Gand. Recueil de travaux publiés par la Faculté de philosophie et lettres. 16e fascicule. H. Engelcke —Gand, J.-B. Istas—Louvain, 1896.

Śrī-Dākārṇava-mahāyoginī-tantrarāja.

INDEXES

1. TIBETAN AND SANSKRIT TECHNICAL TERMS

A. Tibetan

kloṅ, 2 n. 1.
kloṅ-yaṅs, 2 n. 1.
rkyaṅ-ma, 55, 163, 271, 274.
sku, 5 n. 1, 45 n. 1, 119 n. 1, 124, 138, 265, 274.
sku rdo-rje rnal-'byor, 132.
skye-med, 92 n. 1, 276.
khams, 269.
khu-ba, 211 n. 2.
khyad-dga', 78 n. 2.
khyab-byed, 271.
grol-lam, 146.
glaṅ-po' 77.
glaṅ-po-can, 77 n. 1.
dga'-ba, 78 n. 2.
dga'-bral, 78 n. 2.
mgo-bo rduṅ-ba, 31 n. 1.
rgyal-ba rigs-lṅa, 265.
rgyud, 23 n. 1.
rgyen-rgyu, 271.
sgyu-ma, 175.
sgyu-ma lta-bu, 149.
sgyu-lus, 175.
ṅag, 119 n. 1, 270.
ṅo-bo-ñid-kyi sku, 47 n. 5.
sṅags, 112 n. 2.
chos, 129 n. 2.
chos—chos-can—chos-ñid, 129 n. 2.
chos—chos-ñid—blo, 129 n. 2.
chos-ñid, 129 n. 2.
chos-sku, 47 n. 5.
mched-pa, 276.
mchog-dga', 78 n. 2.
ñer-thob, 276.
ñon-moṅs, 71 n. 7.
gñis-med, 123 n. 1.
gñis-med rgyud, 123 n. 1.
gñug-ma, 169 n.
mñam-rgyu, 271.
mñam-pa-ñid-kyi ye-śes, 73 n. 1.
sñan-rgyud, xii.
sñiṅ-stobs, 274.
gti-mug, 271.
gtum, 59.
gtum-mo, 59.
gtum-mo 'bar-'dzag, 68 n. 3.
stoṅ-pa, 118 n. 4, 276.
stoṅ-pa chen-po, 276.
stoṅ-ñid, 8 n. 3.
rten, 64 n. 1.
rten daṅ brten-par bcas-pa, 64 n. 1.
tha-mal-gyi śes-pa, 73 n. 1.
thabs, 123 n. 1.
thabs-byuṅ, 64 n. 1.
thams-cad stoṅ-pa, 275, 276.
thig-le, 25 n. 4, 40 n. 2, 46 n. 1, 58 n. 3, 167, 211 nn. 1, 2, 274.
thugs, 5 n. 1, 45 n. 1, 119 n. 1, 138, 265, 274.
thugs rdo-rje rnal-'byor, 132.
thun-moṅ, 54 n. 2.
thur-sel, 271.
daṅ-po'i saṅs-rgyas, 118 n. 5.
duṅ-can-ma, 77 n. 1.
dran-pa, 25 n. 1, 92 n. 1, 276.
dran-med, 92 n. 1, 276.
gdaṅs, 192.
bdag-por gyur-pa, 265.
'dod-chags, 207 n. 1, 271.
rdul, 274.
rdo-rje, 5 n. 1.
rdo-rje-'chaṅ, 118 n. 5.
rdo-rje rnal-'byor, 265.
rdo-rje-'dzin, 95 n. 2, 118 n. 5.
gnas-pa, 118 n. 4.
gnas-lugs, 48 n. 3.
rnam-par rtog-pa'i rluṅ, 271.
rnam-par rtog-pa med-pa'i rluṅ, 271.
sna-tshogs-can, 77.
snaṅ-ba, 49 n. 1, 276.
snaṅ-ba gsum, 79 n. 1, 271.
snaṅ-ba-la ṅes-pa, 49 n. 1.
snaṅ-ba-la ma-ṅes-pa, 49 n. 1.
padma, 77.
padma-can, 77 n. 1.
sprul-sku, 47 n. 5.
spros-bral, 4 n. 3.
pha-rgyud, 123 n. 1.
pho-ña, 269.
phyag-rgya, 65 n. 1.
phyag-rgya chen-po, 222, 273.
phyag-rgya chen-mo, 222.
bar-do, 48 n. 2.
bud-med, 212 n. 1.

B. Sanskrit

2. SUBJECTS